Advanced
Case Management

Outcomes and Beyond

D1367258

Advanced
Case Management

Outcomes and Beyond

Suzanne K. Powell, RN, BSN, MBA, CCM, CPHQ

Director of Case Management/CQI

Health Services Advisory Group, Inc.

Phoenix, Arizona

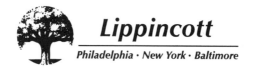

Lippincott

Philadelphia · New York · Baltimore

Editor: Jennifer Brogan
Editorial Assistant: Susan Rainey
Marketing Manager: Michelle Mulqueen
Project Editor: Paula C. Williams

351 West Camden Street
Baltimore, Maryland 21201-2436 USA

227 East Washington Square
Philadelphia, PA 19106

Printed in the United States of America

Library of Congress Cataloging-in-Publication Data

Powell, Suzanne K.
    Advanced case management : outcomes and beyond / Suzanne K.
Powell
        p.   cm.
    Includes bibliographical references and index.
    ISBN 0-7817-2234-9
    1. Disease management.   2. Medical care—Quality control.
3. Outcome assessment (Medical care)   4. Alternative medicine—
Evaluation.   I. Title.
    [DNLM: 1. Case Management.   2. Alternative Medicine—organization
& administration.   3. Disease Management.   4. Outcome Assessment
(Health Care).   5. Total Quality Management—organization &
administration.   WY 100 P886a 1999]
RA399.5.P68   1999
362.1—dc21
DNLM/DLC   99-40665
for Library of Congress   CIP

To purchase additional copies of this book, call our customer service department at **(800) 638-3030** or fax orders to **(301) 824-7390**. International customers should call **(301) 714-2324**.

                                                                          04
                                            2 3 4 5 6 7 8 9 10

To James

A million miles

we have traveled

in this lifetime.

A million smiles

we have kindled

in each other.

You have always been the light to guide me.

Foreword

The seismic event in twentieth century American medicine was the passage of Medicaid and Medicare in 1965. This event was the "big bang" of the health care system. Before 1965, governmental activity in health care was largely restricted to state and local health departments that, except for vital statistics, engaged in preventive activities such as well-baby clinics, health education programs, and x-ray screening for tuberculosis. Government was essentially a case finder for private medicine. There was medical care but no "health care," physicians were still doctors rather than "providers," and caring for the sick was not referred to as the "medical loss ratio." Although concerns over the cost of medical care first surfaced in 1929 and the first published critique of hands-on medical practice appeared in 1956, private medicine had few effective critics. It was largely fee-for-service, solo practice, and well protected by the political power of its professional association, the American Medical Association (AMA). Managed care plans were few and aggressively condemned by the AMA as "socialized medicine." Such medicine was inherently "unethical," presumably because fees passed through a third party rather than moving directly from the patient to the doctor. By this definition, we have now been living under "unethical" medicine for nearly four decades.

Medicaid and Medicare obliterated the sharp demarcation between private medical practice and the health activities of government. Suddenly, if you could not afford private health, you could get public health. The government became the largest single purchaser of health services, and over the next three decades increasingly sought to identify value for money and held physicians responsible for not only the cost of care but also the quality of care. Third-party payments became the rule rather than the exception, and government gradually replaced the AMA as the proverbial "800-pound gorilla" of American medicine.

The passage of legislation in 1973 that created health maintenance organizations (HMOs) encouraged the development of managed care plans whose great promise was their ability to contain costs. Less noted at the time were their capacity to bring standardization to medical practice through the identification and application of best practices and their facilitation of population-based medicine. Although Medicaid and Medicare erased the distinction between private and public health, it was managed care that defined limits and operational qualities of the

Classical public health d  f prevention. Primary prevention is prevent d a disease agent.

Examples include treating water and sewage and, more recently, cleanups of waste materials that pose environmental hazards. Secondary prevention renders people impervious to disease agents should they encounter them. This is achieved through immunization and by avoidance of known risk factors for various diseases. Tertiary prevention refers to measures taken to minimize or eliminate harm done by diseases already present. Back in 1965, and until quite recently, tertiary prevention was the domain of clinical medicine. In 1999, however, tertiary prevention includes clinical as well as population-based medicine. It is this synthesis of clinical care of individuals and measures to affect entire populations that define what is now known as disease management. Under this concept, vaccination against pneumococcal pneumonia and the treatment of pneumonia are simply different loci on the spectrum of community-acquired pneumonia. Similarly, the identification of best practices through population-based research, and the application of these practices to clinical medicine, use population findings to improve quality of care at the individual level.

New discoveries in clinical medicine are now commonplace, and the health care industry is still seeking the optimal administrative form to maximize what the clinician has to offer. New concepts are still seeking adequate definition, and this new book by my colleague, Suzanne Powell, will unravel most of the confusion around the role of disease management in relation to other ideas that impact patient care such as case management, outcomes measurement, continuous quality improvement (CQI), and complementary and alternative medicine (CAM). Coming at this pivotal point in American medicine, Ms. Powell's book will no doubt reach the wide audience it deserves.

Carter L. Marshall, MD, MPH
Director for Clinical Epidemiology
Health Services Advisory Group, Inc., and
Research Professor of Family and Community Medicine
University of Arizona College of Medicine

Preface

I did not intentionally start out writing a second book on case management. I was requested to update and revise the first book, *Nursing Case Management: A Practical Guide to Success in Managed Care*. After several months of adding material, it became apparent that either the book was going to be the size of a "Med–Surg" text, or two books were in order. The book *Advanced Case Management: Outcomes and Beyond* was born. In 1994, when the first book was written, the case management profession was in its infancy and very fragmented. Since that time, the two major case management societies have merged into one consolidated group, The Case Management Society of America (CMSA). CMSA has not only unified case managers but has created a structure that has catapulted case management into an international phenomenon. Case management is no longer the "grassroots" offshoot of the nursing profession it was a few short years ago, but rather is a respected and credible answer to many of the challenges created by managed care. It is gratifying to see how much case management has grown since the first book was written. But the growth happened for good reason; it filled a need. The health care choices are ever expanding, the insurance benefits are often decreasing, and coordination needed to pilot the patient through the health care clouds and storms could only be done by dedicated professionals. Case managers have much to be proud of.

The two books are very different—in content and intent. *Case Management: A Practical Guide to Success in Managed Care* is an essential text detailing the broad scope of case management and providing a basic foundation and structure; it is patient-oriented. *Advanced Case Management: Outcomes and Beyond* is more theoretical, research-oriented, and statistical; it considers such issues as alternative medicine, outcomes management, disease management, and continuous quality improvement (CQI). The advanced book is based on improving care to entire populations of patients (disease-specific management). Population-based case management requires advanced educational components, in addition to the core information in the first book.

In many ways, disease management is case management at its finest; however, even the brightest and most clinically astute case managers may be less successful if the programs that support them are not foundationally sound. Part I comprehensively discusses disease management concepts, starting with its recent history and the driving forces that lead to this system of case management. Components of a successful disease management program, development and design of a disease management program, and the case management/disease management process are addressed from the case management perspective. Example disease management tools are included.

Part II extensively discusses the important issue of outcomes management. The health care field is demanding outcomes; they want to know what is being done to improve patient care, and what is the best method of patient care. In several health care accreditation requirements, outcomes are mandatory. Case management has become an indispensable part of these regulatory requirements. Part II evaluates topics such as the importance of measuring case management outcomes; how to develop a case management/outcomes management program; about the Center for Case Management Accountability (CCMA); study designs for case management intervention evaluation; perspectives to consider when choosing study designs and measurement tools; benchmarking; factors that affect case management outcomes such as risk adjustment, variation/validity, reliability, and interrater reliability; types of case management outcomes domains; understanding quality indicators, process indicators, and outcome indicators; and the essential steps in a quality improvement project. Important charts, tables, and examples are provided.

For case managers to succeed in the current health care environment, the knowledge of outcomes management is essential for survival. Furthermore, it is the knowledge of continuous quality improvement (CQI) concepts and the proper use of CQI tools that will provide the road map to address quality issues, organize outcomes management/quality improvement projects, and demonstrate case management outcomes. Part III, Continuous Quality Improvement (CQI) and Case Management, provides that roadmap in a step-by-step, "how-to" manner. Examples of many CQI tools for process improvement are provided to demonstrate how they can be applied in case management. A problem-solving methodology, specifically geared to case managers, is described. Essential differences exist between patient care meetings and quality improvement/outcomes management meetings; teams and team meetings and decision-making techniques for process improvement are detailed in Part III.

Part IV, Managing Complementary Health Care—A Vision for the Future, illustrates the challenges and the successes behind complementary and alternative medicine (CAM). Complementary medicine is a powerful concern in health care today. Case managers will be increasingly required to manage alternative and Western therapies together, and they must understand CAM's growing influence and applications. Part IV details many "alternative" modalities, their benefits and contraindications, outcome studies done by credible organizations such as NIH, and how CAM and Western medicine work together.

Challenges with the integration of CAM and conventional medicine are plentiful, such as lack of availability of practice guidelines and standards of practice for CAM practitioners; lack of scientific evidence supporting the efficacy of most CAM modalities; finding a reliable source for understanding the indications and contraindications for CAM modalities; locating credentialing guidelines and services for CAM providers; locating or creating outcomes measures for evaluating treatments with CAM; facilitating acceptance of CAM by insurance companies, physicians, and other health care providers; and educating CAM providers and consumers about indications and contraindications of using CAM, managed care, and insurance concepts. These challenges are addressed in Part IV. Case studies that integrate CAM into mainstream health care are provided.

Organizationally, each section includes a list of important terms and concepts, the core topic information, and concludes with resources and references to enhance the text. Study questions are included; however, they are more to provoke thought and assessment than for the purpose of "testing" knowledge. An extensive glossary of terms is offered as a quick reference.

The case managers' role is expanding to include everything from clinical expert to outcomes management expert. This ubiquity is unheard of in any other profession. As The Case Manager's Creed says:

> (case managers) "must understand insurance, electricity, chemistry, physiology, mechanics, architecture, physics, bookkeeping, banking, merchandising, selling, shipping, contracting, claims, adjusting, law, medicine, real estate, horse trading, and human nature. . . must know all, see all, and tell nothing, and be everywhere at the same time." (From Nursefinders, circa 1995)

After perusing this text, the case manager may slap herself on the forehead and exclaim, "What did I get myself into?" More hybrid roles. More techniques. More tools to use as rules. And what about all those CAM modalities? But a case manager is on a "need to know" basis (and more often than not, they "need to know" just about everything!).

These are the issues that today's health care is made of; and knowledge of these specialties may make all the difference in coordinating safe care with good outcomes. Do not underestimate the importance of statistical data (outcomes management), a well-planned improvement project (CQI), disease management programs, or the power of herbs or acupuncture. They are all aspects of that elusive facet of humanity called "quality of life." And it is the "quality of life" that case managers primarily work to improve in their patients; therefore, any idea, philosophy, or new or ancient healing methodology must be objectively considered for us to fulfill our missions.

Acknowledgments

To my husband, James—whose boyish joy makes me laugh; and whose love and support sustains me.

To Dad, who is always in my heart.

To Mom, whose special spirit has made me so much of what I am.

To Dad #2, the 80-year-old, computer wizard, jazz playin' Ph.D. who proofreads my manuscripts. Viva golden oldies!

To Janice Benjamin, R.N., M.S., L.Ac., whose wise insights and compassion have greatly added to the wisdom of this text.

To Dr. Lawrence Shapiro—for believing in me—and pushing me past my "comfort zones."

To Dr. Carter Marshall, with thanks for his sage words and kind contributions to this book.

To Bill Staples, the Zen Graphics Master responsible for many of the charts and figures in this manuscript.

With special thanks to Dr. Herbert Rigberg, Mary Ellen Dalton, Dr. Donald Umlah, Brenda Darling, Dr. Marcia Stevic, Dr. Andrea Silvey, and all my colleagues at Health Services Advisory Group, Inc.

To Sherry L. Aliotta, R.N., B.S.N., C.C.M., C.C.M.A. Chairperson, for her assistance in writing the section on CCMA.

To the Case Management Society of America (CMSA), who has helped case management grow into an international phenomenon that will improve quality of life around the world.

To all the providers who remember when they were referred to as "physicians."

To Aunt Cele, the patients, and their families.

To all the case managers who positively impact the lives of patients.

Contents

Disease Management

"You must be the change you wish to see in the world."

MAHATMA GANDHI

PART I: IMPORTANT TERMS AND CONCEPTS

"At-Risk" Member
Baseline Data
Best Practices
Clinical Outcomes
Component Management Model
Continuous Quality Improvement
 (CQI)
Cross-Functional Team
Data
Demand Management
Disease Management Model
Disease Management Society (DMS)
Disease State Case Management
 (DSCM)
Disease State Management
Economic Barriers
Evidenced-Based Guidelines
Financial Outcomes
Goals
Health Care Financing
 Administration (HCFA)
Health Plan Employer Data and
 Information Set (HEDIS)

Health Status Survey
Humanistic Outcomes
Integrated Data Management
 Systems
Managed Care Organization
 (MCO)
Multidisciplinary Team
National Committee for Quality
 Assurance (NCQA)
Objectives
Outcomes Measurement
Patient Barriers
Patient Outcomes
"Physician Champion"
Pilot Project
Practice Guidelines
Practice Parameters
Provider Barriers
Quality Indicators (QI)
Report Card
SF-36, SF-12
System Barriers
Target Population

CHAPTER 1

Overview of Disease Management

INTRODUCTION

Is case management a component of disease management, or is disease management a component of case management? Perhaps this whole debate is only one of labels and hierarchies. The similarities are striking (Table 1-1), which is why some refer to the process as *disease-specific case management.* However, where case management has been traditionally an individual-based approach, disease management is population-based; where case management has essentially been either acute or post-acute based, disease management is systems based, integrating the patients through multiple levels of care. The essential idea is that disease management is case management at its finest; when case management can be proactive, can follow a disease-specific population across the continuum of care, has time to fully utilize the critical educational element to promote wellness, and therefore generates the improved quality of life case managers seek for their patients—it is termed *disease management.* Thus, disease management is a framework, system, or program; case management is the process through which to utilize disease management programs.

Case management has successfully identified and managed high-cost, long-term-care patients. However, in the early 1990s, it became clear that disease-specific populations of chronically ill patients often remained undetected. Although case managers may get referrals because of a specific disease, these referrals are rendered on an individual, case-by-case basis. Often, only the sickest patients who return to the hospital setting repeatedly were chosen for case management. Cases are rarely referred to case managers for sporadic, short hospital stays in which an exacerbation of a condition only needs to be stabilized. Patients with chronic conditions have an estimated one in three chance of being rehospitalized within 90 days of discharge. Preventive measures to delay or avoid the recurrent illness patterns needed to be found. Disease management strategies began to appear.

Some disease management programs originated from sophisticated case management programs in which physician specialists or primary care physi-

Table 1-1 Comparison of Case Management Process and Disease Management Process

CASE MANAGEMENT PROCESS	DISEASE MANAGEMENT PROCESS
Case selection	Identification of at-risk members
Assessment/problem identification	Assessment/evaluation of members
Development and coordination of the case plan	Development and coordination of disease management plan
Implementation of plan	Implementation of disease management plan
Evaluation and follow-up	Evaluation with outcome measurements
Continuous monitoring, reassessing, reevaluation (not actually a "step"—must be done throughout)	Continuous monitoring, reassessing, reevaluation (not actually a "step"—must be done throughout)

cians (PCPs) teamed up with a specialty case manager. This dynamic team is responsible for all primary medical services, including patient education, tracking, and follow-up. Disease management is an evolving opportunity for case managers, both as managers of patient populations and as administrative leaders developing and facilitating programs. The case manager must understand the driving forces behind the disease management trend, the development and coordination of a disease management program, clinical guidelines and outcome management, and the disease management process.

Although examples are cited and disease management tools shown, it is not the intent of this section to describe specific disease management models in detail. Current models are well detailed in some of the invaluable case management journals that are available. Innovative disease management models are being attempted and documented for many health conditions and disease states; current articles articulate their successes and barriers to success. It is recommended that those who are developing, facilitating, or improving a disease management program review the current literature for the most up-to-date guidelines. However, as a clinical example, diabetes disease management will be used in this chapter. The reasons for this choice are numerous: it is a medically complex condition, and any ideas or assistance that can be imparted here will aide many patients and case managers alike; diabetes disease management programs have been around for a few years, and the guidelines are fairly accepted; early detection and good blood sugar control have proved to allay complications, which can be formidable (blindness, strokes, silent myocardial infarctions, cerebral and peripheral vascular disease, autonomic and sensory nervous system problems, end-stage renal disease, amputations); it is an extremely expensive disease, with some estimates as high as $98 billion in 1997; it is epidemic, with an estimated 15 to 16 million Americans affected, including one out of five people older than 65 years; and finally, case/disease managers can positively impact this disease and the quality of life of the patients and their families. Diabetes is an expensive disease to treat; it is also an expensive disease to develop and implement as a disease management program. The return-on-investment of members' health could take years; and, in those years, the members may potentially change health plans (an inherent risk in all disease management programs).

A second disease example used in this chapter is congestive heart failure (CHF). CHF is another expensive and debilitating disease that severely affects the quality of life. However, in CHF disease management programs, the managed care organization's return-on-investment may be more quickly observed. Readmissions to acute care and emergency department visits typically decrease dramatically in a relatively short timeframe. One study cited an 83% decrease in hospital admissions and a self-reported 44% improvement in quality of life. This disease affects approximately 4.7 million Americans, with 400,000 new cases diagnosed each year (Anonymous, 1998, p. 18).

DEFINITIONS AND THE DISEASE MANAGEMENT SOCIETY

Disease management uses a set of prospectively determined interventions with the intent of altering the course of the disease, improving outcomes and quality of life, and reducing health care costs. The goal is prevention of exacerbation of illness, thereby avoiding or delaying the onset of acute disease. This definition is really a medley of current disease management definitions, because, at this time, there is no standard definition of disease management cited in the literature. Perhaps disease management is in such a fast pace of evolution that no one program has been able to hold on long enough to offer a solid definition. Standards on diseases are being revised and refined as outcome measurements prove "best practices"—then change to newer, improved "best practices." However, there is consensus on some elements.

Some definitions list the components or describe a disease management program. Various providers of disease management services define it from their perspective. Consider those who have a strong continuous quality improvement (CQI) focus: that each disease management process can be evaluated through outcomes research and continuously improved. The continuous changes generated by the CQI approach may cause the elusiveness of the definition of disease management in the first place. Those who advocate a CQI focus state that

> . . . disease management brings together outcomes research and clinical management of diseases to provide efficient care to patient populations in a continuous quality improvement environment. Furthermore, disease management is a continuous process focused on efficiency and applied to selected patient populations. (Nash, 1997, p. 2)

Other literature states that "Disease management will eventually be the core element in continuous quality improvement. Outcomes from medical management programs will eventually influence reimbursement and/or capitation rates" (Todd, 1995, p. 41). Then, those who are actively working to integrate the data information so necessary for accurate outcomes believe the whole definition has changed. Disease management has become "a coordinated, systematic approach using information-management decision-support tools to identify at-risk populations for the implementation of patient-specific interventions to manage total patient care and improve clinical, economic and humanistic outcomes" (Meyers, 1998, p. 32). This definition certainly is an integral part of the disease management process.

The Disease Management Society (DMS) is an organization sponsored by the National Managed Health Care Congress. The DMS's mission is to

> provide health care professionals with vehicles for information sharing that will help them in the development, implementation, assessment and improvement of disease prevention and management strategies...(and) provide members with information on current research, partnerships and processes that underscore the delivery of cost effective, quality care (Disease Management Society [DMS] 70 Blanchard Road, Suite 4000, Burlington, MA 01803 1-888-44-NMHCC).

Even the DMS, however, has not standardized a definition.

The Migliara/Kaplan study in 1996 and 1997 asked respondents to choose their "ideal" disease management definition and a "working" disease management definition. The choice for the "ideal" definition remained constant in both years:

> A clinical management process of care that spans the continuum of care from primary prevention to ongoing long-term maintenance for individuals with chronic health conditions or diagnoses.

The "working" disease management definition choice was less clear, but, according to the DMS, most respondents preferred the following:

> The process of caring for patients using standardized treatment strategies that ensure appropriate utilization and high-quality care across the continuum.

Disease management defined as "proactive case management" may be overly simple, but to seasoned case managers, it is clear, concise, and completely understood. Some disease management definitions incorporate case management as part of the central theme. Mark Zitter, president of The Zitter Group, summarizes disease management as a

> comprehensive, integrated approach to care and reimbursement based on a disease's natural course, focusing on clinical and nonclinical intervention when and where

they are most likely to have the greatest impact. Ideally, disease management prevents exacerbation of a disease and use of expensive resources, making prevention and proactive case management two important areas of emphasis (Rieve, 1998, p. 34).

All definitions imply the continuity of care for the life cycle of the condition, whether it is a chronic disease (as in diabetes), or a self-limiting condition (as in high-risk pregnancy).

One definition that specifically integrates disease management and case management labels this strategy "Disease state case management (DSCM)" (Levitt, Startz, & Higgins, 1998, p. 45):

> Disease state case management (DSCM) is a population-based approach that identifies individuals with chronic diseases, assesses their health status, develops a program or plan of care, and collects data to evaluate the effectiveness of the process. DSCM proactively intervenes with treatment and education so that the individual with a chronic disease can maintain optimal function with the most cost-effective and outcome-effective health care expenditure. The goal of DSCM is to manage at-risk populations across the entire continuum of care.

The definition is certainly changing; will the term *disease management* withstand the test of time and evolution, or will it also change? Some are already considering different terms, because some populations that are managed are not diseases at all, but rather natural conditions, such as pregnancy. Terms such as "disease state case management (DSCM)," "integrated health management," "population-based care," "continuous health care improvement," or "total health (or disease) management" are preferred by some as more accurate. Like the term *case management,* however, *disease management* appears to be fairly entrenched in the managed care world. Although neither term is perfect in every sense, like a comfortable shoe, they have familiarity in a world that is changing at a dizzying pace.

HISTORY

In 1991, Pfizer, Inc. sponsored a pharmaceutical study that was conducted by the Boston Consulting Group. In their report that was released in 1993, the first definition of disease management was unveiled; in 1998, the Disease Management Society cites this definition:

> In the simplest terms, DM is the application of business principles to medical practice. It involves managing and providing care to populations of patients who are at risk of or diagnosed with a specific disease through a comprehensive, integrated system that uses best practices, clinical practice improvement, information technology, and other resources and interventions (Boston Consulting Group, 1993).

Perhaps because of Pfizer's involvement, or because the study was about the pharmaceutical industry, many credit pharmaceutical companies with the inception of the disease management concept. Certainly, this industry had the more sophisticated information systems with the ability to keep a watchful eye on drug interactions and prescription refills, research capabilities, and strong financial backing for educational materials and advertising. And because one large part of managing disease is assuring that the patient receives the right medication, at the right time (early in the disease process or at the preventative level), and in the right dose, this industry had many of the ingredients necessary to put together a solid disease management program.

The pharmacy industry was not without critics. Some were suspicious that disease management programs were thinly disguised attempts to sell more products through educational packaging. Regardless, medication errors (either by prescription, administration, or patient compliance) add billions of dollars to the cost of health care, and it is well documented that the health care system is ailing. Corporate selfishness, secrets, and separation must give way to collaboration if we are to be able to provide quality health care to diverse populations. Simply, pharmacy personnel and capabilities are an important part of the health care team. Often the pharmacist is the one who discovers dangerous drug interactions when a patient is receiving prescriptions from his or her cardiologist, internist, neurologist, and herbalogist.

Disease management history is as old as tuberculosis sanitariums and Hanson's disease clinics; and it is as recent as the 1990s. The crystal ball says that, as more outcome measurements define best practices, the more the management of disease—and health—will develop and mature.

DRIVING FORCES THAT LED TO DISEASE MANAGEMENT PROGRAMS

Fragmentation of Care

Disease management is the result of a major health care paradigm shift. Historically, health care in the United States has been delivered by what some refer to as a "Component Management Model" (Nash & Todd, 1997, p. 1). In this model, the "components" are the various providers that a patient may need along the continuum. Each component, separately and episodically, may strive for cost-effective, quality care. In reality, however, the patient may suffer from the fragmentation caused by the providers viewing care from their own perspective. Component management will pay for expensive hospitalizations, but more often than not, it does not support education or preventive elements with which hospitalizations and emergency care can be reduced. A patient with diabetes may enter the emergency department, where he receives effective care for his exacerbation of the disease. He goes home a happy customer. In the doctor's office, the doctor may not adhere to the latest and greatest guidelines on diabetes management, although she or he does an adequate job and is a great listener. In the pharmacy, the pharmacist may not have explained the finer details of the medications in a way that the patient understood; and it is 5:00 PM Friday and the line at the pharmacy is long. So the patient does his best (also throw in a little noncompliance when no one is looking), and the cycle repeats itself—back to the emergency department. There is little connection between the "components"—patient, physician, emergency department, and pharmacy. Like episodic case management, each component focused on their one slice of care.

Quality of care and cost-efficiency is sacrificed when each part of the health care environment focuses on itself. Studies have shown that "optimizing any component of care separately from other components often generates higher systemwide costs" (Nash, p. 2). One Louisiana study demonstrated this fact when the state's Medicaid program took certain powerful (and expensive) drugs off their formulary; medication costs dropped 13%, but physician services rose 29% and mental health services increased by 39% (Nash, pp. 2–36). This kind of care is not only more expensive, it also has fewer health benefits than an integrated program.

The "Component Management Model" was one driving force that led to the next stage of health care evolution: the "Disease Management Model." Disease management is a more holistic model in which all of the parts are (ideally) working toward the good of the population, or patients with a particular disease state. Component management squeezes parts of the system, thus stressing and damaging the whole; it is not unlike a coronary event, in which, if blood flow is constrained in one part, serious consequences are evident elsewhere.

Financial Pressures

The economics behind disease management are transparent, but for good reason. An analysis in 1994 of every health care dollar spent showed the following estimate:

- Cancer care consumed $.15 of each dollar
- Diabetes and its complications consumed $.12 of each dollar
- Heart disease consumed $.14 of each dollar
- AIDS (acquired immune deficiency syndrome) and infectious diseases consumed $.06 of each dollar

That translates into $.47 per health care dollar (or $423 billion) treating these four diseases.

Furthermore, the year 2000 estimate is as follows:

- Cancer care will consume $.20 of each dollar
- Diabetes and its complications will consume $.16 of each dollar
- Heart disease will consume $.13 of each dollar (note this amount decreased—possibly because of good disease management programs)
- AIDS and infectious diseases will consume $.12 of each dollar

Because one half to two thirds of the nation's health care dollar is exhausted by four conditions, disease management makes sense (Giles, 1998).

Cost containment pressures were, perhaps, the original and most compelling driving force for the development of disease state programs. Those paying for health care were motivated to find the most reliable methods of reducing their costs. The proliferation of capitated contracts moved the financial risk from the insurance company as the sole payor to the provider sector. Disease management has been a growing trend to level the playing field. As good disease management programs demonstrate that they provide quality care at a cost-efficient price, these programs should grow in number; opportunities for nurse case managers will expand proportionately. A capitated reimbursement system is also set up to encourage cost-effective treatment in a variety of settings. When a payor (*e.g.,* a managed care organization) is responsible for the beneficiary across the continuum of care, the incentive is to move toward integration and wellness. Add to this incentive the merger mania that has been occurring. Health systems are merging and levels of care are integrating, causing further incentive to provide holistic cost efficiency.

Quality Improvement Projects
Showing Outcomes of Care

Another incentive pushing health care toward the disease management model is the increasing number of quality improvement projects. Periodically, these projects discovered poor quality of care. Some results were so troubling that projects to change, measure, and improve patient care processes were mandated by the Health Care Financing Administration (HCFA). The seemingly limitless variations of practice patterns for the same disease state or procedure (*e.g.,* prostate cancer or total hip replacement) was also a concern among providers and health care payors. Quality improvement projects were developed to distinguish which processes of care provided the best outcomes; the results often culminated in the development of "best practice" guidelines. In turn, these "best practice" guidelines direct the disease management programs that are developing. Providers are becoming more savvy about health care project management and continuous quality improvement (CQI) techniques and are now more capable of developing and facilitating disease management programs of high caliber.

The evolution of managed care strategies also led to finding appropriate clinical guidelines. In the early 1980s, review of the utilization of resources (*i.e.,* utilization review) was the new wave of managing care. When that proved to be insufficient, management of the utilization of resources (utilization management) became the acceptable practice. The piece that was still missing was a decision tree about what constitutes appropriate care in a given circumstance. In CQI fashion, data were examined, and practice patterns were recommended accordingly.

Accreditation Programs

Accreditation requirements are a driving force and fit nicely into the disease management system. The National Committee for Quality Assurance (NCQA), the accreditation organization that provides certification to Health Maintenance Organizations (HMOs), has developed the Health Plan Employer Data and Information Set (HEDIS). HEDIS is a standardized method to collect HMO-specific data on their performance; in essence, HEDIS measures various aspects of the disease management process. In some respects, HEDIS propelled the disease management movement when, in 1992, the HEDIS asthma standards came on the scene. Although there are no specific disease management standards, payors are required to prove that their providers are working to improve the health of their population. The data then are used as a "report card" and as a comparison between health plans (Nash, 1997, p. 14). This report card shows how well the providers of an HMO are faring in terms of achieving health improvement for the HMO's members. NCQA requirements for patient satisfaction and outcomes data have also steered the disease management movement. On the provider end, Joint Commission on Accreditation of Healthcare Organizations accreditation has also been a driving force.

Computer Systems

Computer technology has been identified as both a driving force in disease management and a barrier. Information technology has assisted disease management programs through the following avenues:

- The growth of sophisticated software assists the disease management steps of patient identification and follow-up.

- Disease-specific decision trees are available and used by telephone triage nurses and demand management companies.
- The crucial outcome measurement element that is responsible for continuous improvement in the management of disease would be impossible without sophisticated and integrated computer systems; the type and volume of data collection that is a current expectation could not have been provided a decade ago.

Some believe that information technology is the key to making disease management work. The health care environment today demands cost–outcome relationships for specific diseases, and integrated computer systems may well be the critical factor that makes disease and health management a success. In some ways, however, the information age has created a structure in which health care is "data rich but information poor." There is an abundance of information everywhere, but putting it together into a useful whole is cost prohibitive and will require collaborative efforts.

Informed Consumers

Consumers are demanding good care. HEDIS report cards and major magazines compare plans; Internet users find disease-specific protocols at their fingertips; pharmacies across the nation pass out free literature about disease, health, and prevention; prime time commercials inform the public of drug uses and side effects; magazines and newspapers regularly talk about new treatments for cancer, human immunodeficiency virus, and other conditions; health fairs in every state saturate the public with important topics. There is no shortage of knowledge in the information age. However, as patient advocates, it is the medical community's (*e.g.,* case/disease manager's) responsibility to assure that the patients in their charge get the most accurate information for health and disease prevention.

Another group of consumers who are moving the health care world are employment benefit consultants. The consultants write RFPs (request for proposals) with specific demands. If a managed care organization is going to bid for this employer's business, they must meet the stringent standards in the RFP; and more are including NCQA accreditation and disease management programs.

COMPONENTS OF A SUCCESSFUL DISEASE MANAGEMENT PROGRAM

There are several important ingredients to building a successful disease management program. Whether a case manager is performing disease management, or is developing or facilitating a disease management program, these key areas are important to understand.

Understanding the Course of the Disease/Practice Guidelines

Good case management has always required clinical excellence; in disease management, every clinical symptom (or potential symptom) and every medication interaction must be acutely understood. This is not new for case managers. What may be new is the strategic method of looking at data and deciding what the cost and quality drivers, causes, and patterns of symptom manifestation may be in any given disease. A cost driver in asthma, for example, may be misdiagnosis. According to the National Jewish Center for Immunology and Respiratory Medicine, up to 20% of chronically ill asthmatics referred to the center for treatment did not have asthma at all, but another illness called vocal cord dysfunction, which presents like asthma but has a very different treatment regimen (Nash, 1997, pp. 5–6). This emphasizes the importance of managing the disease through astute use of physicians. A well-planned disease management program will use both PCPs and specialists wisely. Depending on the patient's requirements, the referral may be for the more specialized evaluation, or the treatment may be appropriately adjusted by the PCP.

Perhaps the most essential reason to understand the sequence of a disease state is for the purpose of preventing the illness from advancing. Through evidenced-based practice guidelines, also known as practice parameters, the disease is "managed" with the intent of slowing progression. Although it is unlikely that treatment guidelines will be appropriate for every patient with the same disease, they can be designed so that most same-disease patients will benefit from following them. With more outcomes data available, these guidelines are likely to be changed and improved. Because of the rapid changes, a physician and case/disease management educational component is essential to keep abreast of "best practices."

Targeting Patients Likely to Benefit from Intervention

Enough data are available today to be knowledgeable about which diagnoses incur high costs. It is also important to target the patients within your organization's disease population that may be most helped from disease management intervention. In one insurance company, 22% of patients with asthma were found to account for 85% of the asthma-related costs; in another company, 4.9% of patients with diabetes accounted for 91.9% of the diabetes-related costs (Nash, 1997, p. 6). Targeting these members may give disease managers satisfaction in improved quality of life and in cost reduction. Oftentimes the case manager must find the candidates for the disease management programs. Hospital case managers are in a natural position for this task; through collaboration with outside case managers, patients are referred into appropriate programs after discharge.

Focusing on Prevention and Resolution

Prevention of acute episodes is an essential function of disease management; when they cannot be prevented, then quick resolution of the acute episode must commence. Prevention in disease management also applies to targeting, and possibly preventing or minimizing, a high-risk individual from becoming ill in the first place. Prevention takes many forms, depending on the disease state that is targeted. However, a common denominator for prevention of disease or exacerbations is education.

Demand management is one method of education that focuses on the general population's ability to use medical resources wisely. A definition of demand management is "the use of self-management and decision support systems to enable, educate, and encourage people to improve their health and make appropriate use of medical care" (Nash & Todd, 1997, p. 331). The educational tools used in demand management may be in the form of mailings, nurse phone triage services, self-care books, newsletters, or electronic media. Essentially, the goal is to provide services that will decrease the excess "demand" for inappropriate medical interventions. Several organizations report success through decreased medical services.

Increasing Patient Compliance Through Education

It is estimated that 15% to 20% of hospital readmissions are attributable to lack of patient compliance with prescribed therapies, and that one half of all chronic disease readmissions are preventable. Education and sometimes counseling provide the basis for prevention in many illnesses. In diabetes, congestive heart failure, or asthma, the disease—and treatment for the disease—is complex. The chronicity of the disease eventually may invoke noncompliant behavior in the best of patients; support groups and counseling can be effective. Educational components should, at the minimum, include:

• Cause and progression of the disease—instruction in how to monitor the disease to avoid exacerbation
• Precipitating reasons and signs and symptoms of impending problems

- Medication time tables, dosages, side effects, what to do about various side effects
- Dietary considerations and other lifestyle modifications
- A discussion about compliance with physician and clinic appointments

Unfortunately, counseling, support groups, education, and many forms of preventive therapy are rarely reimbursed under most insurance benefits. A disease management program, to be successful, must find the balance between services that are not covered—but may be the key to successful behavioral modification of patients—and use of education and nontraditional preventative treatments (see Part IV on Complementary Medicine).

Providing Full Care Continuity

As stated before, the component management model of health care has been found to be less successful than an integrated approach. Many organizations are providing all levels of care, through mergers, partnering with other companies, or carve-outs for specific treatments or diseases. The continuum of care also must be geographically convenient, or the patients simply will not, or will not be able to, access preventive services. Hospitalizations or specialty treatments such as transplantations may take a patient far from home; but chemotherapy, physical/occupation/speech therapies, or disease-specific classes must be within a reasonable distance. The medical services provided also must match the needs of the disease being managed; this must include all of the potential services that the disease requires for optimal wellness.

Successful disease management models use case/disease managers throughout the continuum. Innovative companies have gone one step further by allowing intense follow-up services. The Guthrie Clinic in Pennsylvania discharges their total hip replacement patients directly to home 90% of the time; this is double the national average. They use clinical pathways and aggressive post-acute services to accomplish this benchmark (Nash, 1997, p. 9).

Establishing Integrated Data Management Systems for Outcome Measurements

Measuring outcomes is key to a successful disease management system. Outcomes point the direction for change; they show what works, and what needs improvement. Integrated computer and data management systems are essential for the degree of sophistication necessary in a well-developed disease management program. State-of-the-art software systems that integrate care based on inpatient and outpatient settings are necessary to elicit the best information.

Ideally, everything about the patient, from medical and psychosocial history to clinical encounters across the continuum and pharmacy utilization should be inputted. Not only is this time-consuming to input, but the development of this level of computer sophistication is expensive. Access to data analysts may be important for case managers in the administrative role. Case/disease managers will require computer skill sets, and also must be constantly vigilant to the potential for confidentiality breaches in such a system.

Experts caution that a thorough and accurate assessment of the organization's current data system is critical. Through this time-consuming task, the organization can determine:

- The data that can be available if requested
- The data that is beyond the capabilities of the current system (Minerd & Lee, 1997)

There is no better method of measuring the outcomes of the program than a well-integrated information system. However, if the budget does not allow a major overhaul, partnering with an organization with greater capabilities may be an option.

This overview of disease management has described the definition, the driving forces, and the components of a successful disease management program. Chapter 2 will discuss the development and design of a disease management program and the case management/disease management process.

The Process of Disease Management

For the purposes of this text, there are two parts to this chapter on "The Process of Disease Management." The first section deals with the "Development and Design of a Disease Management Program." The second section describes the actual "Case Management/Disease Management Process."

DEVELOPMENT AND DESIGN OF A DISEASE MANAGEMENT PROGRAM

A critical step before the development and design of a disease management program is to obtain organizational commitment from the top down. Any organization that is about to embark on this time- and resource-intensive process will be seriously undermined if support is missing. There will be many hours of many employees time (from support services to physicians) just in the planning stage; add to that months or, more commonly, years before a financial impact may be felt, depending on the disease chosen. The potential for conflicts, negativity, and indecision is high. Up-front honesty about the probable resources necessary to start the program is important.

Also consider eliciting support from providers outside of your immediate organization. A disease management program, initiated by a managed care organization (MCO), may have to coordinate the support from network physicians, community organizations, outside laboratories, pharmacies, ambulatory services, and radiology services. It is best to include representatives from all important sites in the planning phase. Important links must be planned for in advance. For example, in a diabetes disease management program, the MCO may consider retinal eye examinations a part of the program. Links between the optometrist/ophthalmologist and the primary care provider (PCP) must be forged, or when it comes time to evaluate this quality indicator, no eye examination results may show up in the PCP's office; even if it was done, it was not readily documented. Retinal examinations are a HEDIS 3.0/1998 standard; most know of their importance, but many MCOs have reported special problems coordinating or documenting this task. Computer linkages between providers is optimal, but this solution is often beyond the budget.

Step 1: Define the Target Population

Selection of a disease is the first step when designing a disease management program. Consider your organization's case mix and location. A facility in a rural community, an inner-city facility, and a facility in a retirement community will likely have three different priorities. A rural community may need a diabetes program; an inner city area may benefit from a high-risk maternity program; and a retirement community (high Medicare mix) may find a cardiac program most urgent. Several criteria have been suggested for selection of conditions that can be successfully dealt with using a disease management program. These include:

- High prevalence rates/large population with the condition
- High cost (charges per episode, high prescription drug utilization, etc.)
- High treatment pattern variability (Arrandale, Cave, & Rowles, 1997, p. 76)
- Poor clinical outcomes or a high risk of negative outcomes
- Inefficient systems
- Potential for patient lifestyle changes to improve outcomes

The major question is, "Which disease(s) should be managed?" Well-planned information systems will greatly assist in answering the following questions (Hoffman, 1998, p. 40):

1. How many members represent the major disease groups in your organization?
2. What are the demographics of the populations in #1? Should the organization be focusing on this population at all and, if so, how extensively, with which age-groups and genders, and in which regions? (Meyers, 1998).
3. What are the morbidities and comorbidities associated with the disease groups?
4. What are the treatment costs for the disease, plus comorbidities?
5. What preventative measures are available; how effective are they; how much do they cost?
6. How much health care savings could be anticipated through these preventive measures?
7. Which populations hold the greatest potential to improve patient outcomes and functional status?

These questions are best asked on a regular basis. Disease populations change from year to year, and although you may be concentrating on 1996 data that identify asthma as a leading cause of health care costs, 1999 data may show something different.

Organizations in the past few years have looked at these criteria, and they have chosen many of the same diseases to target, including:

- Asthma
- Cancer (various types)
- Cardiovascular diseases (congestive heart failure, coronary artery disease)
- Chronic obstructive pulmonary disease (COPD)
- Depressive/mental health disorders
- Diabetes
- High-risk pregnancy/neonates
- Human immunodeficiency virus (HIV)/Acquired immune deficiency syndrome (AIDS)
- Hypertension
- Pain management
- Pneumonia/infectious diseases
- Renal failure/hemodialysis
- Transplants

Case managers are familiar with assessing the whole universe of a patient; in this (disease management) universe, an entire population is assessed, compared, and targeted. Start with general characteristics such as age, prevalence of diagnoses, insurance carriers, and cultural background; then add more defining assessments such as clinical outcomes, costs, and system efficiency. If the population is a predominately elderly population, then maternity, well-child, or pediatric asthma programs probably would not be a contender.

Some of this assessment requires computer-based data collection and may require the assistance of data analysts or computer personnel. The ideal system will measure all disease-specific interventions throughout every phase of care and over long periods to facilitate comparisons among diverse populations. This will show which interventions have value, thus avoiding less useful actions; this translates into appropriate use of resources.

An important part of this initial analysis includes an evaluation of the organization's current processes and programs. Perhaps pieces of a disease management program have evolved and are in place. Can these become a useful part of a whole program, or must they be so completely revised that they are better off "relieved of duty"? For a disease management program to be successful, all of the parts must function smoothly with each other yet be independently strong. For example, a diabetes disease management program may have 10 quality indicators that will determine improvement in the quality of care being provided to the diabetic population. All are important as a whole, and all are important individually; but the weakest link determines the strength of the chain. If all of the diabetic services are offered, but the HbA1c is under poor control, no amount of monitoring feet or eyes will prevent complications. In disease management, the whole is greater than the sum of its parts.

When defining the population with which to target, it is all very analytical. However, do not forget to put on the case management patient advocacy hat and really look at the beneficiary. As in case management, ask:

- What does this patient need?
- What is this patient receiving?
- How can the space between the need and the service be reduced or closed?

Decision Point: What are the diagnosis or diagnoses to target?

Step 2: Organize a Multidisciplinary, Cross-Functional Team

The disease management team has a formidable task in front of them. They must:

- Define goals and objectives: What are the expected/desired results?
- Decide what needs to be done, how it will be done, who will do it, how much will it cost.
- Ascertain how the program will fit into accreditation requirements.
- Determine what the potential barriers are that must be overcome, and develop strategic options to minimize these challenges.

Core team members may include case managers, physicians (both PCP and specialists), administrators, outside providers (mammography centers, eye centers, radiology, etc.), pharmacists, data analysts, biostatisticians, quality management, systems management, finance, utilization management, nurses/nurse practitioners, patient educators, home health/skilled nursing facility representatives—essentially, anyone who plays an important role in the chosen disease program. At times, an outside consultant can be useful as an objective observer of processes. And no health care team will move forward quickly without a well-respected and dedicated "champion"—often a "physician champion"—but specialty case managers and pharmacists also can be quite influential in this leadership role. These champions are sometimes needed "to move mountains"—and administration—as only an articulate, convincing, and respected professional can do.

One caution is that teams that are too large often present with additional challenges. It is difficult to get everyone in the same room at the same time, and the varying opinions can be dizzying. One technique is to have a strong core group and call in others as consultants for specific meetings when their input is needed to move forward. (See Teams in Chapter 9).

Facilities using multifunctional teams have another advantage: more accreditation organizations, such as Joint Commission on Accreditation of Healthcare Organizations, require utilization and proof that patient care is being addressed by multidisciplinary team units. When all levels of the health care industry are struggling to do more with less, these teams can also be used for accreditation purposes.

EXAMINE THE DATA

Using the data from Step 1 as a starting point, the team must collect and examine critical pieces of information that will help determine the best direction to place disease management efforts. It is essential to collect baseline data before any disease management intervention is begun. From these baseline data, the organization will be able to compare post-intervention data. This comparison will show whether the intervention is successful, is progressing in the direction hoped for, or needs further improvement. The planning and collecting of pertinent data cannot be understated—and it is no easy task. Choosing the right data to collect may seem like an obvious job duty, but nothing is further from the truth. Make sure, up front, that the data collected will yield the answers to the questions the organization seeks. Harness the skill of professional data analysts. They do not always speak the same language as case managers or administrators, so all of the communication skills we have learned over the years will be invaluable.

ONGOING TRAINING

One critical function for the team is to explore how the training will be done once the program is organized. Nothing causes more frustration and burnout than a poorly trained worker; this was a leading cause of attrition of case managers in the early years. A disease management professional must understand everything from benefits to clinical details. Those performing the data collection must be trained; those monitoring the data collectors must be trained; front and back office personnel often play critical roles in tracking patient care and must have a clear idea of what the program is about; physicians and other providers must be educated as to the goals and objectives of the program and where they fit into the picture. Training and education is time-consuming, ongoing, and will use "non-productive" hours; but perhaps nothing is more important for a successful outcome; it prepares everyone for the changes and reduces "surprises."

BARRIERS TO SUCCESS

The team also must identify barriers that could interfere with a successful program. When assessing and evaluating your organization and its resources, barriers to treatment delivery may be uncovered. This critical assessment provides a starting point for problem-solving. Much back-tracking can be avoided by anticipating the barriers that may hinder your program and by planning detours. Several barriers are listed below, many with viable solutions cited. The sooner a barrier is exposed, the sooner the program will improve; seek out barriers rather than ignoring the signs of trouble. Most barriers cause the greatest trouble when they are not revealed. But do not let *the perfect get in the way of the good*. Through trial-and-error and improvement in outcomes, these programs are making a difference in the quality of care.

Most barriers are the result of system, people (patient or provider), or economic factors.

System Barriers often relate to access of services or processes.

- Many MCOs found that a major barrier was interfacing with the data departments. There is a huge language barrier. Often data people do not talk clinically and the quality people do not talk data. Be very specific in your requests and do not assume anything.
- When asking for medical records for chart audits or monitoring purposes, it is not unusual to receive the wrong records, incomplete records, or illegible records. This can seriously alter time schedules and needs special attention.
- Confidentiality laws sometimes make it difficult to obtain needed information on patients. Conversely, wholesale distribution of confidential information for the sake of disease management programs must be prevented.
- Computer programs are not always devised to elicit the information needed. Systems are often set up for claims and financial data, but not clinical, diagnostic, and treatment data. Programming problems can be modified, but it is time- and resource-intensive.
- Computer integration of systems is a large problem facing the health care industry; various segments of the health care delivery system (inpatient/outpatient, pharmaceutical/medical areas) cannot communicate with one another. In a survey by the National Managed Health Care Congress, 100 medical directors rated inadequate information technology as the biggest obstacle in implementing disease management programs; 77% planned to invest in information technology for the development of disease management programs (Meyers, 1998, p. 30).
- Physician offices often lack an efficient tickler system. Disease management companies noted that computerized offices improved in compliance over the

less sophisticated offices. Again, this problem could be solved, but budgets do not always support this magnitude of problem.

- Poor-quality data such as coding errors create problems. One example of a diabetic disease management coding problem (and there are many types of problem examples) presents when the organization wants to send educational material to diabetic members. When doing a mailing to diabetic members chosen through ICD-9 codes, there is a possibility that some non-diabetics will receive the information. This creates unrest with the nondiabetic member and often spurs them to unhappily telephone the department that sent the information. Some organizations have alleviated this problem by placing a disclaimer on all disease-specific information that is sent to their members. Another potential method to decrease the number of incorrect diagnoses is to send preliminary lists to the PCPs to have them verify whether these patients were, in fact, diabetic.

- Systems are designed for fee-for-service codes. As the MCOs begin to move toward capitated payments, this will create a gap of information for the MCOs. Even simple identification of disease-specific cases becomes more difficult without a fee-for-service coding structure. PCPs will see it as a benefit that they do not have to fill out forms for billing purposes. They are supposed to fill out encounter forms, but there is no financial reward for doing this; thus, it often does not get completed.

- Some disease management programs found that office staff was reluctant to follow-up on noncompliant patients; physicians did not make this a priority. Staffing and time restraints were cited as reasons.

- Health Plan Employer Data and Information Set (HEDIS) has encouraged mammogram monitoring in many organizations. Several system barriers are cited. There is a lack of clarity about who is notifying patients of mammogram results. Because the patient can be notified by the PCP, the obstetrician/gynecologist, the mammography center, or not at all, it was difficult to get reliable data on notification dates and timeframes. Integrated computer systems may be the answer here. There were documentation problems, such as a lack of documented results in the medical record. This is also important for HEDIS accreditation, which requires written documentation of the mammography date and results on the medical record.

- There is a lack of outcome information or personnel who can accurately design studies and interpret this data (Nash & Todd, 1997, p. 49).

- Competing disease management groups within one organization may cause confusion. If a patient with asthma and heart failure has one less emergency department visit than the previous timeframe, does the asthma program get the credit, or the cardiac program (Armstrong, 1996, p. 6)?

- On a larger scale, a barrier can be the lack of integrated levels of care that spans the whole continuum.

PATIENT/PROVIDER BARRIERS

- Keep in mind that change, in general, often leads to resistance.
- Resistance to change and "turf battles" are common personnel barriers.
- Beneficiary turnover is a barrier in some administrators' eyes. This affects the ability to accurately generate large amounts of data on the same population, to gain unequivocal proof of success (Wrinn, 1997, p. 17).
- Itinerant members also make it difficult for some administrators to justify putting in large amounts of money to keep patients healthy who may ultimately become members of another health plan. Of course, the street runs both ways, but the estimated rate of member attrition is 16.5% per year (Nash & Todd, 1997); this translates into an average enrollee period of approximately 24 to 30 months (Kozma, 1998a). There are essentially three areas of risk progression:
  1. General risk
  2. Specific disease risk
  3. Risk for disease progression (Hutcherson, 1995, p. 28)

Most programs focus on the 20% of the population in the "risk for disease progression" category because that is the area that uses the most resources and therefore is shouting the loudest. However, the other two groups (the 80% of the population in the well-known 80/20 rule) most likely will move into the high-utilization group if ignored. In a sense, to only address the high utilizers is a cost-shifting attitude among MCOs: let the future take care of itself because it is unlikely that the 80% will still be in "my" plan when they become high utilizers.

- Sensitivity and confidentiality are important considerations. When sending beneficiaries information about their disease, it must be sent in a nondescriptive envelope. Many beneficiaries do not want anything that identifies them as a diabetic (or other disease), or in need of a prostate examination, advertised to the mail carrier and outside world.
- Because of managed care in the news, the public (and especially Medicare-age beneficiaries) are suspicious. They want to be sure that what you say, do, or send them will not in any way affect their care or coverage. If you ask a member specific questions about a physician or their quality of care or health, they are likely to be less than honest for fear of losing benefits. This has always been identified as a barrier in case management, but it is often

overcome when a trusting relationship is forged. Some disease management programs do not nurture this relationship because of very large caseloads.

- Patient information overload is cited as a barrier (Nash & Todd, 1997, p. 144). In addition, the information is not always clinically accurate or it is conflicting, because the sources may be questionable or camouflaged in marketing purposes.

- Patient attitudes were said to be a barrier. At Pacificare, an Arizona MCO, a mammogram survey of Medicare patients who had not received a recent mammogram showed that the most common attitudes were:
  1. "My physician didn't recommend it." (top reason)
  2. "I'm fine."
  3. "I'm too old."
  4. "It's not necessary."
  5. "I have other health problems."

- *Patient involvement* is key to any disease management success story. Yet the ability to define and understand this process is as elusive to case and disease managers as love is to poets. The process is related to patient compliance and patient education, which is a major focus of case/disease management responsibilities. However, it is one thing to teach a diabetic to monitor blood glucose and diet; it is another matter to have them consistently follow recommendations.

- Finding ways to include members in their care has been a challenge to some programs. Some organizations send members diaries; other use computer diaries to capture day-to-day clinical and care information (Bazzoli, 1997, p. 77).

- Physician attitudes were stated as a barrier. Some physicians believed that their patients wouldn't listen to them (noncompliant); some physicians showed a lack of interest in routine services; many physicians believe that their patient population is unique and do not compare to national data; some organizations believe that many physicians do not actively encourage preventive aspects to disease management programs such as mammograms.

- Physician autonomy, in some respects, has been threatened in disease management programs; many believe this is the classic recipe for "cookbook medicine." A potential solution has been suggested. "This conflict highlights the wisdom of having prescribers (*e.g.,* physicians) participate in the development of goals and objectives for disease state management programs, and the need for flexibility when implementing these programs" (Kozma, Kaa, & Reeder, 1997, p. 5).

- Overwhelming amounts of new medical information is cited as a provider-based barrier. An effective vehicle to overcome information overload includes use of decision-support tools (Nash & Todd, 1997, p. 143). When disease-specific projects included the need to understand complex and fast-changing intricacies of medications such as angiotensin-converting enzyme (ACE) inhibitors, beta-blockers, or the latest recommendation for antibiotics in community-acquired pneumonia, the Arizona Peer Review Organization/ Quality Improvement Organization commissioned a pharmacist to do a thorough literature search and write succinct monographs on the subjects. Organizations were able to use these as teaching tools, thus lessening the need for each physician to perform the same time-consuming academic exercise.

- What are the "best practices" for any given disease state? There is no across-the-board consensus, and the choices are many and conflicting. A consortium of MCOs is so concerned about this, they are willing to shoot fast forward into the next millennium with high-level collaborative efforts; they are endeavoring to pool knowledge and come to a consensus on practice guidelines for specific diseases.

- Related to the above, physicians may choose not to implement the disease management protocols because of suspicion of the validity of the chosen guidelines or treatment plan. Education and support in the form of the previously mentioned monographs—with references to highly respected, peer-reviewed journals—can be the bridge across this barrier.

Economic barriers can be seen when benefits and reimbursement do not match the goals of the disease management program.

- The sheer cost of disease management programs leave some organizations lagging behind. Some resort to either developing programs internally or only buying components of programs such as health risk appraisals. Some organizations do not believe they have the financial ability to implement a disease management program as comprehensively as they would like to (Pinney, 1998).

- A high-quality, well-advertised disease management program may confer some risk on the organization by serving as a magnet for those with the disease. This may seem like contradiction; however, just because an organization has an excellent program for high-cost diseases such as cancer, diabetes, asthma, or acquired immunodeficiency syndrome, it may not be fiscally healthy enough to attract a huge volume of these cases to their health plan (Harris, 1996, p. 840).

- When educational information is mailed, postcards are less expensive to develop and mail. However, as stated in Patient Barriers, take into consideration the privacy (confidentiality) of the recipient of the mailing. Folded cards can be used as an alternative to open postcards.

- Many organizations are facing challenges because benefits are often out of line with what the disease management program is "preaching."
  - If an organization is promoting blood glucose monitoring and not providing test strips or glucometers, that is a barrier.
  - If retinal eye examinations and mammograms are encouraged, think about eliminating the copayments.
  - Outpatient drug benefits are critical for success in many disease management programs; yet the organization does not align drug benefits with need. Although risk-MCOs are beginning to limit drugs and imposing dollar limits on prescriptions, they may want to keep in mind the "special populations," such as diabetics.
  - The referral requirement was cited as a barrier when organizations required them for annual preventive care. It was time consuming to go to the physician for a referral to go to the mammogram center. In response, some benefit designs permit self-referral for mammograms and other preventive measures.
  - There are seldom benefits for educational programs, even when some of these have proven track records of reducing complications of disease. For example, diet and therapy monitoring is often considered "not medically essential."
  - There are seldom benefits for psychosocial support, even though this is often a huge barrier to success. An estimated 30% to 50% of severe asthmatics in the general population have some level of psychosocial condition that interferes with their treatment plan. At National Jewish Center (NJC), known for respiratory treatment, 70% to 95% of pediatric and adolescent asthma patients have psychosocial problems that interfere with the success of their treatment program at the community level. Successful counseling interventions have been attributed to a 45% to 80% reduction in *post-treatment* costs at NJC (Todd, 1995, p. 41).
  - Preventive benefits are often lacking. This is different from the diagnostic preventive benefits such as mammograms, prostate examinations, or colonoscopies. Rather, smoking cessation is encouraged, yet the medications that curb nicotine cravings and the gum and patches are not reimbursable—and are extremely expensive. Neither are stress management or nutritional counseling or special diets (even in morbid obesity) coverable benefits.
- Time constraints are a barrier in nearly every health care setting. Often this is the result of economic restraints. Hospitals are on skeletal staff numbers (which is often why educational opportunities fall through the cracks); physicians must have large rosters of patients to be economically solvent

(this, in turn, reduces the time-per-patient availability); for each level of care, from acute care to physician office, patients are more acutely ill and require more (not less) attention.

- Misalignment of incentives and rewards among plan, provider, and patient are still barriers (Nash & Todd, 1997, p. 49).
- Balancing the cost of designing and administering a disease management program with the delivery of quality medical care remains a concern. Some predict that "as the concept of disease state management evolves, goals may begin to accommodate higher quality health care at increased health care costs. Ultimately, cost and quality decisions will be market driven; society and payors will decide what is acceptable. . ." (Kozma et al., 1997, p. 5).
- ROI (return on investment) in true disease management programs have been estimated to require 5 to 10 years to reach fruition (Lee, 1996, p. 38).

Step 3: Define Core Components, Treatment Protocols, and Monitoring and Evaluation Methods

Defining the core elements of the disease management program, determining how to monitor and evaluate the outcomes, and designing a continuous approach to quality improvement is the essence of the developmental process. They must be based on "best practices" and current, evidence-based guidelines—which, to add another challenge, are moving targets at this time. Like pathways and utilization management guidelines, the guidelines are tools, not rules, that must be adjusted to the needs of the individual population or patient. Furthermore, although the cooperation of the physicians in the use of the chosen protocols is germane, one recent study showed how new information may stifle change in behavior rather than promote it. This study suggested that physicians are more reluctant to prescribe therapy when there are several competing viewpoints about what constitutes the "best practice" (Mazonson, Zagari, & Freston, 1996, p. 72). And there are several viewpoints. There is no shortage of clinical practice guidelines; they can be found in books, in proprietary material, on CD-ROM, on the Internet. The challenge is gaining the consensus of the organization's medical staff on what constitutes up-to-date, credible medical parameters. In a staff model organizational structure, the physicians may have had their "say" about the clinical practice guidelines chosen for a given disease management program. However, in an individual practice association model, it is against the odds that all will be in favor of any given medical protocol. One solution recommended by organizations who have been through the process is to have a well-respected physician "champion" directing the disease management effort.

GOALS AND OBJECTIVES

It is critical for the team to begin with a clear understanding of the disease-based population and the organizational goals and objectives. To decide on treatment protocols without understanding these important elements may lead to poor outcomes. They provide the target with which to aim organizational efforts. Without a clear target, the efforts may go in any trajectory, and a lot of time and resources can be wasted. When the organization *aims* at the specific, chosen target, all actions can be focused in the right direction, and resources are used wisely.

Long-term and short-term goals and objectives are decided on up front. They are used as a compass showing which directions are important to the organization. When deciding on what the goals and objectives will be, examine the data from your organization, current literature, and expert opinion. Also consider external factors such as governmental accreditations and regulations, liability issues, and the impact the program may have on the external providers. Provider cooperation is certainly an important success factor, and including members of the medical community in the initial plans may be strategically sound (Kozma et al., 1997, p. 7).

Writing out goals and objectives will help the team stay focused over the weeks and months of the planning phase. (See Part II for more information on goals and objectives).

EXAMPLES OF WRITTEN GOALS

Cardiovascular Goal

1. To improve and to sustain improvement of acute myocardial infarction (AMI) care for members/beneficiaries.

Diabetes Goal

1. To improve the quality and timeliness of the physician office care provided to patients with diabetes.

EXAMPLES OF WRITTEN OBJECTIVES (NOTE THAT OBJECTIVES ARE MEASURABLE STATEMENTS)

Cardiovascular Objectives

1. To increase utilization of ACE inhibitors in AMI patients with low left ventricular ejection fraction (LVEF) at discharge to the level of the benchmark or above.

2. To increase utilization of beta-blockers in AMI patients at discharge to the level of the benchmark or above.

Diabetes Objectives

1. To increase the percentage of patients who had blood pressure measured at least once during each quarter to the level of the benchmark or above.
2. To increase the percentage of patients with high blood pressure who received an ACE inhibitor to the level of the benchmark or above.
3. To increase the percentage of patients who had a foot examination performed twice a year to the level of the benchmark or above.

Step 4: Pilot the Program on a Small Scale

Once the protocols have been set and everyone instrumental in the process has been trained, it is time to roll out the program on a small scale. A pilot-size trial makes sense because:

- It is easier to control.
- There is less expenditure of resources.
- Changes can be steered more readily on a small scale.
- And most importantly, if a process goes poorly, it may be a minor incident rather than a major disaster.

Tools and guidelines often need tweaking; "just in time" training may be required; and continuous quality improvement (CQI) techniques may save the day. Many references cited the critical need for a well-designed CQI program to allow for positive changes in the program (see CQI chapters). One other word of caution: whether this is a pilot program or time for "the big implementation," the first time an organization tries something of this caliber, it is wise to start small. Perhaps a diabetes program will start with annual retinal examinations, or bi-yearly HbA1c testing, rather than trying to manage 10 diabetic quality indicators right out of the gate. New indicators can be introduced gradually.

Step 5: Measure the Outcomes

In 1910, Dr. Ernest Amory Codman developed the "End Result Idea." This may have been the first inklings of outcomes, when he described the idea that hospitals and physicians follow-up on treatment failures, so that they may be prevented in the future (Dial, 1996, pp. 1, 16). It is essential to measure outcomes before the beginning of the disease management interventions. Only through this exercise of identifying baseline data can the program have a point of comparison to see how well (or poorly) the medical interventions fared. It would be so interesting to have had baseline data in the mid-1980s, before case management became largely mainstream. We know we have made major impacts; this would show both proof and degree.

When deciding which outcomes to measure, look at clinical, humanistic (patient/provider satisfaction), and financial outcomes. Together, they paint a more complete picture than any one separately. Clinical outcomes are often the result of carefully designed tools used specifically for the purpose of collecting the clinical data desired; the Diabetic Tool (Figure 2-1) is an example of one tool that became a permanent part of the patient's medical record. Financial outcomes can be extracted from various encounter and claims databases. The patient/provider, or humanistic outcomes, come directly from the patient/provider themselves. Patient feedback is important; without their participation and cooperation, there would not be a disease management program. Feedback from providers and case managers is equally important; they are often the ones who administer the program.

Outcome measurements require very specialized knowledge of databases and statistics. More physicians and nurses are going back to school for statistical training, a perfect combination for this step. A competent computer systems analyst is also essential for those building their own databases to elicit specific outcome measurements.

However, building one's own database has advantages and disadvantages when looking at disease management from a national and international perspective. If everyone is "doing their own thing," large amounts of national data cannot be compared because, more likely than not, the criteria and data collection for each organization was just a little (or a lot) different; small variations create vast differences when outcome measurements are critically analyzed. The Health Care Financing Administration (HCFA) has, since 1992, sponsored a national project called CCP (Cooperative Cardiovascular Project). This nationwide effort has changed the course of acute myocardial infarction patient care and decreased mortality and morbidity significantly. One goal was to develop a large database to test specific treatment options such as the infusion of thrombolytics within a tight timeframe. A large database could not be gathered if the criteria for measuring the time to infusion of thrombolytics differed among collaborators. If one collaborator measured the time from diagnosis of a myocardial infarction (MI) to infusion of thrombolytics, and another measured the time from the presentation of the patient to the emergency department to infusion of the thrombolytics, two very slight, but very different, measurements would be elicited. Comparison of the data would not be comparing "apples-to-

CLINICAL QUALITY INDICATOR RECORD FOR DIABETES

I. DEMOGRAPHICS

1. NAME _____ _____ ___   2. HIC #: _____
       LAST.   FIRST.   MI   (HEALTH IDENTIFICATION CLAIM #)

3. DOB: __/__/__   4. RACE: CAUC   BLK   HIS   ASN   NAI   OTHER
     (MM/DD/YY)   (CIRCLE ONE)

5. TYPE OF DIABETES: I/II/OTHER   6. AGE OF ONSET: _____   7. GENDER: M / F
     (CIRCLE ONE)   (ENTER AGE OF ONSET)   (CIRCLE ONE)

8. HEIGHT (Inches): _____   9. HMO PLAN: _____

II. COMORBIDITIES
(Circle all that apply)

1. Cancer	5. Coronary Artery Disease	9. PVD
2. Cerebrovascular Disease	6. Hyperlipidemia	10. Renal Disease
3. CHF	7. Hypertension	11. Other
4. COPD	8. Peripheral Neuropathy	

III. PHYSICAL EXAM

	BLOOD PRESSURE (Enter first 4 values obtained each quarter)				ACE INHIBITOR Y / N	WEIGHT (lbs)	I = INSULIN O = ORAL AGENT D = DIET
	/	/	/	/			
	/	/	/	/			
	/	/	/	/			
	/	/	/	/			
	/	/	/	/			

RETINAL EXAM				FOOT EXAM			
QUARTER	EXAMINER IM/FPGP/ OPHTH/ OPTOM/ OTHER	RETINOPATHY N = NORMAL A = ABNORMAL	REFERRED TO EYE CARE PROFESSIONAL Y / N	QUARTER	EXAMINER IM/FPGP/ OTHER	RESULTS N = NORMAL A = ABNORMAL	REFERRED TO VASCULAR SPECIALIST (VS) OR PODIATRIST (P)

Figure 2-1. Clinical quality indicator record for diabetes. (Reference: Diabetes Project; a HCFA cooperative project facilitated by Health Services Advisory Group, Inc. Phoenix, AZ, in collaboration with six Arizona Medicare HMOs.)

apples." Therefore, the disadvantage of everyone making up their own outcome measures is that it does not add to a large, and therefore statistically significant, database.

There is an advantage, however, to experimenting with many different methods in an effort to improve disease-specific treatment protocols. As long as there is a large enough sample of patients to be statistically significant, and the methodology is scientifically sound, comparisons can lead to "best practices" by observing what worked, what worked better, and what worked best. Simply put, one physician said, "I'm washing my hands when I deliver babies."

IV. LABORATORY

GLYCOSYLATED HEMOGLOBIN (Check Appropriate Range)					LIPID PROFILE RESULTS ENTER VALUE				TREATMENT D = DIET M = MEDICATION B = BOTH
QUARTER	6.0 – 6.9%	7.0 – 7.5%	7.6 – 8.5 %	> 8.5%	CHOL	TRI	HDL	LDL	Enter D, M, or B

	PROTEIN DIPSTICK (Check Appropriate Box)			MICROALBUMIN (Check Appropriate Box)		
QUARTER	+	−	ACE INHIBITOR Y = YES N = NO A = ALREADY ON C = CONTRAINDICATED	< 20 MG/L	< 20 MG/L	ACE INHIBITOR Y = YES N = NO A = ALREADY ON C = CONTRAINDICATED

V. EDUCATION
(Check Appropriate Box)

QUARTER	DIET	DIETICIAN REFERRAL Y / N	DIABETIC MEDICATIONS	GLUCOSE TESTING	EXERCISE	SMOKER Y / N	ANTISMOKING ADVICE

PHYSICIAN SIGNATURE _____

Figure 2-1 *(Continued)*.

Another physician said, "I'm not washing my hands when I deliver babies." A comparison elicited the "best practice."

When outcomes have finally been collected and analyzed, it is important to take a step back and match the results to the original organizational goals and objectives, and the needs of the beneficiaries, as stated in Step 3. Do the outcomes show a positive direction when a comparison is made? If they do, the program is on the right track; if they do not, use the Plan-Do-Check-Act Cycle for cyclical improvement. (See the chapters on CQI—the PDCA Cycle, and the chapters on outcomes.)

QUALITY INDICATORS

(See chapters on outcomes for more about quality indicators). When deciding which quality indicators to focus on, look at two important facets:

1. What are the desirable endpoints? A decrease in diabetic amputations may be the endpoint (or goal).
2. What processes must be adhered to to reach that endpoint? These would represent the quality indicators that must be measured. Example quality indicators for the above goal may include those listed below. The Diabetic Tool in Figure 2-1 may be used as a process step to track and monitor the quality indicators.

Diabetic Quality Indicators

Quality Indicator #1: Diabetic patients had a foot examination performed twice a year.

Quality Indicator #2: Diabetic patients had a hemoglobin A1c performed twice a year.

Quality Indicator #3: Diabetic patients had a glycosylated hemoglobin of 8.0 or less.

Quality Indicator #4: Diabetic patients were given diet and medication therapy for diabetes.

Quality Indicator #5: Diabetic patients received education about the effect of exercise on diabetes.

Quality Indicator #6: Diabetic patients received education about self-monitoring of blood glucose.

In another example, if the organization's goal is to decrease morbidity and mortality in AMI patients, the following quality indicators may be measured. The quality indicators represent wise processes (based on current literature and best practices) to reach that goal. That was the goal in 1992 with CCP (Cooperative Cardiovascular Project); this project went nationwide to improve the care of AMI patients and was facilitated by peer review organizations across the United States. Below are some of the quality indicators used:

Cardiovascular Quality Indicators

Quality Indicator #1: Received aspirin during the hospitalization

Quality Indicator #2: Received aspirin on the first day

Quality Indicator #3: Reperfusion: Received thrombolytic or percutaneous transluminal coronary angioplasty within 12 hours of arrival to the hospital

Quality Indicator #4: Received thrombolytic therapy in 1 hour

Quality Indicator #5: Discharged on an ACE inhibitor: ACE inhibitors for low LVEF

Quality Indicator #6: Discharged on aspirin

Quality Indicator #7: Discharged on beta-blocker

Quality Indicator #8: Documentation in the chart of advice or counseling on smoking cessation

Decision Point: How successful is the disease management program? Should the program continue as currently developed, or should it be revised?

Step 6: Implement the Disease Management Program, Plan CQI, and Celebrate!

This is it! It is time to implement the program. Implementation of the disease management program is where case managers typically step in. However, ideally, case managers are brought into the process much earlier:

- In Step 1, case managers have front-line knowledge of the health care gaps that members/beneficiaries must face.
- In Step 2, case managers can be a wealth of information. They know the systems and the barriers, again at the front lines, and can advise and steer planned interventions in more potentially successful avenues. I have seen more than one project get into deep trouble because no one asked the case managers' advice until many resources were used, abused, and wasted.
- In Step 3, case managers can provide useful information in both clinical and beneficiary-focused areas.
- Step 4 is to pilot the program on a small scale. The case manager's perspective is pivotal and can direct small and large changes in the pilot program toward greater success.
- Often data collection is done concurrently with the intervention stages (Steps 5 and 6) and will necessitate case managers as accurate data collectors. When assessing the results of the data, the case management perspective is invaluable—no one else in the health care chain sees the picture like a case manager is trained to do.

In general, disease management interventions focus on two groups: the providers and the beneficiaries (Armstrong, 1996, p. 6). Provider-based interventions usually focus on treatment protocols and guidelines, education, and compliance monitoring. Beneficiary-focused efforts take on a broad range of activities that usually include education, disease-specific clinical monitoring, activities for prevention of progression of the disease, medication compliance, and other processes specific to the disease or wellness program instituted.

Assessing the program and continuous monitoring and revisions will be ongoing. "Disease state management is a continuous process. It is unlikely that all measures necessary to manage a disease will be developed and implemented at the beginning of a program. Moreover, measures selected initially will likely require modification as the disease state management program matures and experience is gained; that is, disease state management programs are likely to be evolutionary, not revolutionary" (Kozma et al., 1997, p. 4). Use the methods and tools in the Continuous Quality Improvement (CQI) chapters to assess, monitor, and evaluate process. Then, as data suggest that there is a better way to do a process, continuously improve using the Plan-Do-Check-Act (PDCA) cycle.

So hire the staff. Train and keep the staff educated. Implement the interventions. Monitor and evaluate. Don't forget to celebrate success!

THE CASE MANAGEMENT/DISEASE MANAGEMENT PROCESS

Step 1: Identification of At-Risk Members

Targeting patients for disease management (or case management) attention is both a science and an art. The case manager/disease manager must take the facts and then become the catalyst for change; therein lies the "art." Many programs reveal patient candidates by looking at encounter data, hospital and outpatient utilization patterns, pharmacy data, or claims data. For some types of organizations, identification of at-risk members is becoming more of a difficult task. When capitation is the financial agreement of choice, there are fewer ICD-9 and other codes with which to identify a specific disease. Encounter forms are not always filled out by physicians, which often eliminates another potential mode of identification. Pharmacy data and claims/billing data, although after-the-fact, are still a means of identifying disease populations, although some think that they are not always reliable, especially claims/billing data. An individual's case identification criteria may include (Nash, 1997, p. 6):

- Patient demographics
- Severity of illness; disease subcategories
- Compliance behavior
- Historical cost profile
- Frequency of recurrence
- Seasonality
- Other epidemiologic markers

Step 2: Assessment and Evaluation of Members

Assessment of psychosocial issues, motivating factors, and competency barriers to optimal self-care behavior affect persons with chronic diseases, whether they are labeled disease management patients or case management patients. Although populations are often identified *en masse,* it then boils down to individual patients with individual balances of psychosocial and financial support and medical severity. Disease-specific clinical details, however, must be added in disease management. For disease management purposes, health risk appraisals must include disease-specific clinical triggers that will alert the case manager to a high-risk situation. Using a congestive heart failure disease management program as an example, the nurse case manager/disease manager would assess the following:

PHYSICAL SYMPTOMS

- Fatigue
- Shortness of breath/dyspnea
- Dizziness
- Chest pain/angina
- Palpitations
- Weight gain
- Increased peripheral edema
- Functional activities—Change in tolerance
- Jugular vein distention
- Cough
- Orthopnea—Difficulty sleeping
- Vital signs
  - Temperature
  - Blood pressure
  - Respiratory rate
  - Pulse
  - Weight
- Dietary practices
  - Low-sodium diet
  - Diet tolerance
  - Fluid restrictions
- Psychosocial stressors/support systems
- Health status survey
- Medications
- Mobility and function

— Activities of daily living
— Activity tolerance
• Compliance with:
— Medication
— Activity
— Dietary
• Medical appointments
— Physician appointments
— Laboratory tests
— Procedures

KNOWLEDGE DEFICITS

Assessment of knowledge deficits is fundamental in disease management programs. Educational deficits are a leading cause of noncompliance in patients. Chronic diseases require long-term, daily attention; therefore, compliance must always be monitored. This is often done telephonically, with monitoring/reminder phone calls. Is the patient taking their medications as ordered? How many times during the holiday season did the patient "cheat" on the diet? Are daily weights (at least) being continued during this holiday season? What do the daily weights tell the patient and case/disease manager? The educational component has a proven track record of improving patient compliance, increasing patient empowerment, decreasing health care costs, and enriching the quality of life. Assess knowledge levels of the disease-specific topics listed below (again, congestive heart failure is used as an example):

• Disease process/symptoms
• Dietary
— Low-sodium diet
— Fluid restriction/Intake and output monitoring
• Medications: Over-the-counter and prescriptive
— Dosages
— Side effects—Drug interactions
— Administration
• Physical changes
— Weight
— Activity tolerance
— Blood pressure
— Fatigue
— Shortness of breath/dyspnea
— Dizziness

— Chest pain/angina
— Palpitations
— Increased peripheral edema
— Jugular vein distention
— Cough
— Orthopnea—Difficulty sleeping
• Prognosis of disease with and without following disease protocols

SEVERITY OF TARGET DISEASE STATE

In disease management programs, it is important to further screen the patients for severity of disease. This will clue the case/disease manager into a big picture of how much attention the individual patient may require. Severity can be broken down into three stratification, or classification, levels:

• PRIORITY 1 PATIENTS: Those members who have a significant potential for exacerbations and emergency room visits or re-hospitalizations; this usually necessitates on-site visits to the member for extensive teaching and monitoring of medication regimen, signs and symptoms of disease exacerbation, and any other needs the case manager assesses for optimal care of the individual. These members may have significant comorbidities, compliance, or psychosocial issues. These patients are generally considered high risk if they exhibit severe acute or chronic illness requiring complex, ongoing coordination of services. Services are often needed frequently or over a long period (Box 2-1).
• PRIORITY 2 PATIENTS: Those whose needs must be monitored on a regular basis but can usually be managed telephonically. These patients are generally considered moderate risk if they have short- to long-term coordination needs. Coordination efforts may be high intensity at the beginning and are expected to level off. Occasional exacerbations of the disease may require higher-intensity interventions (Box 2-2).
• PRIORITY 3 PATIENTS: Those needing minimal attention, whose sole need may be education of the disease process, illness avoidance, or medication therapy. These patients are generally considered low risk if they have one or two health problems and may require minimal or short-term education or coordination of services (Box 2-3).

ASSESSING THE HEALTH CARE BENEFITS

An essential part of a case or disease management assessment is identifying insurance benefits. The insurance benefits should match the disease management program. This is not always the case, as seen in some of the barriers cited

Box 2-1

PRIORITY 1 PATIENTS—HIGH-RISK CHF PATIENTS

(Patients are generally considered **high risk** if they exhibit severe acute or chronic illness requiring complex, ongoing coordination of services. Services are often needed frequently or over a long period.)

Diagnosis of CHF is confirmed—LVEF of 40% or less

Functional capacity*: Rest or minimal exertion causes shortness of breath or fatigue; nocturnal dyspnea always or frequently present; frequent cough; appetite is poor; frequent thirst

Low ejection fraction equal to/less than 25%

2+ to 4+ Peripheral edema; abdomen firm

Breath sounds—rales

Heart sounds—ability to hear S3, S4

3–4 Pillow orthopnea or use of chair to sleep

8–12-cm Jugular vein distention

10–20-Pound fluid weight gain over 2–3 weeks

Severe comorbidities

Prognosis of 1-year life expectancy or less

Complex or new medication regimen

Multiple emergency room visits or rehospitalizations

Chronic noncompliance with medical treatment plan

Significant psychosocial issues—or "Yes" to 3 depression questions on the SF 36 Survey

Health Status scores (SF 36 or SF 12)—PSC and MHC <52

Use of durable medical equipment/oxygen

Use of physician specialist(s)

POTENTIAL INTENSITY OF CASE/DISEASE MANAGEMENT SERVICES

- Authorization for 4–6 home health visits may be requested for these patients, with further authorization possible based on individual patient circumstances
- Number of visits depends on educability of patient/family (may require more visits) and stability of medical condition
- Case/disease management monitors home health progress with patient
- During periods of stability, the case/disease manager will contact the patient as needed (minimally every 1–2 weeks); exacerbations will require higher-intensity interventions.

*Functional capacity is based on subjective symptoms and is not a classification of the degree of ventricular dysfunction or congestive heart failure.
Reference: CHF CASS (Congestive Heart Failure—Continuity Across Selected Sites); a HCFA cooperative project facilitated by Health Services Advisory Group, Inc, Phoenix, AZ, in collaboration with 6 Arizona Medicare HMOs.

Box 2-2

PRIORITY 2 PATIENTS—MODERATE-RISK CHF PATIENTS

(Patients are generally considered **moderate risk** if they have short- to long-term coordination needs. Coordination efforts may be high-intensity at the beginning, and are expected to level off. Occasional exacerbations of the disease may require higher-intensity interventions.)

Diagnosis of CHF is confirmed—LVEF of 40% or less

Functional capacity: Moderate exertion causes shortness of breath or fatigue; nocturnal dyspnea occasionally present; cough with exertion; appetite fair; thirsty sometimes

Ejection fraction between 25% and 40%

1+ To trace peripheral edema; abdomen soft, distended

Breath sounds—basilar rales

Heart sounds—murmur (any type)

2–3 Pillow orthopnea

6–8-cm Jugular vein distention

5-Pound fluid weight gain over 2–3 weeks

Knowledge deficits about cardiovascular disease processes

High recidivism rate for emergency room or hospitalizations

Complex or new medication regimen

Moderate comorbidities

Noncompliance issues

Psychosocial issues, or "Yes" to 2 of 3 depression questions on the SF 36 Survey

Health Status Survey (SF 36 or SF 12) scores—PSC or MHC <52

May use durable medical equipment/oxygen

May use a physician specialist

POTENTIAL INTENSITY OF CASE/DISEASE MANAGEMENT SERVICES

- Authorization for 4–6 home health visits may be requested for these patients
- Number of visits depends on educability of patient/family (may require more visits) and stability of medical condition
- Case/disease management monitors home health progress with patient
- During periods of stability, the case/disease manager will
  contact the patient at least monthly (more as needed);
  exacerbations will require higher-intensity interventions.

---

*Functional capacity is based on subjective symptoms and is not a classification of the degree of ventricular dysfunction or congestive heart failure.

Reference: CHF CASS (Congestive Heart Failure—Continuity Across Selected Sites); a HCFA cooperative project facilitated by Health Services Advisory Group, Inc, Phoenix, AZ, in collaboration with 6 Arizona Medicare HMOs.

Box 2-3

PRIORITY 3 PATIENTS—LOW-RISK CHF PATIENTS

(Patients are generally considered **low risk** if they have one or two health problems and may require minimal or short-term education or coordination of services.)

Diagnosis of CHF is confirmed—LVEF of 40% or less

Functional capacity: Few complaints about shortness of breath or fatigue, nocturnal dyspnea, cough, thirst, or appetite

New onset congestive heart failure

Knowledge deficits about cardiovascular disease processes/lifestyle changes

New medication regimen

Peripheral edema rarely present; abdomen nondistended

Breath sounds—clear

Heart sounds—S1–S2

1–2-Pillow orthopnea

Minimal or no fluid weight gain

Potential for multiple emergency room visits or hospitalizations

Few or none—comorbidities

Few or none—noncompliance issues

Few psychosocial issues—and "Yes" to 0–1 of 3 depression questions on the SF 36 Survey

Health Status (SF 36 or SF 12) scores—within 10 points of national norm

POTENTIAL INTENSITY OF CASE/DISEASE MANAGEMENT SERVICES

- Authorization for 2–3 home health visits may be requested for these patients
- Number of visits depends on educability of patient/family (may require more visits) and stability of medical condition
- Case/disease management monitors home health progress with patient
- The case/disease manager will contact the patient intermittently (every 1–2 months) to assess for impending problems

---

*Functional capacity is based on subjective symptoms and is not a classification of the degree of ventricular dysfunction or congestive heart failure.

Reference: CHF CASS (Congestive Heart Failure—Continuity Across Selected Sites); a HCFA cooperative project facilitated by Health Services Advisory Group, Inc, Phoenix, AZ, in collaboration with 6 Arizona Medicare HMOs.

previously. If a patient needs a particular benefit that is not available, but is encouraged by the disease management program, that part of the program needs to go back to the drawing board, and, in CQI fashion, be reevaluated. As stated above, alignment of program goals and objectives with the benefit structure is important if the program is to be successful. Hospital-based and post–acute-based disease management programs may not be afforded the luxury of suggesting that the benefits of the various patient groups match their program. Still, it is the case/disease manager's responsibility to assess the patient's benefits and attempt to find alternatives if the benefits do not meet the needs.

Step 3: Development and Coordination of Disease Management Plans

(**NOTE:** Step 3—Development and Coordination of Disease Management Plan, and Step 4—Implementation of Disease Management Plans, incorporate many of the same elements in case management as in disease management.)

Medically sound quality indicators are the foundation for disease management programs. Disease-specific protocols are used as a road map for optimal care, and case/disease managers work with the patients to improve treatment compliance with the recommendations for care given in these disease management guidelines. Disease management directions are further individualized according to the individual needs of the patient. This requires collaboration with the physician and other providers and is nothing new to case management; merely add the elements of treatment guidelines and disease-specific modalities to the case management process. Coordination of multidisciplinary services is a mainstay of case management programs. In some ways, it is where case managers have received the most appreciation and attention. It is equally important in disease management organizations.

Step 4: Implementation of Disease Management Plans

It is important for the patient to be involved in their own implementation of the disease management program. This gives the patient a sense of control over the disease process, enhances self-esteem, and encourages a collaborative relationship with the health care team. Patients should be educated in monitoring symptoms and taking appropriate preventive measures. For example, congestive heart failure patients would be taught to monitor for changes in weight or respiratory comfort; rapid weight gain or shortness of breath may trigger a visit from the disease management team or a home health nurse. Diabetic members are educated about the many aspects of diabetes, including monitoring blood glucose levels and appropriate adjustments of insulin dosage and diet. Ninety-five percent of diabetes care is provided by the patients themselves (Childs, 1998); therefore, education about self-management of diabetes can save the managed care organizations significantly. In one study, it was found that approximately 50% of hospitalized diabetic patients had some element of educational deficit as a direct cause of the admission (Peragallo-Dittko, 1997).

Many of the diseases chosen for disease management programs are complex, chronic, and require sharp problem-solving skills. The patient often must synchronize blood tests (glucose, for example), diet, exercise, stress, and a host of other factors that impact the disease. Chronic disease protocols are not easily adhered to, and compliance can be problematic even when the educational component has been well-taught and comprehended. Compliance training includes all of the reasons why it is essential to follow disease protocols. Sometimes that is all the incentive that is needed; more often, it is not. Follow-up is the essential ingredient that is both expected in disease management programs and can make the difference between repeat hospitalizations versus a successful program. As in case management, the case/disease manager is the link to needed services and becomes the patient advocate if the services are not in the benefits or affordable. The advocacy role of the case/disease manager must also take the patient's innate ability into consideration; not everyone is mentally or emotionally equipped to cope with major, chronic illnesses.

Step 5: Evaluation: Outcome Measurements

Several categories of outcomes are important to objectively assess and measure the benefits of a disease management program. Outcomes can be viewed as the end result of the medical intervention. Were the goals attained? These goals can be clinical, financial, or humanistic. It is important to balance the types of outcomes measured; ignoring quality over financial outcomes can offer some major lessons. Some indicators are evaluated by the PCP, a specialist, or a case/disease manager, and will usually be tracked by the case/disease manager; others will be tracked on information systems, clinical and financial databases, pharmaceutical systems, billing/claims databases, and so forth. In some ways, this is the critical piece for the future of disease management. "The programs will be judged by cost and by statistically validated outcomes that enhance the quality of life and slow the progression of disease" (Goldstein, 1998, p. 102). By definition, some organizations believe that disease management is synonymous with outcomes management. High compliance rates in clinical, financial, or patient (humanistic) indicators evidence a successful program.

CLINICAL OUTCOMES

Examples of Congestive Heart Failure Clinical Indicators

The patient shows evidence of stability or improvement in the following areas:

- Monitoring of weight changes and fluid balance (including rales, jugular venous distention, edema, weight gain)
- Diet instruction and monitoring (includes fluid restrictions monitoring)
- Anti-smoking education
- Activity tolerance—Change in functional abilities
- Cardiac diagnostics (including LVEF assessment)
- Medication monitoring and management (*e.g.,* ACE inhibitors, digitalis, coumadin)
- Monitoring of vital signs
- Monitoring of respiratory status (including symptoms of pulmonary edema)
- Lifestyle assessment (assessed through use of Health Risk Appraisal Tools)

FINANCIAL OUTCOMES

The intent of disease management is to manage the patient care to optimize health and minimize complications and exacerbations. With good outcomes, there should be a significant decrease in physician office visits, emergency room visits, and hospitalizations. Because complications and recidivism are decreased with disease management strategies, when hospitalizations do occur, the length of stays are shortened because of less severity of illness on admission. These visits and any inpatient or ambulatory services are often tracked using sophisticated information technology.

Judicious use of home health care is another disease management strategy (See Priority 1, 2, and 3 Patients). Studies have shown that overly stringent use of home health services has translated into higher bills from emergency departments, hospitals, and frequent physician office visits.

PATIENT OUTCOMES (ALSO KNOWN AS HUMANISTIC OUTCOMES)

Patient outcomes are often viewed from patient satisfaction, quality of life, and patient compliance issues. A Patient Satisfaction Survey is administered intermittently to measure member satisfaction with the disease management program. This provides a forum for evaluation and improvement in services. Some questions include:

- Was the care easy to access?
- Was the case manager caring and helpful?

- Was the family unit/patient appropriately involved in the disease management program?
- Was continuity of care an issue?
- Was quality of care an issue?
- Were the patient's/family's health care goals achieved?
- Were the patient's/family's privacy and dignity respected?
- Is the patient/family coping better because of the efforts of the disease management program?

A patient-reported Health Status Survey (also referred to a Quality of Life [QOL] assessment) is another disease management strategy. The use of the Health Status Survey (SF-12 or SF-36) has gained credibility in the health care arena. The Health Status Survey is a patient's self-assessment of perceived QOL issues and has proved to be a predictive tool that may indicate the member has a potential for a hospital admission in the next 6 to 12 months. By early use of this tool, and early identification of possible problems, a disease management plan can be implemented to attempt to avoid or delay increased use of emergency department visits or hospitalization. This tool can be administered early in the disease management process; it can then be readministered at 6-month intervals to assess the patient's perception of their health curve. When data are collated with medical resource use, this tool can show outcomes of how well the program is working.

THE FUTURE OF DISEASE MANAGEMENT

Disease management—population-based medicine—is an important idea whose time has come. Many organizations believe that, as long as outcome measures provide good news, disease management programs will continue. In a slightly different bend, some believe that outcomes are the cornerstone of disease management as they continue to provide health care with new insights into better methods of disease treatment.

Technological advances will continue to drive disease management. Those with advanced and integrated technological systems, and the interventions that are proven through positive outcomes, will become the survivors; other organizations may likely become extinct. These integrated information systems will be "a dream come true" for any case manager who has ever wished that all patient history was in one place; only the most recent events need be updated. These systems will also have standards and treatment parameters readily available.

The attention to comorbidities will increase in the near future. If disease management is only for those with a "pure" disease, there is not as much to gain from the exercise. Studies show that singular diseases are rarely the case. One study looked at diagnostic codes in asthma patients over a 1-year period. Of the 222 cases, 208 had unique combinations of diagnosis codes (Kozma, 1998, p. 65). Comorbidity challenges arise when a patient presents with diabetes and congestive heart failure and pneumonia. If 2 hospital days are saved, which disease management program gets the credit? Outcome measurements are difficult enough without muddying the waters with comorbid thoughts. One potential answer lies in developing more sophisticated information systems that really aggregate identifying factors about the disease population as a whole. Patients with asthma or diabetes will still be treated with the most state-of-the-art care. However, as disease management programs evolve, the understanding of how to handle comorbidities must be addressed (Kozma, 1998, p. 66).

Another change whose time has come is a message that case managers have been encouraging for years: that collaboration is germane to good patient outcomes. Managed care organizations are, for the most part, competitors. Mergers force some of them together like planned marriages in ancient traditions, sometimes causing subtle behaviors that can have a negative impact on the reputation of health care. But something new is emerging: not in every state, and not with every organization. Collaboration is being attempted among competitors in various degrees. The Arizona Peer Review Organization/Quality Improvement Organization (PRO/QIO) has facilitated this type of collaboration for several years. The diabetic tool (Figure 2-1) is a result of some of the collaboration on diabetic quality indicators. The competitive MCOs who initially collaborated on this project went back to their organizations and tried various methods to improve diabetic care; there were successes and barriers; tools were tried and revised; processes were measured and amended. Then, a few years later, a "think tank" was facilitated by the PRO/QIO. The original, competing MCOs were invited; they brought tools and tales to share (literally photocopied and distributed); barriers were exposed, often with successful interventions following "failures." They realized that it is a waste of resources for each organization to have to reinvent the disease management wheel. This is only the exciting beginning.

A legal change that requires food for thought are the portability laws. Those chronically ill patients that are on "the other HMO's plan" may be on "your" plan in the coming months—or years. Weeding out the sickest and refusing membership is no longer in option in most cases. Collaboration among providers and insurers to keep the chronically ill populations from deteriorating medically serves everyone—the providers, the insurers, and mostly, the patients.

Treatment guidelines, although "tools, not rules," will become less consensus-based and more evidence-based. The technology, the quality improvement projects, and the trials of multiple organizations in trying to optimize their members' health and utilization statistics all contribute to the fund of disease management knowledge that will create these protocols. As stated earlier, they are a moving target; as new medications and drug protocols are discovered, as more complementary-medical synergies become apparent, better treatment guidelines will replace the "best" practices of the past.

There is a growing trend in the direction of more preventive health measures. Actually, the terms "health care," "health insurance," or "health benefits" are misnomers; America has never focused on "health," but rather "disease." That is changing. And given the current trend of public support for alternative therapies, it is possible that, for disease management to be fully integrated into customer service, the whole concept of disease management will transform. Disease management programs that do not consider the large population that supports alternative medicine, proven by their willingness to invest billions of out-of-pocket dollars, will be left in the dust. Consumers will decide what "quality" means to them, and they seem willing to pay for it. As new as outcome measurements are in the world of traditional medicine, they are even more recent in the alternative medicine arena. But alternative outcomes are being studied, and by organizations as credible as the National Institutes of Health's Office of Alternative Medicine, and several major medical universities and centers. Together, they make a marriage the likes of which the world has not seen. (See chapters on Complementary and Alternative Medicine.) It may be that disease-specific clinics in the near future will include physicians, herbalogists, acupuncturists, and homeopathic practitioners. Physical therapy locations may include sports medicine physicians, physical therapists, chiropractors, rolfers, and polarity/energetic healers.

In the book *Disease Management: A Systems Approach to Improving Health Outcomes* (Nash & Todd, 1997), two forward-thinking authors looked beyond disease management. Components of a true prospective health management system include:

- Economic risk analysis
- Screening and early detection
- Health risk assessment
- Behavioral approaches to risk reduction and health optimization
- Economic and other incentives

- Demand management and self-care
- Anti-aging and mind-body-spirit medicine
- Occupational medicine/corporate health

The World Health Organization's definition of health is "a state of complete physical, mental and spiritual well being, not merely the absence of disease." In parts of China, the people do not pay Chinese doctors if they are ill; they are paid in times of health. In the West, innovative thinkers state that "From a continuous quality improvement (CQI) perspective, every medical diagnosis and every episode of medical care represent a failure—a failure of prevention" (Nash & Todd, 1997, p. 309). The kaleidoscope turns; the paradigm shifts.

How do case managers fit into all of this? Case management is evolving in the right direction. We must become even more astute in our clinical expertise when working within disease management systems. We must understand the concepts that are important to managed care organizations such as outcomes management and continuous quality improvement. And we must understand what is important to the ultimate customer: the patient. What is important is an acceptable quality of life, whether that translates into conventional medicine or alternative treatments; the case manager must understand the clinical condition and all types of potential treatment to truly be a patient advocate. Episodic case management has left many professionals feeling less than satisfied. For those who enjoy impacting health through education, following patients from the preventive and wellness phase, and into all environments, working with patient-centered coordinated care teams, then disease management may be a perfect fit.

PART I: REFERENCES, RESOURCES, AND BIBLIOGRAPHY

Anonymous. (1998). DM program reports 83% drop in CHF patient admissions. *The Case Manager, 9*(2), 18.

Anonymous. (1996). The business of disease management. *Medical Interface, 9*(7), 118–119.

Anonymous. (1996). Assessing the role of drug companies. *Health Data Management, 4*(1), 34.

Armstrong, E. (1996). Disease state management and its influence on health systems today. *Drug Benefit Trends, 8*(7), 18–20, 25, 29.

Arrandale, K., Cave, D., & Rowles, M. (1997). Patient care management: Maximizing efficiency through use of prevalence rates. *Managed Care Interface, 10*(11), 75–78.

Bazzoli, F. (1996). Putting the pieces together. *Health Data Management, 4*(1), 29–37.

Bazzoli, F. (1997). Disease management. *Health Data Management, 5*(6), 69–72.

Behrendt, D. (1998). Home care and clinical paths: Steps toward more effective care. *Home Care Innovations, 8*(1), 23–26.

Boston Consulting Group. (1993). *The changing environment for US pharmaceuticals.* Boston: Author.

Childs, B. (1998). Diabetes care. *Case Review, 4*(3), 14–20, 60.

Conlon, P. (1997). Diabetes: Managing the macrovascular complication of diabetes. *Disease Management Digest, 1*(2), 2–3.

Dial, W. (1996). Disease management: A byword in search of a definition. *Managed Health Care News, 12*(1), 1, 16–17.

Dial, W. (1997). Disease management: Coming of age, or apart at the seams? *Managed Health Care News, 13*(5), 1, 12.

Fazio, A., Hynes, J., & Keefe, J. (1998). Retention of patients with a diagnosis of diabetes in selected managed care plans. *Managed Care Interface, 11*(6), 68–72.

Genuth, S. (1998). Diabetes: Managing the retinal, renal, and neurologic complication of diabetes. *Disease Management Digest, 2*(1), 12–13.

Giles, K. (1998). Disease management: A better alternative to the managed care process. Retrieved 1998 from the World Wide Web: http://www.assoc-cancer-ctrs.org/disease.html.

Goldstein, R. (1998). The disease management approach to cost containment. *Nursing Case Management, 3*(3), 99-103.

Grahl, C. (1998). An expert's summary of disease management essentials. Retrieved 1998 from the World Wide Web: http://www.modernmedicine.com/mhc/dsm10sb2.html.

Gurnee, M., & Da Silva, R. (1997). Constructing disease management programs. Retrieved 1999 from the World Wide Web: http://www.managedcaremag.com/archivemc/9706.disease_man.shtml.

Haas, L. (1998). Diabetes: The early detection of diabetes mellitus: advantages for patients and society. *Disease Management Digest, 2*(2), 10–11.

Harris, J. (1996). Disease management: New wine in new bottles? *Annals of Internal Medicine, 124*(9), 838–842.

Hazelwood, F., Rodriguez, D., & Cypress, M. (1998). Exploring the roles of case managers in diabetes care. *The Case Manager, 9*(2), 57–61.

Hoffman, W. (1998). Making dollars and sense. *Managed Health Care News, 14*(4), 40–41.

Hutcherson, A. (1995). Disease management demystified: What can it do? *Health Care Innovations, 5*(6), 25–28.

James, M. (1998). At the heart of the disease management revolution. *The Case Manager, 9*(2), 47–50.

Johnson, S. (1996). The state of disease state management. *Case Review, 2*(4), 53–57.

Kozma, C. (1996). Evaluating disease state management interventions. *Medical Interface, 9*(6), 110–111.

Kozma, C. (1997). From disease management of disease to disease state management. *Medical Interface, 10*(1), 107–108.

Kozma, C. (1998a). Enrollee retention and disease state management. *Managed Care Interface, 11*(6), 66, 72.

Kozma, C. (1998b). The role of comorbidities in disease state management. *Managed Care Interface, 11*(7), 65–66.

Kozma, C., Kaa, K., & Reeder, C.E. (1997). A model for comprehensive disease state management. *The Journal of Outcomes Management, 4*(1), 4–8.

Lashley, M. (1995). CM and DM team up for effective management of high-cost care. *The Case Manager, 6*(3), 71–78.

Lee, S. (1996). New trends in disease management. *Continuing Care, 15*(7), 37–39.

Levitt, D., Startz, T, & Higgins, R. (1998). Disease state case management in an academic medical center utilizing osteoarthritis-of-the-knee model. *The Journal of Care Management, 4*(5), 45–55.

Lewis, A. (1996). Disease management carve-outs: Caveat Emptor. *Medical Interface, 9*(10), 88–90.

Mazonson, P., Zagari, M., & Freston, J. (1996). Shortening the time between availability of new medical information and its adoption in general practice. *Medical Interface, 9*(3), 71–77.

McCarthy, R. (1995, December). Disease management: A critical look. *Medical Utilization Management,* 4–8.

McKinnon, B. (1996). Chronic disease management gains favor in pharmacology. *Continuing Care, 15*(1), 23–24.

Meyers, J. (1998). Beyond intervention: Data warehousing and the new disease management. *Managed Health Care, 8*(1), 28–34.

Minerd, R., & Lee, S. (1997). Using business process reengineering to develop disease management programs. *Inside Case Management, 4*(9), 8–9.

Nash, D. (1997). Disease management: A bumpy road ahead. *The Journal of Outcomes Management, 4*(1), 2.

Nash, D., & Todd, W. (Eds.). (1997). *Disease management: A systems approach to improving patient outcomes.* Chicago: American Hospital Publishing, Inc.

Owen, M. (1997). Disease management's role in health care increases. *Inside Case Management, 4*(8), 6–8.

Patterson, R. (1995). Disease management. *Case Review, 1*(2), 59–62.

Peragallo-Dittko, V. (1997). Diabetes: Newer approaches to diabetes education. *Disease Management Digest, 1*(3), 14–15.

Pinney Associates, Inc. (1998). Barriers to implementing disease management programs. Retrieved 1998 from the World Wide Web: http://www.medscape.com/scp/dbt/19...9.n02/d503.pinney.html.

Rhinehart, E. (1998). DM payoffs include lower costs and better utilization. *Managed Health Care, 8*(6), 20.

Rieve, J. (1998). Disease management concerns. *The Case Manager, 9*(2), 34–36.

Rodriguez, D. (1998). Diabetes: Medical nutrition therapy in diabetes care: contributions of the registered dietitian and the case manager. *Disease Management Digest, 2*(3), 8–9.

Schofield, G. (1998). Developing a disease management program to improve outcomes and efficiencies. *Health Care Innovations, 8*(1), 11–29.

Sylvestri, M., & Marro, E. (1996). Disease management: Partnering for better patient care. *Medical Interface, 9*(7), 100–104.

Todd, W. (1995). New mindsets in asthma: Interventions and disease management. *Journal of Care Management, 1*(1), 37–44, 52.

Ward, M., & Rieve, J. (1995). Disease management: Case management's return to patient-centered care. *Journal of Care Management, 1*(4), 7–12.

Wehrwein, P. (1997). Disease management gains a degree of respectability. Retrieved 1999 from the World Wide Web: http://www.managedcaremag.com/archivemc/9708/9708.mainstream.html.

Wrinn, M. (1997). Focusing on education to reduce costs. *Continuing Care, 16*(9), 16–21.

PART I: STUDY QUESTIONS

1. What does "disease management" mean to your organization? Write a definition of disease management that meets the needs of your type of patient/member population.

2. Evaluate your patient/member population. Prioritize a list of at least three diagnoses that would benefit from a disease management program in your organization.

3. Your organization will be starting disease management programs for the three diagnoses listed in number 2. Evaluate each of the components of a successful disease management program as a preparation for a successful program.
   - Understanding the Course of the Disease/ Practice Guidelines
   - Targeting Patients Likely to Benefit from Intervention (done in number 2)
   - Focusing on Prevention and Resolution

(continued)

- Increasing Patient Compliance Through Education
- Providing Full Care Continuity
- Establishing Integrated Data Management Systems for Outcome Measurements
4. Discuss the barriers in your organization for each component.
5. Discuss the strengths in your organization for each component.
6. Plan a disease management program using the following steps:
   a. Define the target population.
   b. Organize a cross-functional, multidisciplinary team.
   c. Define core components, treatment protocols, and monitoring and evaluation methods.
   d. Pilot the program on a small scale.
   e. Measure the outcomes.
   f. Implement the disease management program, plan continuous improvement (CQI), and celebrate!
7. Use the principles of case management in your disease management program:
   a. Identification of at-risk members
   b. Assessment and evaluation of members
   c. Development and coordination of disease management plans
   d. Implementation of disease management plans
   e. Evaluation—outcome measurement of the program
8. Discuss how the future of disease management/case management will affect your organization.

Outcomes Management

"In God We Trust. All others must use data."

ANONYMOUS

PART II: IMPORTANT TERMS AND CONCEPTS

Abstractor
Accountability
Baseline Measurement
Benchmark
Center for Case Management
  Accountability (CCMA)
Client Variation
Comparative Data/Feedback
Data
Data Analysis
Data Collection
Descriptive Design
Eligibility Criteria
Evaluation
Experimental Design
Exploratory Design
External Benchmark
Generic Benchmark
Goals
Group Benchmark
Health Care Quality
Health Status Survey
Internal Benchmark
Interim Measurement

Interrater Reliability
Interventions
Minimum Data Set (MDS)
Numerator/Denominator Format
Objectives
Operational Variation
Outcome Indicator
Outcomes Management
Outcomes Research
Population
Practice Guidelines
Practitioner Variation
Process
Process Indicator
Protocols
Quality Indicator
Quasi-experimental Design
Reliability
Risk Adjustment
Short-Form 36 (SF-36, 12)
Standards of Care
Study Design
Validity
Variation

Overview of Outcomes Management

INTRODUCTION

Case managers are adding a new role to their already hybrid profession: that of **Outcomes Manager**. This component of accreditation, and health care in general, is growing in importance; this chapter will help the case manager understand components of a quality improvement project that are essential to measure and report health outcomes.

Outcomes have been examined for a long time. In the nursing profession, Florence Nightingale sat in the battlefield and observed which conditions led to faster versus slower healing of the soldiers' wounds. In a simplistic sense, this was outcomes research. In his classic 1988 article on outcomes, Ellwood defines outcomes management as "a technology of patient experience designed to help patients, payors, and providers make rational medical care-related choices based on better insight into the effect of these choices on the patient's life" (Ellwood, 1988). In an almost predictive way, Ellwood continues explaining outcomes technology consisting of a "patient-understood language of health outcomes; a national data base containing information and analysis on clinical, financial, and health outcomes that estimates as best we can the relation between medical intervention and health outcomes, as well as the relation between health outcomes and money; and an opportunity for each decision-maker to have access to the analyses that are relevant to the choices they must make" (Ellwood, 1988). This is essentially where outcomes management has progressed more than a decade later.

This Outcomes Management chapter begins with three definitions. When taken down to their essential characteristics, they lose their mystique and can then be practically applied:

- **Outcomes** are simply results, or endpoints.
- A **process** is the intervention taken to achieve the outcome.
- **Accountability** is being responsible.

Therefore, **case managers are accountable (responsible) for case management outcomes (results); and case management interventions (processes)**

drive outcomes. Furthermore, outcomes are a measurement of a process. The measurement results (outcomes) will determine whether something should be done about the process that caused the outcome. Outcomes that are less than favorable give case managers the opportunity to improve; here is where continuous quality improvement (CQI) comes in. CQI provides the tools and team techniques needed to assess processes and evaluate problems. An important point to consider when forming multidisciplinary teams for outcomes management purposes is to use experts in the field. Case managers have always functioned as a leader in a multidisciplinary environment, yet few professionals in any discipline understand the intricacies of statistical analysis, methodology, data collection and analysis, risk adjustment, and project coordination. For outcomes measurement and CQI purposes, expand the multidisciplinary team to include biostatisticians, epidemiologists, data analysts, and other necessary experts.

According to the Institute of Medicine, *health care quality* is "the degree to which services for individuals and populations increase the likelihood of desired health outcomes and are consistent with current professional knowledge." Therefore, the relationship between outcomes and quality, and the ultimate goal of case management, is to provide good patient outcomes. Successful organizations have used their outcomes data as an excellent marketing tool; it is also the stuff that case management articles are made of.

WHY MEASURE CASE MANAGEMENT OUTCOMES?

Outcomes has become a predominant topic in recent years. Measuring outcomes is complicated, frustrating, time-intensive, and costly. Then why do it? The answer lies in the *purpose* of measuring outcomes: to quantify and qualify the impact of case management services. The health care industry is demanding evidence of quality care, customer/patient satisfaction, and efficiency of care delivery; and case managers are key health care professionals in every domain being tested. Hands-on case managers are being asked to, at the very least, collect the information used for this analysis; therefore, it is important to see the big picture to appreciate the importance (and immenseness) of this task. Administrative case managers may be required to develop quality improvement projects; in that instance, this information (and the information in the chapters on Disease Management and CQI) is even more essential.

Case management incentives for measuring outcomes include the following:

- To assess the effectiveness of alternative case management interventions, which will answer the question: Which case management intervention provides the best outcome in a specific population?

- To prove and document the value of case management in measurable terms; this includes cost and quality measurement. The results also may be used as a marketing tool for case managers when payors require hard data to justify the cost of case management.
- To demonstrate the contribution of case management when health care organizations are obtaining required accreditations
- To identify opportunities for improvement
- To help standardize case management processes and establish "best practices" for the profession of case management
- To continuously improve the current "best case management practices"
- To assist in the continual improvement of case management standards and guidelines
- To measure case manager performance
- To identify problems by measuring such factors as patient/customer satisfaction; with this information, case managers will have a direction with which to point CQI efforts (see chapter on CQI). This leads to improved case management services.
- To develop a large database of results to elicit stronger statistical significance of our efforts, and to predict needed skills for professional development
- To identify gaps in services in organizations, which may lead to poorer quality and increased costs
- To track costs and predict future costs
- To help develop, monitor, and adapt case management accreditation standards

CENTER FOR CASE MANAGEMENT ACCOUNTABILITY (CCMA)

Through the sponsorship of the Case Management Society of America (CMSA), an outcomes initiative was created in 1996: The Center for Case Management Accountability (CCMA). With the assistance of prominent and respected scientists in the field of quality and outcomes research, CCMA is establishing evidence-based measures consistent with the Standards of Practice for Case Management and providing a mechanism for the measurement, evaluation, and reporting of case management outcomes. CCMA's goals are to:

- Demonstrate the impact of case management on health care
- Develop a consistent framework for measuring and reporting case management outcomes
- Add to the body of knowledge on case management practice and outcomes

- Identify methods to increase case managers' capacity to participate in quality improvement and outcomes measurement (CCMA Brochure, 1998)

CCMA has developed a task force of leaders to advance the CCMA initiatives. The task force is now defining priority quality indicators; identifying appropriate tools to measure these indicators; designing data collection methods; designing a database to analyze preliminary data collection and its integrity; and developing a pilot study to test all of the former steps (CCMA Brochure, 1998). This is a dynamic process that will necessitate continued refinement; therefore, future activities under consideration include:

1. Development and refinement of measurement tools. Wherever possible, CCMA will encourage the use of existing measures. However, when outcomes measurements that are deemed high priority are not yet developed, CCMA will develop new quality indicators that meet the specific needs of case management (CMSA, 1998).

    This is an important function; for pooled data to be significant, two requirements must be met (AHCPR, 1995):

    a. *Identical measures of outcomes must be used.* There must be agreed-on definitions and rules for the gathering of each piece of data, or the outcomes will not reflect the same measurement. For example, in the national HCFA project (Cooperative Cardiovascular Project—CCP) on acute myocardial infarctions, one quality indicator measured the time to thrombolytic administration in the emergency department (ED). Clearly, if some hospitals used the time of the patient's *presentation to the ED* (to the time thrombolytics were administered), and other hospitals used the time of *diagnosis of the myocardial infarction* (to the time thrombolytics were administered), the two unlike timeframes would result in incomparable outcome data. The hospitals may believe they are measuring the same thing, but they are not.

    b. *There must be similar methodologies for data collection.* The same reasoning as above stands here. For comparable data, comparable methodologies must be used.

2. Educational Components:

    a. Build a research library. CCMA plans a centralized resource of published and unpublished studies investigating the impact of case management on key dimensions of accountability (CMSA, 1998).

    b. CCMA will become the "expert resource" for recommending how the key concepts, indicators, and measures might be used in case management practice. This would include "best practice" information considering the various case management practice settings, practitioners, and disease states.

   c. Expand a continuing education curriculum.

3. Develop an accountability database. To support large-scale research and comparative benchmarking, CCMA plans to design a centralized accountability database with supporting data capture, analysis, and reporting capabilities (CMSA, 1998). This will encompass data across the continuum of case management roles and levels of care/settings.

   CCMA could serve to organize measures that will provide case management with statistically significant outcomes. This is an essential task. Designing a national (or international) database is necessary because, for any outcome measurement to have statistical significance, an adequately large sample size must be included in the population. There are a few methods of generating a satisfactory sample size (AHCPR, 1995):

   a. The data may be collected over an extended period.

   b. The population may come from an aggregate of case management departments/organizations.

   c. Both 1 and 2

4. Facilitate collaborative improvement projects. CCMA plans multisite projects designed to achieve measurable and significant performance improvement on key dimensions of case management accountability, including health outcomes, quality of care, and cost containment (CMSA, 1998).

5. Identify linkages to quality, cost, and health status.

These are formidable tasks, but they are essential for the survival and growth of case management as a profession. A recent history lesson from managed care illustrates why CCMA is so important. It is well known that managed care is demanding outcomes to confirm the value of systems and processes. Not many years ago, this demand was placed on health care providers. Consumers wanted to know which insurance companies provided the best care. In turn, insurance companies demanded to know which physicians and other providers had the best and most cost-efficient outcomes.

In answer to this, many insurance companies hastened to design tools, collect data, evaluate data, and "prove their worth" so the consumers would pick them as their representative insurance company. And many of the physician groups scrambled to design tools, collect data, evaluate data, and "prove their worth" so the insurance companies would pick the physician groups as part of their network.

It sounds like a reasonable survival technique, but everyone was "doing their own thing." For example, each insurance company would devise their own patient satisfaction survey. It is impossible, methodologically speaking, to compare satisfaction from two (or more) different companies when the tools/questions are different. One cannot compare apples to tangerines. Realizing this problem, standard tools for measuring everything from satisfaction to prenatal care were created. Now comparisons are "apples to apples."

Case management has already realized this dilemma, and CCMA was created. As a group, case managers must agree on what it is they want to measure, a standard methodology of data measurement and analysis, and standardized measurement tools. This must all be fed into a giant database so we can compare case management "apples" with case management "apples." CCMA can establish an international clearinghouse that would disseminate the data results from the standardized tools and methodologies. This is an essential goal for case management survival.

Do case managers always need to "stick together" when measuring outcomes? Absolutely not. Although case management (perhaps through the efforts of CCMA) should measure the same outcomes, using consistent measuring tools, the processes to achieve the outcomes may be different. For example, two case management organizations may choose to measure their own outcomes on a new disease management process they are creating and evaluating. After initiation of the new disease management process, the case managers from Company 1 may get an overall patient satisfaction rating of "excellent" through use of the XXX process; the case managers from Company 2 may get an overall patient satisfaction rating of "good" through use of the YYY process. *The difference is in the process details; therefore, case management as a group can learn something by comparing the two processes and evaluating the differences.* As different case management processes are attempted, we can continuously improve and refine the case management profession; that is the essence of CQI. These studies will become the magazine articles of the future—and potentially the next level of CQI in case management.

In the future, case management must also define what constitutes a "poor," "good," or "excellent" outcome. These ranges must come from previous outcomes studies and must be specific and well-defined to level the playing field. Measurable ranges will have to be determined and agreed on as a profession.

Another aspect of outcomes management that needs monitoring relates to the fact that case management practice, like all clinical practice, changes over time. For example, some of the quality indicators in the CCP project have been updated since 1994, after discovery of better procedures or medications for AMIs. How to account for the most up-to-date practice patterns and still maintain sound methodology will be a challenge for case managers. Through

CCMA, with the assistance of experts in the field, case managers will be assured that important elements will be known and monitored.

OUTCOMES MANAGEMENT VERSUS OUTCOMES RESEARCH— AND WHERE DOES ALL THIS FIT INTO DISEASE MANAGEMENT AND CONTINUOUS QUALITY IMPROVEMENT?

The lines of distinction between outcomes management, disease management, and CQI are both communal and tangential. The flowchart in Figure 3-1 displays the relationship between outcomes research, outcomes management, disease management, and continuous quality improvement. *Outcomes research* is a complex discipline requiring exact methodologic, analytic, and research skills; this does not necessarily require the skills of a case manager. But case management skills are fundamental in *disease management* and *outcomes management.* (NOTE: Case management interventions fall in the same category as "Disease Management Strategy.") Through study of the Disease Management and Continuous Quality Improvement chapters, the case manager will appreciate how vital our contribution is to the whole outcomes effort.

Interest in health care outcomes is driven by several factors:

- Public policy
- Computerized medical records
- Purchaser demand
- Clinical research
- Quality assurance

These factors are pushing outcomes in two directions: outcomes research and outcomes management (Davies, Doyle, Lansky, Rutt, Stevie, & Doyle, 1994). Both directions share common attributes, as well as unique factors in each modality.

Outcomes Research

The goal of outcomes research is to methodically and precisely define alternative interventions that are most effective in producing selected outcomes. This goal is important, because it supports conducting clinical research to address effectiveness. Outcomes research is based on well-established, traditional research methods (Jennings & Staggers, 1997). Outcomes research demands a unique knowledge base of statistical analysis and design methodology that is usually reserved for specific Master's and Ph.D. level skill sets.

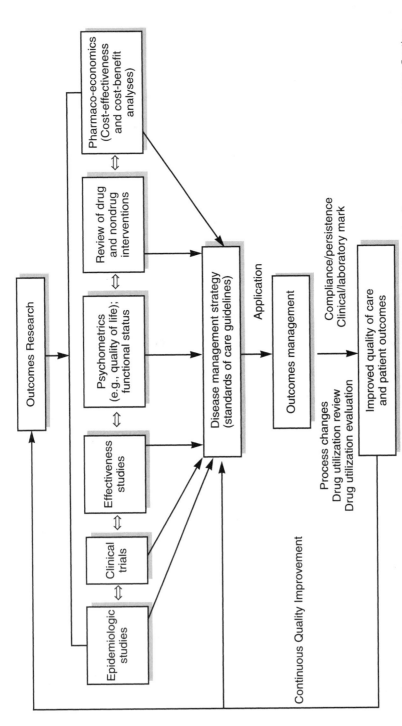

Figure 3-1. The multidisciplinary scientific basis of outcomes research and the manner in which it flows into disease management programs. Continuous quality improvement of outcomes is the ultimate goal. Reprinted with permission from Epstein, R. & Sherwood, L. (1996). From Outcomes research to disease management: A guide for the perplexed. *Ann Intern Med, 124*(9), 832–837.

Outcomes Management

Outcomes management seeks to produce desirable outcomes in a clinical setting and is therefore the application of outcomes research to practice (Epstein & Sherwood, 1996). Historically, outcome measures have "evolved from simple dichotomous ones such as survival or occurrence of a clinical event, to patient-oriented measures such as satisfaction, quality of life, and functional status" (Epstein & Sherwood, 1996, p. 832). Outcomes management techniques appeared in response to changes in the standards and survey methods used by the Joint Commission on the Accreditation of Healthcare Organizations (JCAHO). As a result of JCAHO accreditation changes, hospital quality management or outcomes management programs are now examining outcomes and the results (outcomes) of care. *The goal of outcomes management* is efficiency or examining patient outcomes relative to processes and resources used (Jennings & Staggers, 1997).

Outcomes research and outcomes management differ in several ways:

1. The goals are different, as stated above.
2. The language of outcomes research is standard within research as a mode of scientific inquiry; however, the language of outcomes management is currently being formed, often causing ambiguous communication (a new lexicon).
3. The outcomes research model is relatively stable; the model guiding outcomes management is still changing.
4. Research-based studies are likely to be conducted with a better understanding of mathematical tenets underlying the statistical analyses. Poor analysis promotes poor conclusions (Jennings & Staggers, 1997, pp. 18–19). Or, as these authors say, it creates the "garbage in, gospel out" phenomenon (p. 22).

Outcomes management is based on the assumption that by remedying problems, inefficiencies, and unintended variation within the care delivery process, improvement in the end result of health care interventions will be evident. These assumptions are based on the following rationale:

1. *Outcomes are evidence of quality* (Jennings & Staggers, 1997): The evidence may demonstrate poor quality or good quality, depending on data results. The bottom line is, what will be done with the outcomes data once it is known?
2. *Quality and cost are not mutually exclusive* (Jennings & Staggers, 1997): The relationship between cost and quality is still in debate. Obviously, if financial costs go down, but so does quality, then the care becomes a quality issue.

However, "there is no inherent incompatibility between maximizing health and minimizing costs: eliminating inefficiencies can simultaneously reduce cost and improve quality of care" (Todd & Nash, 1997, p. 84). Many disease management programs have proven that quality care *is* cost effective care.

3. *Minimizing unintended variation and inefficiencies will contribute to cost-effective, quality care delivery* (Jennings & Staggers, 1997): A case management outcome achieved on one occasion does not predict future case management outcomes, unless the processes that led to those outcomes are stable. The concept of variation is important, in that the more variation in a case management process, the less stable that process is (therefore, the outcome is less predictable). For a detailed discussion on the power of variation to affect quality of care, see sections on Variation in this chapter, and see Statistical Process Control Charts in the CQI chapters.

PROTOCOLS, STANDARDS, AND PRACTICE GUIDELINES

The pace of the changes occurring in the health care industry is creating a terminology problem; some basic terminology in areas such as utilization management and outcomes management have not yet been clearly defined. Case management went through that phase when definitions of case management had more to do with specific models of case management than what a case manager is and does. The same is true for terms such as practice guidelines (also called clinical guidelines), protocols, and standards. Because so much of outcomes measurement uses these tools as a foundation for research, an attempt will be made to define and clarify these terms.

Protocols and practice guidelines, like clinical pathways, have been considered the best thing since sliced bread, or the most ominous thing since managed care itself. Most doctors have loved them or hated them; there is little middle ground. Those that are against them say they are a legal hazard and they represent cookbook medicine. Those physicians who are using them are now becoming their authors; and physician-driven, evidence-based guidelines, protocols, and pathways are the rule rather than the exception in many organizations.

Protocols

Protocols are essentially "standing orders" similar to those nurses have been using for many years. "Protocols are orders that prescribe diagnosis or procedure specific activities that have traditionally required a written order in the medical record. They do not have a sequencing timeline or an outcome assessment" (Mateo, Matzke, & Newton, 1998, p. 3). Standard orders protocols are often physician specific at this medical evolutionary stage. Unlike clinical paths, there is no real timing directive for the orders. A set of standing orders for a postoperative coronary artery bypass graft (CABG) patient may have telemetry orders, medication orders, vital sign orders, intravenous fluid type and rates, and emergency orders; no sequencing is prescribed, and it often appears that everything is supposed to be done "at once."

Standards of Care

A standard of care can be described as that degree of care, skill, or learning expected of a reasonable, prudent health care provider in the profession or class to which he or she belongs within the state acting in the same or similar circumstances. In the legal sense, standards of care can be used as a "sword or a shield." In malpractice case court proceedings, there is an attempt to determine whether a patient suffered harm because of negligent violation of a standard of care. The standard of care for the case is detailed by questioning expert witnesses who have studied the facts of the case and have relevant professional knowledge of the situation. When experts in a professional field have come together and written out standards (such as the Standards of Practice for Case Management), then the document is also a measure to which the case manager may be held accountable in a court of law.

Some experts have drawn a line between the use of standards and the use of guidelines in this way:

- Standards are to be used every time the standard applies.
- Guidelines ought to be used most of the time, with professional judgment making the final determination.

Practice Guidelines

Clinical practice guidelines are systematically developed statements, or algorithms, for assisting practitioners to make patient decisions about appropriate health care for specific clinical circumstances (AHCPR). They are usually developed by multidisciplinary teams that consist of appropriate clinicians from multiple specialties, including experts in the field; they should be based upon scientific evidence. Guidelines usually do not follow a strict timeline. Therefore, case management guidelines can be described as systematically developed statements to assist case managers in practice decisions that will result in improved quality of life for patients and family, excellent quality of care for the health condition of the patient, and appropriate use of resources.

Many credible organizations have a hand in developing practice guidelines using expert panels and evidenced-based literature. The Agency for Health Care Policy and Research is a government-funded organization whose mission is to promote, support, and disseminate national practice guidelines. National Committee for Quality Assurance (NCQA), JCAHO, and other national regulatory organizations also help provide clinical guidelines. The practice guidelines are tested against stringent validity and reliability determinations. A guideline is valid if the guideline stands for what it claims for itself; that is, if the guideline is carefully followed, it will lead to the health and cost outcomes projected for it (Gosfield, 1997).

The National Guideline Clearinghouse (NGC), developed by the *Agency for Health Care Policy and Research (AHCPR)* in partnership with the *American Medical Association (AMA)* and the *American Association of Health Plans*, is an Internet-based repository for evidence-based clinical practice guidelines. This online service gives clinicians free and easy access to the latest health care information from a variety of sources as they make treatment decisions with their patients. The NGC identifies and features evidence-based clinical practice guidelines presented with standardized abstracts and tables that allow for comparison of guidelines on similar topics. The tables provide information on the major areas of agreement and disagreement among guidelines, which will help users make informed selections. The NGC will continuously update the website by receiving guideline submissions on an ongoing basis.

Thousands of clinical practice guidelines have been created by medical and professional societies, managed care organizations, hospitals, state and federal agencies, and others. However, case managers and other clinicians often have had difficulty gaining access to a full range of guidelines; and more importantly, had challenges identifying which guidelines are evidence-based. The plethora of guidelines has also been a major cause of increased variation in patient care. An important consideration when considering the use of guidelines is that they are an effective method to reduce inappropriate variation in case management and clinical practice patterns, thereby increasing process stability. Reduction in variation translates into a more stable process, necessary for quality case management practice. According to John M. Eisenberg, M.D., AHCPR administrator, "It is well known that variation in health care results partly from uncertainty and a lack of evidence for clinical treatment. The NGC will help reduce variation and improve health care quality by giving clinicians and other health professionals a source of information on evidence-based treatment to help guide their decisions."

However, to many health care practitioners, guidelines translate into a loss of professional autonomy. Do not become so overreliant on guidelines, or outcomes, that patient care becomes automatic. This may lead to a case manager's feeling of loss of autonomy, and underutilization of creativity (an essential case management skill). Just as case managers use utilization management as tools, not rules, so should guidelines be treated as descriptions rather than prescriptions. The NGC is an important tool in clinical decision making as case managers continue to address the problems of underuse, overuse, misuse, and uncertainty in health care quality. Access the website at the address below:

**NATIONAL GUIDELINE
CLEARINGHOUSE (NGC)**

www.guideline.gov

STUDY DESIGNS FOR CASE MANAGEMENT INTERVENTION EVALUATION

A **study design** refers to the approach and methods used to organize and conduct the study and evaluate the case management interventions. Selection of a study design method depends on what is being examined and the perspective of the target audience. A basic understanding of study designs that can be used to conduct evaluation will help round out the case manager's knowledge. The choice of the design can affect how programs are organized, implemented, modified, and how the results are interpreted.

When considering a choice of the following designs, take into consideration a challenge posed by Epstein and Sherwood:

> In disease management, clinical trials are not always possible. When a health plan has developed a new clinical program, members may not feel comfortable having an intervention withheld, and employers may be unwilling to conduct a trial before disseminating the program. However, if the program is implemented without a concurrent comparison, what remains is a *before-and-after comparison*; within a rapidly changing health care environment, the aging of the population and other factors can confound results. This issue is an especially important methodologic challenge of program evaluation. (Epstein & Sherwood, 1996, p. 834)

Case management **"before-and-after comparisons"** would have been especially valuable had the case management "before" started when case management first became a significant managed care method in the late 1980s. The "and-after" comparisons of today would be impressive! We have lost that window of opportunity; however, there are still many "before-and-after comparisons" left to be discovered. When starting any phase of a new case management process, or a new disease management program, collect data before the change and after the change.

Another type of design is to compare a variable *"with and without case management."* This is the standard use of a "control group," but from this perspective, the impact of case management can be successfully measured.

- Compare cost of care with and without case management.
- Compare cost of (disease-specific) patient care in a mixed case management caseload versus a disease-specific case management caseload.
- Compare a patient's health status with and without case management.
- Compare a payor's cost with and without case management.
- Compare a patient's clinical status with and without case management.
- Compare readmissions to the emergency department for a specific disease with and without case management.
- Compare length of stay with and without preoperative physical therapy teaching for total hip replacement patients.
- Compare SF-12 scores with and without preoperative physical therapy teaching for total hip replacement patients.

There is no shortage of variables to measure. Consider the *Types of Case Management Outcome Domains* listed at the beginning of Chapter 4. For the outcomes listed, put the word "compare" before the outcome; put "with and without case management" after the outcome. However, the challenge posed by Epstein and Sherwood is valid here; this is one intervention (case management) that few complex patients should do without.

Case managers have several other design options for evaluating their interventions:

1. Faith
2. Change and watch
3. Exploratory
4. Descriptive
5. Quasi-experimental
6. Experimental

Faith is based on the assumption that a given case management intervention will improve quality or outcomes, or reduce costs, especially if the process before the intervention has known waste and inefficiency. No real evidence is required (Kozma, 1996).

Change and watch is a nonexperimental approach and is frequently used with disease management programs. First, various utilization rates are measured. The intervention is the commencement of the disease management program (the change). Then, utilization rates are remeasured after a period of watching. Although this design is often used, it is not possible to attribute changes directly to the interventions (Kozma, 1996). Other factors may have contributed to the utilization change.

Exploratory design is used when the purpose of the evaluation is to explore or discover a new aspect of case management. Exploratory designs are often based on case management observations and act as building blocks for other designs. Interviewing techniques are commonly used in this design (Lamb, Donaldson, & Kellogg, 1998).

Descriptive designs are used when the purpose of the evaluation is to describe some aspect of case management practice or demonstrate a relationship between two or more aspects of case management practice (Lamb et al., 1998). Descriptive designs focus on counting or relating events (are number oriented), are objective, and can use existing data. Because there is no attempt to control factors in descriptive designs, there are limitations in the conclusions that may be drawn, and cannot "prove" case management effectiveness. Examples of descriptive aspects of case management include:

- Numbers of case management cases
- Population characteristics such as age, functional status, comorbidities, diagnosis, etc.
- Changes in use of health care services, functional abilities, etc.
- Frequency of various case management services
- Types of case management interventions such as assessment, monitoring, coordination, etc. (Lamb et al., 1998)

Quasi-experimental designs and **experimental designs** are used when the goal is to establish a cause-and-effect relationship between case management intervention and the outcomes of that intervention. The goal is to be able to conclude with some certainty that the outcomes are attributable to the interventions (Lamb et al., 1998). Each design uses a different method to control for extraneous factors and, therefore, differ in the degree to which attribution of causation can be determined.

Quasi-experimental designs use techniques such as comparison groups and repeated measurements over time. Comparisons can be made between two groups: those having congestive heart failure who are case managed, and those having congestive heart failure who are not case managed. The degree of causation of the results has much to do with the degree to which both groups are similar in important characteristics; this can be a shortcoming of this style of design (Kozma, 1996).

Experimental designs will also use patients who are randomly selected, that is, drawn from the universe of cases by a statistically valid method. Based on probability theory, external variables that may affect what is observed should be evenly divided between the groups; therefore, the observed differences are likely caused by the case management intervention. "The danger in not using experimental approaches is that we may attribute cause incorrectly, and this may lead to inefficiencies. Programs may be developed, funded, and appear to work (or not work) when the outcome is not caused by the program itself but by the design used to evaluate the program" (Kozma, 1996, p. 111). But randomization of patients hosts a number of ethical, operational, and financial problems; therefore, quasi-experimental designs are often selected.

Quasi-experimental designs and experimental designs are characterized by a focus on cause-and-effect relationships, are controlled and standardized, require sufficient numbers for statistical power in which to draw conclusions, require extensive monitoring, and are time consuming (Lamb et al., 1998). However, they are a highly respected and credible design. Examples that demonstrate a causal relationship in case management include (Lamb et al., 1998)

- Symptom management interventions and perceived health status
- Authorization decisions and service use and cost
- Disability case management interventions and worker's compensation costs

Perspectives to Consider When Choosing Study Designs and Measurement Tools

Case managers are familiar with diverging perspectives: Clinical versus economic. Objective versus subjective. External customers versus internal customers. Many times we have felt ethical conflicts between the needs of our employer versus those of the patients versus the claims payor stating the benefits versus the physician orders.

There has been no clear method to satisfy the outcome needs of all the health care players: providers, employers, case managers, managed care organizations, accreditation organizations, payors, and patients. What one group wants or expects may not fit the expectations of another group. What is clear is that clinicians need information that will allow the best outcomes for their patients; patients want subjective outcomes and want to believe that their quality of life has improved. Case managers require information so they can provide optimal information to their patients, employers, payors, and providers. Payors need information that will allow contract decisions that make fiscal sense; business coalitions want information that will compare provider performance, so they can contract with those who provide the best "value"; and managed care organizations want outcomes that reflect comparative data on utilization, costs, and quality of care. Administrators are interested in objective, hard data; they need to know what interventions decrease costs while maintaining or improving health care quality. Regulatory agencies and accreditation commissions need clinical performance measures to develop and enforce accreditation policy; they are interested in the outcomes as a method to check the organization's adherence to specific standards.

Differing perspectives in outcomes management can be a barrier to improvement. From a provider perspective, it seems as though they must perform several similar quality improvement projects just to satisfy the many who require outcomes. This is often overwhelming and sometimes leaves resistance in its wake. However, case managers are not new to juggling different perspectives, and this provides another opportunity for case managers to shine and to demonstrate case management negotiation and diplomacy skills.

Tools—MDS and SF-36

Another important perspective consideration is choosing tools that will be used for outcomes measurement. This can be illustrated using a current situation in the skilled nursing facility (SNF) level of care. The changes being implemented with the Balanced Budget Act of 1997 are, perhaps, the most far-reaching health care changes in over a decade. Home health and skilled nursing facility regulations are being particularly hard hit. Most, as of this writing, do not know how the changes will all play out and therefore are having difficulty formulating strategies for survival. However, one change that is imminent is the expanded use of case managers in the SNF level of care.

The **MDS (Minimum Data Set)** assessment tool for SNF residents may be of some use in determining case management outcomes in SNFs. Essentially, the MDS is a functional assessment tool that must be used at several intervals during the patient's SNF stay: at initial admission to the facility, quarterly, after admission, annually (fourth quarter) after admission, on significant change in health or functional status, and readmission after a temporary discharge to a hospital, other treatment facility, or home. Also, other assessments may be performed for miscellaneous reasons. Different assessment questions may be required for each of these SNF assessments (CHSRA, 1998).

The MDS can be used to collect some outcomes, although some limitations do apply. For example, the initial, baseline assessment is more apt to show care in a previous setting than in the current SNF. Subsequent assessments can provide information about the care in the current SNF, except for one type of assessment; any assessment done after a temporary discharge to another care facility may represent either care in the SNF or care in the facility from which the patient was transferred. Therefore, the relationship between quality care and a quality indicator will be more obscure because the two facilities "shared" the care; did care in the SNF cause the need to transfer to the acute level?

The importance of considering "perspectives" has been documented with the use of another tool, the *Health Status Survey* (SF-12 or SF-36), developed by John E. Ware, Jr., Ph.D., and the Health Outcomes Trust. The Health Status Survey is used to determine the *patient's perspective* on the status of their health, in eight functional dimensions that are considered critical to quality of life. Data taken from many years of using this tool have determined that there is a definite correlation between a person's perception of their health, and the potential for hospital admission within 6 to 12 months' time. However, many outcomes measures were developed for use in population surveys and not for use in monitoring individual patients; the Health Status Survey results are said to be more reliable when determining "population," rather than individual, resource consumption.

There are various "health status" tools. The SF tools, are perhaps, the most commonly used in health care. SF stands for "short form." The numbers, 12 or 36, describe the number of questions on the survey for the patient to answer (an SF-8 is being tested as of this writing). The SF-12 takes about 2 minutes to complete. According to experts, the SF-12, although shorter, is as predictive as the SF-36 in determining future health care resource use. Scoring of the results is most easily done by a proprietary computer program, but it can be done manually for smaller groups. Manuals to accurately score results can be found on the Health Institute at the New England Medical Center's web site listed in "Resources" later in this section.

The eight domains of health assessed in the health status survey include:

1. *Physical Functioning:* assesses a range of physical activities such as self-care, walking, climbing stairs, and vigorous activities
2. *Role Physical:* assesses the impact of physical health on the patient's life roles and regular daily activities
3. *Bodily Pain:* assesses the severity of bodily pain and its interference with work inside or outside the home
4. *General Health:* assesses perception of general health, health outlook, and resistance to illness

5. *Vitality:* assesses the frequency of feeling tired versus energetic
6. *Social Functioning:* assesses the extent and frequency of limitations in social activities attributable to health problems
7. *Role Emotional:* assesses the impact of emotional problems on the patient's life roles and regular daily activities
8. *Mental Health:* assesses anxiety, depression, and loss of behavioral/ emotional control versus psychological well-being

Case managers can use health status tools in several ways. They are an important addition to a case manager's toolbox, and new applications, such as follows, may be found:

1. To demonstrate patient satisfaction and the value of case management services to clients and administration. A generic program would include the following steps:
   a. Collecting baseline scores
   b. Initiating case management services
   c. Remeasuring scores at 6 months or 12 months after initiation of case management
   d. Comparing the baseline and remeasurement scores and evaluating the results
2. To use the SF-12 or SF-36 scores to predict future health care resource use
3. To assist in disease management program evaluation. Design a health status tool that is disease-specific by modifying the instrument (Stewart, 1995). Stewart suggests that an organization choose the condition to be monitored. For example, if a study of back pain is chosen, add the prefix "Because of my back" to the generic tool questions. Caution should be advised when trying this technique for copyright reasons and for reasons of reliability/validity of the results. Disease-specific health status tools are available; however, they may be copyright protected.
4. To bring the patient more fully into the case management assessment process

BENCHMARKS

The Japanese word *dantotsu* expresses the essence of benchmarking; it means striving to be the "best of the best" (Camp & Tweet, 1994). The principle behind benchmarks is simple; benchmarking is the "continuous process of measuring products, services and practices against the toughest competitors or those known as leaders in their field" (*Journal of Quality Assurance,* 1991, p. 17). Benchmarking is not merely the "best performance" but also consists of how the organization accomplished the excellent outcomes. The purpose of benchmarking is to set an orientation point for a case management organization to aim for; it is a direction-setting process that also depicts the practices needed to reach new goals (Camp & Tweet, 1994).

Benchmarking is a powerful tool. All health care organizations have ongoing quality improvement projects; it is almost impossible to bypass this task and acquire any kind of accreditation. In working with quality improvement projects all over the state of Arizona, it is clear that "data drives doctors"—and organizations. No one wants to be "average." One of the strongest of the "movers and shakers" is the use of competitors' data; and often this is translated into state benchmarks. The Health Care Financing Administration (HCFA) has six national projects. These national projects will eventually elicit national data—and national benchmarks—in areas such as heart failure, acute myocardial infarction, diabetes, stroke, mammography, and community-acquired pneumonia.

Several plausible methods identify "best practices" (Camp & Tweet, 1994):

- *Internal benchmarks:* Compare similar processes within the organization. This is a good place for an organization to start.
- *External benchmarks* (also called *competitive benchmarks*): Compare processes of one organization with competitor's data. Eventually, the "gap" between the organization and the competitor should close.
- *Group benchmarks:* Compare with the best practices in the industry, although not necessarily one's direct competitors. The national HCFA quality improvement projects will eventually provide some group benchmarks.
- *Generic benchmarks:* Compare with a documented plan for a process. This may include use of performance guidelines that are credible.

Benchmarks have changed the face of health care. If one hospital can safely get postoperative CABG patients off ventilators in 7 hours, others will find out how it was done and use the benchmark as a goal. The benchmark process has four stages (McLaughlin & Kaluzny, 1994):

1. Plan which processes to study, identify best practices (who/where they are done), and study your own process.
2. Visit other sites; gather data on process performance and identify factors that drive superior performance.
3. Analyze the "gap" between what others have done and what your organization does.
4. Interpret, adapt, improve, and adopt what was learned; and fit it to your organization.

This is simplistic, and each step is time consuming, resource consumptive, and may require collaboration with other organizations. Determining the data collection methods, collecting and analyzing data, establishing functional goals and action plans, implementing plans, and monitoring results all take a multi-disciplinary team effort. Lastly, *recalibrate the benchmark to your organization.* Benchmarking is not about copying other organizations. Each organization in every state and every country has different requirements for patient care. Rural Mississippi is very different from rural Arizona; and New Zealand is very different from America. The differences in cultures, accreditation requirements, information technology sophistication, and insurance types all contribute to how patient care is performed—and the subsequent benchmarks.

Some summarizing criteria for benchmarks come from a lecture by Dr. Norman Weissman, Ph.D.:

- Benchmarks should represent a level of excellence
- Benchmarks should be demonstrably attainable
- Providers with high performance should be selected from among all providers in a predefined, data-driven way
- All providers with high performance should contribute to the benchmark level
- Providers with high performance but a small number of cases should not unduly influence the level of the benchmark (NOTE: this "risk adjustment" is considered in the statistical analyses of benchmarks). (Kiefe, Weissman, Farmer, Weaver, Allison, & Williams, 1998)

Benchmarking is still a science in progress. The actual statistical mathematics for benchmarking data is currently being tested and is in an evolutionary stage. Furthermore, outcomes in case management is still in its toddler stage and has few external benchmarks to choose from. But that is quickly changing and, with the work of CCMA, we will soon be comparing outcomes, patient satisfaction, functional and clinical improvement, costs, and quality for similar services, clients, and patients.

FACTORS THAT AFFECT CASE MANAGEMENT OUTCOMES

"The primary goal of a case management evaluation study, indeed of any systematic evaluation, is to be able to make general conclusions about a population or a phenomenon based on observations of a small group of individuals that represent the population and/or phenomenon being studied" (Lamb et al., 1998, p. 29). However, for the outcome evaluation studies to be accurate and useful, there are attributes to examine and cautions along the way.

Several factors must be considered when using quality indicators to measure outcomes.

Variation

The essential outcomes question is, "Did *case management* impact this case or disease, or did another variable?" A critical ingredient in outcomes measurement is assessing the degree to which processes that led to the outcome are stable. When answering the question, coming to a solid conclusion may be dependent on this one factor. Case management, and health care in general, is fraught with multiple opportunities for variability. *Stability* in a process depicts a process that is well defined and consistent in methods used. *Variability* in a process is just the opposite; variable processes are inconsistent and changeable. It is difficult to attribute outcomes to processes that are unstable. In the CQI chapters, statistical process control charts (SPCC) are discussed. These charts can be used to monitor and display variability, and thus stability, of a process. They also assist in determining the cause of the variation by looking for patterns of "special" or "common" causes (See CQI chapters, special and common causes). If the chart demonstrates a wide degree of variation, this means there is little control over what is happening, and this will result in management nightmares; the desired state is to decrease the amount of variation, thus making the process more stable.

> A stable process is a predictable process; an unstable process is an unpredictable process.

Expressed from a slightly different perspective, outcomes are measured so that outcomes can be managed. The goal is to manage outcomes in such a way that unintended variation is reduced; therefore, **the ultimate goal of outcomes management is reduction in unintended variation.** By reducing unintended variation, resources are more effectively managed, and quality can be improved. This is an important concept for case managers interested in outcomes management to understand. However, because case managers customize their case management plans to the needs of the patient/family unit and the resources available, variation in case management practice is the "norm" rather than the "exception." This further complicates the requirement for consistent case management practice and is cause for concern when developing outcomes management programs: "Significant variation in the delivery of a targeted intervention either with the same case manager or between case managers dilutes the effectiveness of the intervention and the link between interventions and outcomes" (Lamb et al., 1998, p. 53).

There are three principal sources of variation that could affect case management outcomes:

1. *Operational Variation:* Includes system problems such as poor work flow, communication flow, confusing chain of command, or equipment shortages. Interfacility problems are also in this category (Lamb et al., 1998).
2. *Client Variation:* Includes an almost limitless variety of client factors such as variation in client's stage of disease or condition on admission, compliance issues, motivation, or capacity for change (Lamb et al., 1998). Also consider client insurance, financial, and psychosocial support.
3. *Practitioner Variation:* Includes provider omissions, errors, delays, and consistency and use of current "best practices" (Lamb et al., 1998).

(NOTE: The concept of variation and process stability is further discussed in the CQI chapters in the section on Statistical Process Control Charts (SPCC). The function of that CQI tool is to study variation over time; it is also an excellent patient teaching tool. It is recommended that case managers evaluate ways to use SPCC in their case management practice.)

Risk Adjustment

"But MY patients are sicker." It is one of the most common complaints heard when providers are given comparative data and their numbers are not among the best. Risk adjustment is a method of "leveling the playing field" when comparing quality across organizations. Comparisons of case management organizations/departments, the patient's health status, or whatever is being measured, must be as similar as possible. To attain this similarity, adjusting for age, gender, severity of illness, and other variables is a necessity.

The purpose of measuring outcomes is to ascertain a strong causal link between the action (case management intervention) and the result (outcome). It is difficult to make the leap between "intervention and outcome" when variability abounds. One method to decrease variability is *risk adjustment,* or *severity adjustment.* It is a method of adjusting the outcome to remove the effect of confounders such as age, severity of disease progression, or specific comorbidities; this is risk adjustment by patient population. In clinical improvement projects, risk adjustment also can be part of the definition of the quality indicator being measured. For example, in a community-acquired pneumonia project, bacterial pneumonia can be ruled in; viral pneumonia can be ruled out. This is a simple form of risk adjustment used in projects, sometimes called *eligibility criteria*.

Without risk adjustment, a single outcome can be attributed to several factors, confusing the true reason for the outcome. For example, if two groups of case managers both work with congestive heart failure (CHF) patients, but one group clearly has lower emergency department, readmission, and hospitalization rates, ask whether the groups were risk adjusted for severity of the disease and comorbidities. Did the more successful case managers have CHF patients with less advanced disease? Or, did they have better methods of case managing the CHF patients? If the two groups were risk adjusted before the comparison, the first question need not be asked; for that factor, both groups would be equal.

One caution is that the definition of *severity* is not standardized in health care; this becomes another point of variability when measuring outcomes. Two case management organizations may have CHF programs, yet each has their own definition of what constitutes a mild, moderate, or severe disease state. When risk factors are as concrete as age, education level, or financial status, the delineations are clear; however, risk adjustment is very difficult to achieve with less defined measures. Clear definitions of risk-adjusted data are necessary for an accurate conclusion. Defining risk adjustment criteria, therefore, is a work in progress in an early stage of development. JCAHO, NCQA, and the *American Medical Accreditation Program (AMAP)* are consolidating their efforts to coordinate performance measurement activities across the entire health care system. This collaboration established the *Performance Measurement Coordinating Council (PMCC)*. Realizing that risk adjustment is a key issue for measuring performance at the physician, facility, and health plan levels, one goal of PMCC is to address the standardization of risk adjustment techniques (JCAHO, 1998).

For case managers who are visually oriented, risk adjustment concepts can be viewed by using mathematical equations. Try these two equations on, and see how they fit. Risk adjustment placed into a mathematical, numerator/denominator format, can look like this:

$$\frac{\text{the number of patients who actually experienced a particular outcome}}{\text{the number of cases that were eligible for the outcome}\\ \textbf{with the same degree of risk}}$$

One organization stated the relationship between risk adjustment and quality indicators by use of an equation:

Quality Indicator = quality of care + risk + error (CHSRA, 1998)

Variables may need to be "ruled in" or "ruled out" of the operational definition of the quality indicator to make successful comparisons among distinct case management systems. Consider the following examples of factors that may require risk adjusting:

PATIENT-SPECIFIC FACTORS

Risk adjust for age, gender, race, education, geographic region, severity of illness, comorbidities, patient preferences of treatment choices, patient compliance, patient involvement in their care, socioeconomic level, occupation, family support, payment source/insurance support.

CLINICIAN PRACTICE-SPECIFIC RISK FACTORS

Assess clinician's level of expertise and experience, diagnostic skills, judgment, "bedside manner."

INSURANCE/PROVIDER NETWORK-RELATED RISK FACTORS

Assess availability of qualified staff, availability of all levels of care and support services geographically near the enrollees, interfacility comparisons, organization's systems and processes for governance, management stability.

COMMUNITY-RELATED RISK FACTORS

Assess integration of health care resources, availability of resources to fill gaps in coverage issues, environment, pollution, workplace safety, safe neighborhoods, water safety, lead levels for children.

Validity

Validity is defined as "how well a particular characteristic is measured (*i.e.,* the effectiveness of a measure in achieving a specific purpose)" (Lamb et al., 1998, p. 161). Validity is not always a "0% or 100%" measure; validity can measure the extent, or degree, to which a particular characteristic is "valid."

Validity in quality indicators is stated slightly differently than validity in practice guidelines:

- Validity is the degree to which a *quality indicator* measures what it is intended to measure.

- Validity is the degree to which the *practice guideline* accomplishes its purpose. Practice guidelines are valid if, when followed, they lead to the health and cost outcomes projected for them (JCAHO, 1998).

For practice guidelines, the guideline is likely to be valid if three conditions are met (AHCPR, 1995):

1. The relationship between the process and the outcome is known
2. That relationship formed the basis for the practice guideline
3. The review criteria have been derived "faithfully" from the guideline

Reliability

A reliable tool will consistently reproduce the same results when repeatedly applied to the same population; it can be trusted to measure what it was designed to measure. This attribute of a measure is important for ensuring comparability of results. If two case management organizations use a reliable measurement tool (sometimes called an *abstraction tool*), then the comparison will likely be a good one, assuming the improvement project is well designed. A reliable tool also will be useful when the study design calls for measurement over time; a reliable comparison can be made with a "*before* case management interventions" and "*after* case management interventions" design.

Reliability in practice guidelines is stated slightly differently from reliability in measurement tools. Practice guidelines are considered reliable and reproducible if two conditions are met (AHCPR, 1995):

1. If, given the same evidence and methods for guidelines development, another set of experts would produce essentially the same statements, and
2. If, given the same clinical circumstances, the guidelines are interpreted and applied consistently by practitioners or other appropriate parties

This concurs with one attorney's test of a reliable guideline: that any group of experts could look at the same issues and develop the same components of the guideline; and, when applying the guideline over time, a group of experts would come to the same conclusions regarding the care reviewed (Gosfield, 1997).

There are three categories of reliability assessment (McGlynn & Asch, 1998):

1. *Internal Consistency:* This method of determining reliability is used for scores from multiple items.
2. *Test–Retest:* This method of determining reliability is used for survey measures.

3. *Interrater Reliability:* This method of determining reliability is used for medical record abstraction.

Case managers will often hear the term *interrater reliability* on their outcomes management travels. When data are being collected to measure outcomes, humans are often the ones performing the collection (also know as "abstracting the data.") Humans are known to be afflicted with "human error." Therefore, *abstractors* who review the events to measure the quality indicator must meet certain standards of accuracy. *Interrater reliability* is a monitoring method to ensure that the data collected are correct and reliably. This is essential for the integrity of a project; without accurate data abstraction, the final data will be inaccurate, leading to erroneous conclusions. Simply, the goal of interrater reliability is for two abstractors to obtain the same answers (*i.e.,* data). Abstractors must meet a predetermined rate of accuracy in their data collection answers; organizations usually aspire to a 95% accuracy rate, although some agree to 90%. A lower interrater reliability score may indicate that the abstractors may need more training, or the abstraction tool is ambiguous. A high interrater reliability score will help to ensure that ambiguity or misinterpretation of data definitions is minimized.

Population Size

If you have a caseload of 45 patients, you will likely use the entire group as the population of your study. A **population** is the group of people from which the study sample will be chosen. However, if the group is 100,000, you will want to study a sample of the population. A **sample** is the subset of a population or the group of cases to whom a performance measure will be applied. Another related concept is called a **random sample**. A random sample is a group selected for study that is drawn at random from the universe of cases by a statistically valid method. The opposite of random sampling is "cherry picking," a form of "cheating" in a quality improvement project.

Chapter 3 has presented an overview of outcomes management, including study designs, perspectives, benchmarks, and variables. Chapter 4 will discuss various types of case management outcome domains, and essential components of a case management/outcomes management program.

A Case Management/Outcomes Management Program

TYPES OF CASE MANAGEMENT OUTCOMES DOMAINS

Case managers are accountable (responsible) for case management outcomes (results). This is how case management will "prove its worth." There are hundreds of potential outcomes in case management. As managed care changes (as we know it will), the broad categories may remain stable, but the details may reshape to address the demands of the times. The following lists are extensive and often applicable in more than one of the outcome domains:

• Clinical outcomes
• Financial/economic outcomes
• Humanistic outcomes
• Quality outcomes
• Organizational/administrative/systems outcomes

As a group, case managers may choose to divvy up the homework into groups, with each group concentrating on a specific outcome domain or specific measurement. Many of the broad categories listed below have already been measured, although not on a consistent or national scale. Research the progress in case management outcomes for ideas. Then improve on those ideas and customize them for your organization.

An important recommendation when starting outcomes management projects is to start small and build on successes. Do not attempt to measure everything; begin by looking at one or two outcomes. First attempts should be easily and concretely measurable. Cost savings has been the most common measurement used for case management outcomes. It should be noted that *hard savings* are more tangible and easily measured; *soft savings* are more obscure. Quality-of-life issues are also more nebulous and will require careful consideration when turning them into something that is measurable.

Developing indicators of quality in which to measure is an essential process in an outcomes program. The case management outcomes domains listed below are general and need further definition. However, they are the stuff that quality indicators are made of and are a good place to start. Develop the outcomes below through the following sequence. Quality indicators and the numerator/denominator format are described in the following sections.

1. Choose an outcomes domain to evaluate.
2. Next, select a more specific topic of interest. Some potential ideas are listed below the main outcomes domains, although the list can be further expanded by customizing a need specific to your organization.
3. Then construct a measurable outcome. This is done by designing the chosen outcome in quality indicator, numerator/denominator format, *so it can be measured.*

Clinical Outcomes for Case Managers

Case Manager facilitated appropriate clinical outcomes in collaboration with multidisciplinary team:

- Management of the therapeutic regimen (case manager, provider) (goal = improved)
- Appropriateness of clinical care (goal = improved)
- Necessity for emergency department visits (goal = decreased visits)
- Disease-specific complications, exacerbations, comorbidities (goal = decreased)
- Adverse drug reactions/adverse blood product reaction (goal = decreased)
- Infection rate (goal = decreased)
- Unscheduled returns to the emergency room within 72 hours (goal = decreased)
- Delay in diagnosing condition (can also be a system problem) (goal = decreased)
- Readmissions within 15 days of discharge from acute or post acute services (goal = decreased)
- Complications of procedures/therapy (goal = decreased)
- Disease condition present in acute care or skilled nursing facility (SNF) that was not present on admission (goal = decreased)

Financial/Economic Outcomes for Case Managers

- Case Manager facilitated appropriate resource utilization and management:
  — Length of stay (LOS)
  — Number of intensive care unit days

— Number of emergency department visits
— Number of readmission rates
• Case Manager facilitated change in level of care/LOS
• Case Manager facilitated change to contracted (PPO) provider/facility
• Case Manager facilitated appropriate number of acute/postacute/SNF/home health days
• Case Manager facilitated productivity (goal = reduced lost work days)
• Case Manager facilitated reduction of disease exacerbations
• Case Manager facilitated adherence to the therapeutic regimen (patient compliance)
• Case Manager negotiated rates of service or equipment/supplies
• Case Manager negotiated intensity of services/equipment
• Case Manager negotiated frequency or duration of service or equipment
• Case Manager provided accurate assessment of equipment "rent versus buy"
• Case Manager avoided inappropriate/ineffective services
• Case Manager avoided insurance denials (goal = 0%)
• Case management costs to system:
— Equipment/supplies (computers, software, mobile phones, beepers, office supplies)
— Wage (salary, overtime, administrative costs, sick/vacation, travel expenses)
— Productivity

Humanistic Outcomes for Case Managers

• Case Manager facilitated recovery of functional status
• Case Manager facilitated improved patient comfort through effective pain management/symptom management
• Case Manager facilitated improved quality of life for the patient, as evidenced by satisfaction with case management services
• Case Manager facilitated caregiver well-being
• Case Manager facilitated improved level of physical independence
• Case Manager facilitated improved cognitive performance
• Case Manager facilitated employability
• Case Manager facilitated psychosocial adjustment/coping with life changes
• Case Manager facilitated patient/family satisfaction (in such areas as clinical outcomes, pain management, education of disease process/management, case management, access to health care)
• Case Manager facilitated provider satisfaction (with case management interdisciplinary collaborative efforts, case coordination, autonomy, their patient's access to health care)

- Case Manager facilitated payor satisfaction (in case managers' negotiation skills)
- Case Management Satisfaction in areas such as:
  — Job satisfaction
  — Roles
  — Case load size
  — Autonomy
  — Minimal ethical dilemmas
  — Challenging cases
  — Adequate training

Quality Outcomes for Case Managers

- Case Manager facilitated access to health care/avoidance of delay in services
- Case Manager facilitated reduced mortality and morbidity
- Case Manager facilitated prevention of adverse occurrences
- Case Manager facilitated improved compliance with organizational standards/guidelines
- Case Manager facilitated decreased fragmentation of care/services
- Case Manager recognized important psychosocial needs/risks
- Case Manager recognized important clinical needs/risks
- Case Manager facilitated health-seeking behavior in patient
- Case Manager facilitated compliance issues (in both patient and provider)
- Case Manager facilitated patient self-care

Case Management Organizational/Administrative/ Systems Outcomes

CASE MANAGEMENT OUTCOMES

- Case Manager facilitated assessment of patient/family support/financial/ psychosocial/insurance benefits
- Case Manager facilitated coordination and development of case management plans and services
- Case Manager facilitated education of patient/significant other/family
- Case Manager facilitated appropriate monitoring, reassessment, and reevaluation of cases
- Case Manager facilitated appropriate discharge planning/changing levels of care
- Case Manager facilitated appropriate utilization management/resource management
- Case Manager facilitated appropriate clinical activities for each patient

- Case Manager facilitated improved organizational communication on outcomes data, plans for improvement
- Case Manager facilitated appropriate use of on-site versus telephonic case management services
- Case Manager facilitated the reconsideration process when necessary
- Case Manager facilitated expedited appeals process when necessary
- Case Manager facilitated standard appeals process when necessary
- Case Manager facilitated appropriate referrals to hospice, SNF, rehabilitation, home health
- Case Manager facilitated increased health plan membership retention rate (related to customer satisfaction)
- Case Manager facilitated member satisfaction with networks provided
- Case Manager facilitated patient access to providers/services
- Case management patient records are accurate and complete
- Case Manager facilitated appropriate length of case management services
- Case Manager facilitated high confidentiality standards
- Case Manager facilitated appropriate case management problem identification
- Case Manager facilitated appropriate case management assessment of educational needs
- Case Manager provided appropriate case management educational material/instruction, such as:
  — Adequacy of dietary counseling/teaching
  — Adequacy of medications counseling/teaching
  — Adequate patient education for safe self-care
- Case Manager facilitated availability of inpatient and outpatient services (rehabilitation)
- Case Manager reduced delay in diagnosing condition (can also be a clinical or system problem)
- Case Manager facilitated timeliness of case management interventions
- Case Manager facilitated appropriate use of "reasons for case closure"
- Case Manager facilitated appropriateness of discharges or referrals
- Case Manager facilitated beneficiary retention

ORGANIZATIONAL SUPPORT TO CASE MANAGEMENT SERVICES

- Insurance benefits match disease management incentives
- Organization supports use of outcomes to evaluate case management staffing (appropriate number of case managers)
- Organization supports appropriate specialty case management programs based on enrollee diagnoses rates

- Organization supports availability and accessibility to appropriate specialists and services for enrollees
- Organization has an established panel of available, credentialed physician advisors (various specialties) for case management support
- Organization supports information systems that are useful in case management and outcomes management
- Organization supports programs for prevention of disease
- Organization supports a continuous quality improvement (CQI) program or Quality Council to address quality of care and access to benefits/care issues
- Organization supports a case management evaluation process
- Organization supports case management credentialing/certification
- Organization supports case management accreditation
- Organization supports case management continuing educational opportunities
- Organization has written policies and procedures on such issues as:
  — Confidentiality
  — Timeframes for various case management responsibilities
  — Grievance, reconsideration, and appeals

A CASE MANAGEMENT/OUTCOMES MANAGEMENT PROGRAM—GETTING STARTED

Outcomes management represents a young and growing area of research that has significant opportunities to improve patient care, reduce unnecessary services, preserve medical resources, and improve satisfaction to all who use or work in the medical field. It is, however, complex and resource consumptive. In an effort to make it more understandable, this chapter will enhance the understanding of quality indicators. *Steps in an Improvement Project* will be discussed in Chapter 5.

Important concepts about quality indicators include:

- The definition
- The difference and relationship between process and outcomes
- The quality indicator numerator/denominator format
- The relationship between goals, objectives, quality indicators, and case management interventions

Outcomes management and quality improvement projects are intimately connected; once an outcome in need of improvement is recognized, a quality improvement project—a focused effort to address a specific opportunity for improvement—is the next step. The remaining section will show where the quality indicator fits into the whole program and the sequence of the critical steps involved in a quality improvement project. The steps to a project are also explained in further detail in the chapters on CQI (see the section on the PDCA [Plan-Do-Check-Act] Cycle).

UNDERSTANDING QUALITY INDICATORS

Quality Indicators: The Definition

A quality indicator is a statement about a process or outcome of care; they are *pointers* that indicate either good quality or potential problem areas needing further investigation. Quality indicators are a tool to measure the quality of case management components such as appropriateness of clinical care, provider or patient satisfaction, or cost. It is important to understand that indicators are not direct measures of quality and should not be used to make final judgments. Rather, they can be used as red flags that direct the case management attention to areas needing further assessment and improvement. "Case managers can think of quality measurement tools as a compass; where you are headed is more important than how fast you are going. Quality measurement tools provide direction to prevent case managers, other members of the health care team, and patients from getting lost in the health care maze" (Rieve, 1997c, p. 38).

Case management improvement projects should be based on quality indicators, which are disease-, condition-, or situation-specific statements that are related to *processes* or *outcomes* of care. They can incorporate guidelines, standards of care, or practice parameters and must be grounded in literature where available (Health Care Financing Administration [HCFA]). Through the use of quality indicators, which are sometimes referred to as *clinical performance measures, outcome indicators,* or *outcome measures,* case managers will be able to measure outcomes; that is, if the quality indicators are written in a way that is measurable (*i.e.,* numerator/denominator format) (Box 4-1).

It is recommended that, when initiating the first case management improvement projects, one should use only one or two quality indicators to measure the case management intervention. It is easier to make changes on a small scale, therefore increasing the chance to be successful. Early success in case management improvement projects is important; it provides motivation to continue the efforts and often increases administrative support for the extensive use of resources that these projects require.

Box 4-1

QUALITY INDICATOR CRITERIA

Quality Indicators:

- Are measurable variables derived from practice guidelines or other credible sources
- Are used to measure processes and outcomes of care
- Are usually expressed as numerators and denominators
- Should identify significant steps in the process of care that have the greatest potential for improvement
- Should be measurable through claims data, primary data collection, or other sources
- Use criteria, a set of rules by which the data collector or analyst determines whether an indicator has been met; specific criteria assure uniformity in the data collection process.

From the Health Care Financing Administration (HCFA).

Process Indicators and Outcome Indicators: Understanding the Difference

Indicators are often broken down into the types of events they measure. Therefore, it is important for case managers to broadly appreciate the relationship between process and outcomes and the differences between process indicators and outcome indicators.

Essentially, there are two approaches to performance measurement:

1. Identifying clinical intervention **processes** that link to desired health outcomes, and measuring them
2. Identifying **outcomes** that reflect the biopsychosocial status of the member

According to the Joint Commission on Accreditation of Healthcare Organizations (JCAHO), an **outcome indicator** may measure a result of care that either is desirable or undesirable. When an outcome indicator is used,

> (it) measures what happens (or does not happen) to the patient after something is done (or not done) to the patient. . . **A process indicator** measures a care activity done for a patient. Process indicators generally seek to measure discrete steps in the patient care process that are important. The best process indicators focus on processes of care that are closely linked to patient outcomes, meaning that a scientific basis exists for believing that the care provided (or not provided) will lead to a specific outcome." (JCAHO, 1989, p. 332)

Through diabetic case management educational efforts, independence in monitoring and controlling blood sugars is desirable, thus lowering HbA1c levels; less control and higher HbA1c levels are undesirable. Here, the educational effort is the process; the lower (or higher) HbA1c is the outcome.

The Center for Case Management Accountability (CCMA) has this to say about the relationship between process, outcomes, and case management accountability:

> The core functions of case management rely on excellent work processes performed consistently well. CCMA encourages consistency in process measurement as a component of professional standards of care for case management. Measuring the relationships between process and outcome is also essential for quality improvement. However, processes are the means for achieving results, and the results are what customers want to see. Consequently, accountability should be based on outcomes rather than processes. (CMSA, 1998)

Process Indicators

Processes are case management interventions—what they do, and how they work with patients, families, insurance companies, and other case managers. Processes result in outcomes. Process indicators are essentially diagnostic in their description (tests, medications, procedures, surgeries) and tell what outcome indicators should be measured. The process indicator approach has limitations; good processes cannot always guarantee good outcomes, because patients often have their own agendas, and diseases are dynamic. However, process measures provide significant insight into the quality of care. Increased utilization of scientifically based processes should lead to improved patient care; conversely, suboptimal outcomes are often rooted in poor or variable processes of care. Process indicators should be chosen for their contribution to good case management care. In the CQI chapters, the flowchart tool is used for evaluating processes; "a process is not worth doing for its own sake. Unless it makes a measurable contribution to the whole, it probably is wasteful and should be abandoned" (Kongstvedt, 1993). This philosophy is recaptured in the CQI section on flowcharts, where redundancy or unnecessary steps to a process are weeded out.

Process indicators are generally thought to be easier than outcome indicators to construct, require less data collection and analysis to produce, and are easier to understand. Many measures of performance, such as the Health Plan Employer Data Information Set (HEDIS), are built on process indicators (American College of Emergency Physicians, 1998).

Examples of clinical process indicators include:

Blood pressure quarterly
Lipid profile annually
Annual mammograms for breast cancer screening
Foot examinations twice a year in diabetic patients
Retinal examinations annually in diabetic patients

Outcome Indicators

Outcomes are the result, effect, or impact of the case management interventions conducted. Outcome indicators answer the questions: How did the patient respond to case management clinically, financially, functionally, emotionally, or spiritually? What effect did case management have on the cost of care? What effect did case management have on the satisfaction levels of the patients, families, providers, or payors?

Some experts in outcome projects have determined that it is more difficult to get positive data movement using outcome indicators. However, outcome measurement is potentially the most efficient strategy for measuring performance, because it reflects the person's current biopsychosocial status. It must be determined if accepting improvement in a specific process necessarily translates into improvement in outcomes; and this may take some time to make a determination. Outcome measurement of clinical performance is still in its infancy, although organizations such as the Agency for Health Care Policy and Research and HCFA have been active in promoting research to identify these measures. With such measurements, the case managers and public will be able to objectively compare health plans, outpatient treatment centers, home health agencies, SNFs, physician specialists, and so forth. And organizations will certainly compare case managers' effectiveness as well.

Examples of clinical outcome indicators include:

To increase treatment for hyperlipidemia by 10% over the next 12 months
To increase use of angiotensin-converting enzyme (ACE) inhibitor if
    hypertensive by 10% over the next 12 months
To increase use of ACE inhibitor if proteinuria by 10% over the next 12 months
Ophthalmologic referral if abnormal retinal examination in 100% of diabetic patients
Beta-blockers after myocardial infarction in 100% of acute myocardial
    infarction patient discharges

Table 4-1 (Examples of Case Management Process Indicators and Outcome Indicators) depicts a few of the many process and outcome indicators that case managers can use to "prove our worth." It is important to understand how an indicator must be written to yield **measurable** results. For that critical piece, see the section on how to write indicators in numerator/denominator format in this chapter.

Just to muddy the waters a bit more, remember that what may be a *process* to one case manager may be an *outcome* to another. For example, a discharge to an appropriate rehabilitation center for a head-injured patient may be the outcome to the hospital case manager. The efficient admission of the patient to a rehabilitation case manager would be a process that will lead to increased patient satisfaction (the outcome). The ultimate outcome of the total case (inclusive of all case managers and facilities) would be optimizing the quality of life of the patient using the most cost-efficient methods. To measure this ultimate goal, the procedure will take a variety of process indicators and outcome indicators, in anatomically correct "numerator/denominator" fashion.

NUMERATOR/DENOMINATOR FORMAT

An essential component of a quality improvement project is a *measurable outcome*. What is measured is the *change* that has occurred. This measurable change may be from a process change, a system change, or a health behavior change that is expected to lead to improved health outcomes, improved quality of life, or increased satisfaction with appropriate use of services. For the outcome to be measured, the quality indicator must be in a format that allows this measurement: the numerator/denominator format.

An indicator expresses information as an event or a ratio (or rate) of events within a defined universe (JCAHO, 1989). The use of raw numbers should be avoided; they are vague and do not lend themselves to consistent comparisons. The standard approach to constructing quality indicators is to state them in a numerator/denominator format. In general, the *numerator* states the total number who met what is being measured; the *denominator* defines the total number who have the condition or procedure the indicator is measuring (eligible population). Two studies can be accurately compared if the same numerator and denominator are used; the same denominator, even in different organizations, levels the playing field.

The Numerator/Denominator Format of a Quality Indicator

Putting the quality indicator in numerator/denominator format is the first step; it is also essential to choose the correct numerator and denominator. Consider the difference in the following example:

TABLE 4-1 Examples of Case Management Process Indicators and Outcome Indicators

PROCESS INDICATORS	OUTCOME INDICATORS
Process Indicator Case management educational efforts (self-monitoring of blood glucose) in 100% of diabetic patients	**Outcome Indicator** HbA1c levels equal to or less than 7.5 in case-managed diabetic patients
Process Indicator Case management educational efforts (dietary and weight monitoring) in 100% of CHF patients	**Outcome Indicator** Reduction in readmission rates for CHF patients by 40%
Process Indicator Case management educational efforts (correct peak flow meter use) in 100% of asthmatic patients	**Outcome Indicator** 50% less emergency department visits in case-managed asthmatic patients
Process Indicator Negotiation of price for DME (durable medical equipment) when using non-PPO agencies in 100% of non-PPO use	**Outcome Indicator** Savings of 20% in DME when using non-PPO agencies
Process Indicator Adheres to case management reports schedule (time frame per contract) in 100% of contracted case management cases	**Outcome Indicator** Reduction in "late" case management reports to clients by 95%
Process Indicator Case management of 100% of on-the-job back injured employees	**Outcome Indicator** Reduction of lost work days by 50% in case-managed employees
Process Indicator Case management calls contract contact person monthly 100% of the time	**Outcome Indicator** Case management contracts renewed 95% of the time
Process Indicator Negotiated and PPO rates decrease payor costs by an average of 25%	**Outcome Indicator** Payor satisfaction with case management 95% of the time
Process Indicator Use of appropriate community resources in stroke cases 100% of the time	**Outcome Indicator** Decrease post-hospital costs by 15% in stroke cases
Process Indicator Obtaining approval for (specify service/ procedure/DME) in 100% of the cases	**Outcome Indicator** Achieves 95% patient/provider/payor satisfaction
Process Indicator Advance directives are discussed in 100% of appropriate case management cases	**Outcome Indicator** Families are satisfied with "code" decisions 90% of the time
Process Indicator Initiates case management contact on new cases with 1 business day of referral	**Outcome Indicator** One step closer to obtaining case management accreditation!

Numerator: How Many Met What Is Being Measured

Denominator: How Many Were **Eligible to Meet** What
is Being Measured

An organization collects information to assess the percentage of abdominal surgical wound infections. During data collection:

- The organization performed 800 surgeries.
- The organization performed 80 abdominal surgeries.
- There were 8 postoperative wound infections.

Incorrect:

$$\frac{\text{abdominal surgical wound infections}}{\text{number of surgeries}} \quad \frac{8}{800} \quad =1\%$$

Correct:

$$\frac{\text{abdominal surgical wound infections}}{\text{number of \textbf{abdominal} surgeries}} \quad \frac{8}{80} \quad =10\%$$

Notice that the incorrect denominator included all surgeries. This is inaccurate for two reasons:

1. Only abdominal surgeries should be included in the definition of the denominator (How Many Were Eligible to Meet What Is Being Measured). Total hip replacements or head surgeries have no place in the denominator. Another example is that, if HbA1c results were being measured in an HMO case management department, it would be incorrect to include the total population of enrollees, even those without diabetes.
2. By including the wrong population in the denominator, the percentages will be wrong, leading the conclusion down the wrong road. In the preceding example, the incorrect percentage was 1%; the correct percentage was 10%. Whereas a 1% surgical postoperative infection rate may be within reason, a 10% rate may be unacceptable. By including the full 800 surgeries in the denominator, case managers may be led to believe that "all is well."

Consider carefully what the organization wants to measure before writing out the numerator and denominator. Case management examples may include the following:

$$\frac{\text{patient satisfaction with case management}}{\text{number on case management case load}}$$

$$\frac{\text{number of cases who received a (specific) case management service}}{\text{number of cases eligible to have the case management service}}$$

Numerator/Denominator Format in Settings with Phases

Designing numerator/denominator format in settings in which there are phases, such as cardiac or other forms of rehabilitation, is done essentially the same way. The denominator still includes all those who are eligible to meet what is being measured, or the number of patients who are in the phase of the rehabilitation being measured.

Cardiac and other systems of rehabilitation are often denied by insurance companies, primary care physicians, and even cardiologists. Outcomes management projects could be the answer to changing some of those practices. Many disease management programs are focusing efforts on cardiac care. Coronary heart disease is the leading cause of morbidity and mortality in the United States. Each year, it is estimated that 1.5 million Americans will sustain a myocardial infarction (MI); of that number, almost 500,000 are fatal. Research studies have confirmed that there is a 20% to 25% reduction of death in those patients who received cardiac rehabilitation after an MI; there is also a 37% reduction in the incidence of sudden death during the first year (Kopin, 1997). Many other diagnoses are also appropriate for cardiac rehabilitation: postoperative coronary artery graft bypass (CABG) patients, percutaneous transluminal coronary angioplasty (PTCA) patients, some forms of angina, and a medley of other cardiac failure patients. For these reasons, cardiac rehabilitation will be used as an example of numerator/denominator format in settings with phases.

Cardiac rehabilitation is typically in three phases (Kopin, 1997):

Phase I begins immediately after the cardiac event and follows through the hospitalization. The emphasis of phase I is gradual progression of activities and exercise tolerance. There is an important educational component to helping patients and families understand heart disease, risk factors, and possibilities for a healthier lifestyle.

Phase II begins at discharge from the hospital and continues as an outpatient program. The primary goal of phase II is to recondition the patient to a physically active state. Progressive heart training is done with medical supervision and telemetry monitoring. The educational component continues with more about dietary and lifestyle changes, and psychological support. Phase II generally lasts for 12 weeks, with three visits per week recommended.

Phase III begins after the patient completes phase II. The primary goal is to instill in the patient the importance of a lifetime maintenance program that encourages heart-healthy behaviors. The exercise program is also offered to individuals without a history of heart disease as a primary prevention effort.

Outcomes of cardiac rehabilitation include examples such as educational tasks, physiologically measurable exercise gains, intake assessment, and cost. A generic formula for a quality indicator for a phased intervention is:

$$\frac{\textit{Total number of patients who met what was being measured}}{\textit{Total number of patients } \textbf{in x phase}}$$

PHASED NUMERATOR/DENOMINATOR FORMAT

The organization interested in cardiac outcomes may choose to see whether their patients are at or near a benchmark for that phase. For example, if a benchmark for patient strength improvement is 25% in phase II, a numerator/denominator may look like this:

$$\frac{\textbf{Number of patients with 25\% increase in strength in phase II}}{\text{Total number of patients in phase II}}$$

If the goal, or benchmark for graduation from phase II, is 12 weeks, a numerator/denominator may look like this:

$$\frac{\textbf{Total number of patients who move out of phase II in 12 weeks}}{\text{Total number of patients in phase II}}$$

Other suggestions for outcomes projects in cardiac rehabilitation include improvement in symptoms, decrease in blood lipids, decrease in blood pressure (if hypertensive), improvement in psychological well-being, reduction in smoking, improvement in diet choices, decrease in weight (if overweight), improvement in blood glucose levels (if diabetic), or measurement of return-to-work time. (See Table 4-2 for examples of quality indicators in numerator/denominator format.)

Whether the quality indicator will measure a process or an outcome, it is critical to explicitly define the eligible population. This is part of "risk adjustment" and will also assure that everyone will use the same criteria when mea-

TABLE 4-2 Example Case Management Quality Indicators in Numerator/Denominator Format

QUALITY INDICATOR	NUMERATOR	DENOMINATOR
Percentage of HbA1c levels equal to or less than 7.5 In case-managed diabetic patients	Total number of case-managed diabetic patients with HbA1c levels equal to or less than 7.5	Total number of case-managed diabetic patients
Percentage of case management reports completed in (*time frame per contract*)14 days	Total number of case management reports completed in 14 days	Total number of case management reports completed (requiring same time frame)
Percentage of reduction in readmission rates for case-managed CHF patients (NOTE: This would require baseline and remeasurement comparisons)	Total number of readmissions of case-managed CHF patients	Total number of case-managed CHF patients
Percentage of reduction in emergency department visits in case-managed asthmatic patients (NOTE: This would require baseline and remeasurement comparisons)	Total number of emergency department visits in case-managed asthmatic patients	Total number of case-managed asthmatic patients
Percentage of reduction of lost work days in case-managed employees (NOTE: This would require baseline and remeasurement comparisons)	Total number of lost work days in case-managed employees	Total number of case-managed employees
Average number of hours per case management case	Total number of case management hours	Total number of cases
Percent of case-managed (*specify diagnosis*) diabetic patients (*specify what was done, facilitated, or received*) who received education about a diabetic diet (NOTE: This formula will work for many types of disease management percentages)	Total number of case-managed diabetic patients who were given education about the diabetic diet at least once during the review period	The total number of case-managed diabetic patients

continued

TABLE 4-2 *(Continued)* **Example Case Management Quality Indicators in Numerator/Denominator Format**

QUALITY INDICATOR	NUMERATOR	DENOMINATOR
Percent of case-managed *(specify diagnosis)* CHF patients *(specify what was done, facilitated, or received)* who received education about fluid weight gain prevention (NOTE: This formula will work for many types of disease management percentages)	Total number of case-managed CHF patients who were given education about fluid weight gain prevention at least once during the review period	The total number of case-managed CHF patients
Percentage of improved SF 12 scores on remeasurement of case-managed oncology patients	Total number of improved SF 12 scores in case-managed oncology patients	Total number of SF 12 scores in case-managed oncology patients

suring the quality indicators. This, in turn, leads to consistent application of the measure. Eligibility criteria may be different for each quality indicator, and both the numerator and the denominator will require assessment. Ask whether there are any "rules" to be placed on the gathering of the data for this part of the quality indicator. For example, perhaps the outcomes project will be solely for Medicaid or Medicare patients, or pediatric patients from 7 to 14 years of age. Or, if medications (for example, beta-blockers or ACE inhibitors) are in the quality indicators, consider which patients should or should not be considered in the study.

A common complaint heard when providers or facilities are given comparative data is that there is no scientific validity with small denominators. This is true. Because the denominator represents the sample size, and small sample size can lessen the statistical power of the outcome, conclusions based on the use of small denominators must be used with caution. However, currently there is benchmarking mathematical work in progress to adjust for small denominators. Through the efforts of CCMA, it is hoped that case managers will not run into this problem, although it should be accounted for in single-department projects.

THE RELATIONSHIP BETWEEN GOALS, OBJECTIVES, QUALITY INDICATORS, AND INTERVENTIONS

At times, the various components of an outcomes management program may whirl about, hardly appearing to relate at all. However, rest assured, there is a connection. This section will show the flow from writing the case management goals and objectives to developing the corresponding quality indicators with their case management interventions. Diabetes will be used as an example.

1. The Goal Statement

Initially, a case management organization must understand and define what it wants to accomplish; this can be written as a goal. According to the National Association for Healthcare Quality (NAHQ), a **goal** is defined as "a broadly stated or long term outcome written as an overall statement relating to a philosophy, purpose or desired outcome." Example goal statements may be written as:

- To decrease hospital admissions in diabetic patients
- To improve the processes of care for diabetic patients
- To improve the quality of life and satisfaction of diabetic patients
- To reduce costs related to hospitalizations in the diabetic population

2. The Objectives

After the goal statement is written, the case management department/organization will develop specific, measurable objectives that will provide evidence of deficiencies. According to the NAHQ, an **objective** is defined as "specific action-oriented statements written in measurable and observable terms that define how the goals will be attained." Example objectives that relate to the above goals may be written as follows:

- To increase the percentage of diabetic patients who have a HbA1c monitored every 6 months from 50% to 75% in the next 12 months.
- To increase the percentage of diabetic patients with an abnormal result of a retinal examination who were referred to an eye care specialist by 20% in the next 12 months
- To increase the percentage of diabetic patients who receive education about self-monitoring of blood glucose to 100% in the next 12 months.

3. The Quality Indicators

Once outcomes-based objectives have been determined, it is time to write the quality indicator(s) in numerator/denominator format.

1. The percentage of diabetic patients who have an HbA1c monitored every 6 months:

Number of patients that had a HbAlc
performed during the 6-month period
Total number of diabetic patients

2. The percentage of diabetic patients with abnormal results of a retinal examination who were referred to an eye care specialist:

Number of patients with abnormal results of a retinal examination
who were referred to an eye care specialist during the 12-month period

Total number of diabetic patients who had abnormal results
of a retinal examination

3. The percentage of diabetic patients who received education about self-monitoring of blood glucose:

Number of patients who were given education about self-
monitoring of blood glucose at least once during the 12-month period
Total number of diabetic patients

4. The Action Plan:
The Case Management Interventions

Finally, each quality indicator requires the development of an action plan, which comprises the interventions that address the objectives. Interventions may be directed at the patients, providers, pharmacists, laboratories, diabetic educators, diabetic case managers, dietitians, family members, specialists, or others included in the medical team. Interventions may be in the form of mailings, written booklets and guidelines, community seminars, clinics, home-based teaching—the opportunities for interventions are ripe for the creative case management imagination.

GOALS, OBJECTIVES, QUALITY INDICATORS, AND INTERVENTIONS—THE SEQUENCE

1. Understand what the case management organization desires to change, and write a *goal statement*.
2. From the goal statement, write *objectives*.
3. From the objectives, write *quality indicators* in numerator/denominator format.
4. Write an action plan that provides the case management organization with *interventions* that will improve the care, and meet the measurable objectives.

CHAPTER 5

Quality Improvement Projects

STEPS IN AN IMPROVEMENT PROJECT

The critical steps in an improvement project are few and appear deceptively simple. The actual effort necessary to perform each step, so that meaningful results are generated, is genuinely difficult and requires the special knowledge of various professionals. The sequence of the critical steps in an improvement project include five benign-looking components:

1. Baseline measurement
2. Initiation of case management interventions
3. Early interim measurement to assess success of interventions
4. Remeasurement
5. Evaluation

However, before any of these steps can take place, assessment and planning of all aspects of the project must be carefully considered. Like managing a patient's case, proactive assessment and planning can avert numerous hazards during the intervention phase; and when the proper steps have been given the attention needed, the analysis phases will be clearer and generate meaningful results. Planning and assessment domains for outcomes management projects are discussed in the following section. This is a multidisciplinary effort, so assemble a team of people with the knowledge to proceed (see CQI chapter on teams).

PLANNING AND ASSESSMENT—DEVELOPING A FOCUSED INTERVENTION PLAN

What Will the Organization Measure?
What Is Important to the Organization?

The first planning and assessment consideration for the organization is to decide what they are interested in measuring. It is important to align case management goals with the larger goals of the organization. A basic continuous quality improvement (CQI) tenet is that the administration of the organization must be supportive of, and in agreement with, any major projects or changes planned; without this support, success is questionable. To determine what is important to the organization, ask such questions as:

- What does the organization want to learn about its case management processes and performance?
- What are the most common/most costly disease conditions?
- What processes are likely to reveal opportunities for improvement?
- Is this in fulfillment of accreditation requirements such as JCAHO/ORYX, NCQA/HEDIS, or case management accreditation?
- What is unique about your case management environment, your community, or your patient population? Adjust your outcomes plans accordingly.

Define a Budget

It is also important to assess what resources will be needed, and define a budget for the project that is acceptable to the organization. Measuring outcomes is an important marketing tool but requires resources of time, money, and personnel. Consider:

- What resources are *available* to plan, select, modify or develop, and implement an effective case management intervention?
- What resources are *required* to plan, select, modify or develop, and implement a case management intervention?
- In some projects, other people/organizations are asked to commit resources to the project. In those instances, determine what resources will be required of others. Are they willing and able to provide the resources? Some resources to consider are provider staffing, physician time, or beneficiary copayments or deductibles.
- Can the improved outcome be translated into projected cost savings? If the cost of the case management intervention will exceed the amount of projected cost savings, is this still acceptable to the organization?
- Data collection and analysis is complex and costly. Does the case management organization have the necessary resources and information systems to execute these tasks? Or can the organization secure appropriate data elements from other avenues that will provide information necessary to record outcome measurements? Put a dollar amount on this and assess whether it is feasible.

The familiar concept of *prioritization* is another important consideration during the budget assessment. If the *entire* project is too costly, consider whether there are distinct aspects of the project that are an organizational priority, and trim down the expectations according to those decisions.

What/Who Is the Target Population of the Measurement?

Identifying and getting to know customer desires and expectations is another key assessment piece. Who are the case management customers? Consider internal customers and external customers:

- **Internal customers** are those within the case management organization. Answering the questions above will help define internal customer needs.
- **External customers** may consist of many different people, organizations, or departments. Examples include the patient/family unit, physicians, other providers, pharmacists/pharmacies, home health agencies, hospice agencies, skilled nursing facilities, rehabilitation facilities, hospitals, managed care organizations, payors, employers, or other case managers.

Given the extensive possibilities and diverse groups of a **target population** (also known as a **target audience**) for the case management interventions, it is understandable why this target must be chosen before going much further in project planning. The type of assessment, project timeline, data measurement strategies, experimental design, intervention strategies, and evaluation will depend on who (or what) is the target.

When assessing the target of the case management interventions, consider the following:

- Concentrate on outcomes your customer regards as most important.
- Look at the system of the targeted intervention: Does a *behavior* need changing or is it something in the *system* that needs changing to become more effective?
- Assess the potential for change; what is the potential that the case management intervention will have a measurable effect on behavior? Does the customer or target population have the capacity to change?
- Assess all the factors labeled in the risk-adjustment section, such as age, diagnoses, comorbidities, and gender.
- Assess the customer's present knowledge level about the intervention and provide education if required.
- Keep everyone well-informed. If a managed care plan sends diabetic beneficiaries educational materials stating that their primary care provider (PCP) should be checking their feet, the HbA1c level, their eyes, etc., inform the PCPs that this is being done.

- Obtain detailed data about the target population of the intervention through activities such as literature reviews, data collection, surveys, focus groups, or assessing practice patterns. Some useful information about the customer/patient includes:
  — Knowledge about the customer's/patient's *perception* of the intervention
  — Knowledge about the customer's/patient's perception of the *need* for change and the *intent* to change. Ability to change, and intention to change, are major predictors of actual change. The customer/patient may value the current behavior.
  — Knowledge about the barriers that may prevent a positive outcome, such as lack of resources (financial, transportation) or lack of skills, communication barriers, or cultural barriers. Interventions must be appropriate for the target population.
- Consider what customers and patients of health care truly want, such as:
  — Effective communication
  — Nonadversarial problem-solving
  — Coordination of services
  — Educational programs
  — Patient advocacy
  — Consensus building
  — Timely follow-through
  — Formal grievance procedures
  — Feedback mechanism
  — Other patient support functions (Carneal, 1998)

Clarify Case Management Goals and Objectives

Part of project planning is a written list of goals and objectives, and a written timetable. Once this has been accomplished, it has been decided which processes or outcomes to measure (cost, quality, system), and who the target of the measurement will be, the next planning and assessment key task is to identify where case management can perform interventions that will result in a significant and measurable change. Set case management goals, and then develop measurable objectives.

Determine Quality Indicators

Whenever possible, it is always better to use "tried and true" outcome measurements. However, that is not always possible. Unlike other areas of health care, case management outcomes projects are in an early stage of development. It may require a few years of experience, and the work of the Center for Case

Management Accountability (CCMA), to amass an index of meaningful and statistically accurate case management quality indicators.

First, decide what clinical, process, system, or other area you want to measure. For the choice to be meaningful, it should be one in which there is either too much variability or known substandard outcomes. *Get facts.* A project team may think a certain process or system is a problem; however, until research is performed on the situation, it will be unknown whether the "problem" is real or piggybacked onto some other challenging situation. Sometimes the real solution is hidden behind a layer or two; or sometimes the "problem" may simply be a team member's hidden agenda. Use some of the CQI tools for process improvement to discern the root cause(s).

Once an area to measure has been chosen, conduct a literature review and consider partnering with other case management organizations to increase the brain pool of possibilities. Contact CCMA. Ask whether existing intervention tools can be modified to reduce the cost of the project without compromising its integrity. Evaluate the scientific strength of any prewritten measure your organization is considering. Ask whether the nature of the intervention is such that it can be measured. If not, rethink the intervention. (See Chapter 4, "Relationship Between Goals, Objectives, Quality Indicators, and Interventions.")

How Will the Data Be Selected, Collected, and Measured? Does the Organization Have the Capacity or Connections/Resources to Collect and Measure the Data?

At this point in the project planning stage, a system for data collection and management must be established. A good data collection protocol is clearly stated, complete, and can be replicated by others. Every effort must be made to assure that data collection is simple and can be integrated into practice with minimal cost and burden on case managers and their patients (CMSA, 1998). The organization must clarify protocols for finding sources for the data or generating new data sources, and planning methods of data collection and measurement, including the development of a data abstraction tool if necessary.

Planning the details of data collection and measurement in advance is not optional. Precise planning leads to consistent and accurate data collection; a haphazard approach can ultimately lead to serious errors in decision-making. Inaccurate conclusions can come from using poor data, or misusing good data. According to some experts, most organizations do not measure processes, clearly define their measurement goals, analyze their data, or use their data for decision-making (Rieve, 1997a). This allows the loss of tremendous opportunities for improvement.

DATA COLLECTION METHODS AND DESIGNS

When determining data collection methods, consider whether individual data or aggregate data will meet your needs. Individual data, which is data collection depicted by organization, client, case manager, or patient population, can provide essential information on the impact of case management services on a controlled group. Aggregate data are pooled data on groups of similar organizations, clients, case managers, or patient populations. Aggregate data make it possible to examine patterns and variations between similar groups. This can be looked at from a variety of perspectives by sorting the data in different ways: by diagnosis, by payor, by provider, etc. (Lamb et al., 1998). Determining the overall study design for the improvement project also should be assessed (see section on "Study Designs for Case Management Evaluations" in Chapter 3).

DETERMINING DATA SOURCES

After the quality indicators have been chosen, examine what type of data will provide the information necessary to measure them. Evaluate current data sources (such as medical records, case management records), what experimental design has been chosen (cross-sectional, experimental, longitudinal), the sample size, and timeframes for measurement. Then, determine whether systems currently used are feasible for collecting the data, or whether the organization can secure appropriate data elements from other avenues that will provide information necessary to record outcome measurements. This must be assessed from both a budgetary standpoint and a feasibility standpoint.

When determining data sources, look for computerized sources whenever possible; this decreases the burden of having to "hand abstract" documentation and often supplies more valid data. However, because most information systems currently are not sophisticated enough to be "all things to all organizations," data on specific quality indicators will often need to be hand-abstracted with abstraction tools developed explicitly for the purpose. The four data types most commonly used for quality assessment include enrollment, administration, clinical, and survey data (McGlynn & Asch, 1998).

Enrollment Data

- Used to identify the target population under a specific insurance plan
- Can be used to identify a target population for preventative services

- *Problem with using enrollment data:* rarely contains information that is not required for insurance verification, such as race, education, income, health status

Administrative (Claims) Data

- Generated to support reimbursement activities in noncapitated or indemnity health plans
- Can be used to identify a population based on a health care event (such as a surgery or procedure) or diagnosis
- *Problems with using administrative data* for quality projects include unreliability due to coding problems; inability to determine timing of diagnosis/tests/follow-up; no test results, and there is no information unless there are encounters documented in the system. Many types of encounters are not typically documented in capitated environments; therefore, this type of data is not always usable unless the patient is in an indemnity-type plan.

Clinical Data (*i.e.,* Medical Records)

- Offer the most complete source of data for information on diagnoses, treatment, medications, surgeries, clinical outcomes of care, or test results
- *Problem with using clinical data:* When there are multiple providers, tracking of clinical data is difficult. Even something as simple as whether a mammogram was completed is difficult to ascertain if the patient can self-refer to an OB-GYN, who orders the test, and the results are not sent to the PCP. Ophthalmic examinations pose the same problem, as do all other "specialty" referrals.

Patient Survey Data

- Assess knowledge, preferences, perceptions, attitudes, receipt of services, and behavior; survey data are considered the gold standard for "patient satisfaction" scores.
- *Problems with using survey data* include the potential for bias, costs associated with and time needed for collection and analyzing the results.

DATA ANALYSIS

Analyzing data is a skill many case managers have had little practice in. Data must first be accurately analyzed before they can be translated into meaningful conclusions. Consider putting a data analyst and an information systems specialist on the project planning team, especially for this assessment domain, and when deciding on the quality indicators. It will save countless headaches at the back end. Right up front, these professionals will be able to assess whether the case management data collection plans are feasible, whether the quality indicators will elicit the information desired, and whether the current information systems can support the project. Data provided by case managers will be analyzed and summarized to detect trends and draw conclusions about case management performance and value to customers. Good analysis methods are statistically sound, easy to understand, reproducible, and focus on providing information of relevance to customers' decision making. This domain should describe methods used for data analysis, including data aggregation techniques and statistical tests (CMSA, 1998).

What Are the Known Risks of Applying/Withholding the Intervention?

Depending on the design chosen for the study, the quality indicators used, the processes applied or withheld, or the outcomes hypothesized, the project team should spend some thoughtful consideration to assess whether there are any known risks or ethical issues inherent in the project. Some prudent questions to ask may include:

- Will resistance be encountered? Are there financial risks, clinical risks, autonomy risks? Can they be reduced or eliminated? If not, are they acceptable?
- Will the success of the intervention have negative ramifications for other health care issues? For example, if a recommended medication must be prescribed as brand name only, but a plan's pharmacy benefit will cover only a generic known to perform inferiorly, will the ultimate outcome require extra testing, threaten medical stability, or otherwise inconvenience or endanger the health of patients?
- Are there potential confidentiality issues? Ask what is going to be done with the information? Who will see the information? Is the patient data assured confidentiality?
- If the study design calls for a control group, will administration, payors, or patients potentially be harmed by withholding the intervention?
- Other questions specific to the project planned

Draft a Communication Strategy

As in every phase of case management, communication is germane to good outcomes. During project planning and assessment, communication is essential to gather accurate information. During the actual project, good communication is necessary to keep all important contacts up-to-date. Success requires inter-organizational communication strategies, and, depending on the customers or partners involved in the project, intra-organizational communication strategies. Do not forget to include the patients/beneficiaries or other pertinent people in the outlined communication strategies.

Another important phase that requires a communication strategy is for dissemination of data and results to everyone who participated in the project, to those impacted by the project, and to others interested in gathering a library of case management outcomes projects, studies, and results. Data results are often the impetus for change—and therefore, ultimately improve outcomes. However, for this to occur, dissemination of the results needs to occur. Data are a powerful force for change in the health care arena. Data comparing health plans or physicians have changed more behavior than nearly any other "change" method; no one wants to be "last."

Data alone will not draw one's attention. How the data are presented will make the difference in whether the message is "heard." Reports for dissemination of project results can be written or presented formally. Present the data to the appropriate audience in clear, simple, accurate terms. Well-designed reports summarize the dimensions of accountability, state the rationale for their selection and importance, and incorporate essential information for interpretation of the results, including methods used for data collection and analysis. Formats used to display case management outcomes should be selected for their simplicity, clarity, and ability to illuminate what is meaningful in the data (CCMA, 1998). Consider using some of the CQI tools for process improvement (Chapter 7); this is a succinct method to share information, and very useful when presenting to a "visual" audience.

Take the data one step further, and offer suggestions on how these data can be used as the impetus for a further quality improvement initiative. Case managers have yet another opportunity to be leaders.

PRESENTING THE DATA

When presenting data to a group, consider the following:

- Begin with an overview of the project. Whenever possible, include the target of the presentation in the overview to involve the audience in a personal manner.
- Visuals are a good idea, because they keep everyone on the same idea. Keep them clear and simple. Provide handouts of the visuals and other pertinent information.

- If the audience is administratively represented, keep the presentation strategically based and statistically credible; if the audience is clinical, details on the clinical aspects of the quality indicators may be more meaningful.
- Considering the above point, assure that you have the appropriate people presenting, who can relate to the audience and answer questions accurately. In different situations, this may include physicians, data personnel, pharmacists, case managers, nurses, or biostatisticians. Make sure each person who is represented has a specific role.
- Include individual data and comparative feedback. Everyone wants to see their own data; and everyone wants to know where they rate within the group being studied. Code the comparative feedback data by number or letter to ensure confidentiality.
- Discuss the implications of the results. This is the bottom line. As "experts," the audience will likely want to know your thoughts on the outcomes. They will also draw their own conclusions.
- Allow a question-and-answer period. However, be aware that at times, this may become a "gripe session" about the lack of accurate data abstraction, statistical power, or validity of the data. It is wise to hear them out; it is also good strategy to plan answers to potential disagreements before the meeting.
- When organizations have done well in the study, find out what they did "right." This is where the information for future improvement is obtained. Let them "brag" until they are finished; then wait about 10 more seconds, when oftentimes the best information is revealed.
- Lastly, and perhaps most importantly, keep it brief and succinct.

SEQUENCING THE STEPS IN AN IMPROVEMENT PROJECT

Project planning and assessment is now complete. The remaining project steps listed earlier include:

1. Baseline measurement
2. Initiation of case management interventions
3. Early interim measurement to assess success of interventions
4. Remeasurement
5. Evaluation

Many of these tasks require data collection and analysis activities, which are distinct from, yet interconnected with, other project tasks. Data collection and analysis tasks are part of baseline measurement, interim measurement, and remeasurement activities. Other project activities include the planning and assessment tasks, the implementation of the case management interventions, and the critical evaluation component. A discussion of the five steps will demonstrate how they interrelate:

I. Baseline Measurement

The case management organization or department has identified opportunities to effect measurable improvement. For the case management organization to know whether an improvement has occurred, a baseline measurement of the quality indicator(s) must be verified and documented before the initiation of any new case management interventions. Baseline data is a critical measurement that determines how well the case management department is performing in the chosen area. Remeasurement, Stage IV, will determine how the newly initiated case management interventions affected the process: did the process/outcome improve, deteriorate, or remain constant? This is the bottom-line method for case management to "prove its worth."

II. Initiation of Case Management Interventions

Interventions are at the heart of any project, just as they are the essential component of case management. Interventions are what a case manager *does*; they are "actions intended to have an effect on outcomes" (Issel, 1997, p. 133), or a catalyst to stimulate change. Some general **case management interventions,** in line with the case management process, include the following activities:

- Assessment of patient/family support/financial/psychosocial/insurance benefits
- Coordination and development of case management plans and services
- Education of patient/significant other/family
- Monitoring, reassessment, reevaluation
- Discharge planning; facilitating appropriate levels of care
- Utilization management/resource management
- Clinical activities

A case management **project** is a set of related case management activities that is designed to achieve measurable improvement in case management processes and outcomes of patient care relative to a baseline value. Improvements are achieved through **interventions** undertaken by the case manager. The target of the intervention may be health care providers, patients, other case managers, or anyone involved in the total care of the patient. If the objective of the project is to improve a case management system, then the target of the intervention may be more administratively directed. Interventions should be based on the best applicable science from various disciplines, when available, and on expert opinion or relevant prior case management experience when it is not. Given that, the relationship between outcomes and interventions is simply that outcomes are the consequences of interventions.

Two important aspects of an intervention must be considered for the intervention to be a meaningful contribution to the outcomes management process:

1. The degree to which the processes that led to these outcomes are stable and conform to scientifically based knowledge
2. What was done by the case manager that led to improved patient outcomes (AHCPR, 1995)

Linking the case management intervention to the improved patient outcome is not always a "cause-and-effect" matter. The impact interventions have on behavior in any discipline has been the subject of debate for decades. The experience of the Center for Substance Abuse Prevention (CSAP) and the National Institute for Drug Abuse (NIDA) illustrate the complexity of the issue. CSAP and NIDA have been working to find ways to change individual and community behavior for over 40 years. In the 1950s, pressure and scare tactics (e.g., "Reefer Madness") were attempted. When that did not work, they switched to information and educational tactics in the late 1960s. Still not achieving the results they wanted, they switched to self-esteem building, therapeutic interventions, and alternative programs (e.g., midnight basketball).

The latest conclusion is that different approaches work in different ways with different populations. CSAP and NIDA have a six-level model along a continuum of intensity of interventions, ranging from education to direct process intervention and change. They emphasize multi-level interventions targeting different population subgroups with customized programs. This is not unlike the trend in case management/disease management: each population group is differentiated by disease, then further defined by categories of risk. In addition, the case manager's intervention is customized to meet the needs of the individual patient. These are case management, multi-level interventions. Current case management outcomes research is directed at finding out what works best for each population. The Center for Case Management Accountability (CCMA) is leading the way:

> It is the premise of CCMA that case managers' value must be measured where they have direct influence. Measuring the intermediate outcomes will clearly establish the value of case management to the organization. It is only by identifying those interventions that are within the scope of the case manager's control, measuring and then analyzing them that the true value of case management can be demonstrated. (CMSA, 1998)

Outcomes measurement can be used to assess case management interventions in several ways:

- Outcomes can be used to assess the effectiveness of alternative case management interventions. For example, more than one case management organization/department intervenes in a specific disease; and often each organization has their unique method of intervention. Did one method improve outcomes better than the other? Does one type of educational method produce greater compliance in patients? What is the most valid (and simplest) method to monitor various case management activities?
- As case management guidelines are written, outcomes measurements can be used to evaluate the effectiveness of the case management intervention recommendations. The basic tenet of CQI is that *anything that can be done, can be done better.* Case managers are always striving to improve on current methods of patient care.
- Case management guidelines may have recommended interventions for the frequency of case management encounters (or other measures of frequency). Outcomes measurement may provide ongoing verification of the recommended frequency. At some time in the future, case management encounters may be monitored, just as case managers monitor the number of home health visits.

FEASIBILITY OF THE PROJECT

The concept of **feasibility** is critical to consider in all aspects of an outcome management project, and especially when focusing on interventions. An intervention is feasible when it is capable of being put in effect, or being accomplished. Conversely, an intervention is not feasible if the barriers are too great to overcome, or require more resources than can be compiled. This takes careful assessment—a skill that is no stranger to case managers. Case managers have always assessed what is a feasible intervention for their patients, given the available financial, spiritual, social, and insurance support. If there is not considerable control over variables in the case or the project, it is probably not feasible. Some variables to assess include:

- *Resources:* Depending on the outcome indicators, resource needs could range from insurance benefits available to information systems. For example, if complex data collection is necessary to carry out the project and the computer system available is incapable of the sophistication needed, the organization must make a decision: can it afford to upgrade the equipment, or must the organization set its sights on other improvement efforts? It is feasible if it is in budget; it is not feasible if the expense cannot be met.

- *The potential for change:* As in compliance issues in case management, the behavioral component must be assessed in projects as well. What are the environmental factors that cause a specific behavior (that you want modified)? What is the potential for modifying the behavior(s)? Can the environmental factors be impacted? Is there control over the necessary variables (reimbursement/benefits limitations, for example)? Why is the behavior at the current level? Is it due to:
  — *Functional limitations*—people, organizations, lack of skill lack or knowledge
  — *Resource limitations*—time, money, staff, family support
  — *Environmental issues*—the system rewards this behavior
- *Check potential barriers to success and challenges:* The potential challenges are numerous. It is wise to know what may occur, before the problem rears its ugly head. As in the case management process, plan for problems and detours. Some potential barriers include:
  a. During accreditation time, human resources and timeframes are tight
  b. Identification of "turf" issues and addressing them ahead of time
  c. Identification of intervention criteria and assessing barriers in the criteria
  d. Identification of how to get baseline data, and whether remeasurement data are available post-intervention
  e. Identification of project-specific/facility-specific/behavior-specific barriers
  f. Identification of how to demonstrate measurable impact of the intervention

Interventions that are *feasible* have a higher chance of success. Ingredients for success include interventions that:

- *Are based in science.* For example, if the case management organization/department wants to obtain evidence that case management can improve HbA1c results in diabetic patients, there is scientific evidence that demonstrates that this goal is worthy of pursuit (*i.e.,* higher HbA1c results can lead to conditions such as blindness, cardiovascular complications, increased amputation rates)
- *Are appropriate to the population or target audience.* A high-risk pregnancy disease management program will not significantly affect a population that is predominately older than 50 years. Diabetes clinics will not be used if the patients cannot get to the facility because of rural surroundings and poor transportation support.

- *Are cost-effective.* The cost of the intervention should not outweigh the benefits likely to result from the intervention. Existing resources (case managers, expert knowledge, information systems) can be used effectively.
- *Support a national priority (e.g.,* CCMA);
- *Contain well-planned evaluation components:* The components should enable evaluation of the intervention's impact, identify areas for improving the intervention, and facilitate the sustainability of the improvement elicited by the intervention.
- *Have a plan for sustaining the improvement:* This is as important as planning the initial intervention. In CQI terminology, it is called "holding the gains." Case managers want educational efforts to have long-lasting compliance in our patients; we give patients the tools and the knowledge—to build their capacity—to sustain the health improvements made during our case management efforts. We want them to be as independent as possible. The same is true for projects. Once case managers have improved an outcome, the goal is to sustain the improvement. Interventions should be planned so that the impact of the targeted change will be sustained. In projects, as in case management, this may take educational and monitoring efforts—until the behavior (of the target of the intervention) becomes second nature. The short-term focus is that the intervention produces positive changes; the major goal and long-term focus is the transferring of the skills to teach the community, patient, or organization to continue the positive changes.

When initiating the case management interventions chosen for the project, it is recommended that a small pilot test on a target population be done before pulling out all stops and doing a full-scale project. Perform a small interim measurement on the quality indicators. If the intervention is not successful, or partially successful, changes made on a small scale are much less difficult to correct than once a large number of systems and people are involved. If the pilot project is successful, then enlarge the project; if the enlarged project is successful, implement the case management intervention(s) into standardized practice (see PDCA Cycle, CQI chapters for more details).

III. Early Interim Measurement to Assess Success of Interventions

After the chosen case management interventions have been in place a short time (although long enough to have impacted on the quality indicators), collect a small sample of data to test whether the interventions are causing a change in the desired direction. The interim measurement may demonstrate that:

1. The interventions created a positive impact on the outcomes; the interim measurement demonstrated improvement over the baseline data.
2. The interventions did not create any impact on the outcomes; the interim measurement data remained the same as in the baseline data.
3. The interventions created a negative impact on the outcomes; the interim measurement demonstrated that the interventions made things worse!

If the interventions demonstrated that improvement was occurring, continue the case management interventions. If the interventions did not create any impact on the outcomes, it may be that the intervention did not yet have time to affect the quality indicators; or it may be a weak or inappropriate intervention that is not a precise match capable of affecting the desired change. If the interventions created a negative impact on the outcomes, reevaluate the project, the quality indicators, and the interventions. Examine where the problems may be. Identify possible causes for the problems. Use the PDCA Cycle to guide you through the process.

IV. Remeasurement of Baseline Data

For outcomes to be meaningful, they must be measured and compared against another set of data. A comparison can be accomplished by collecting data on two or more case management organizations, hospitals, home health agencies, skilled nursing facilities, processes, etc. These data can be compared but will simply show how well peer groups are rating during a specific point in time. A second method of comparison that can be made is by collecting data twice from the same organization over a span of time. However, this will not be particularly meaningful unless there is a reason to collect data twice, that is, a change has occurred such as a new case management intervention. By collecting baseline data, initiating case management interventions, then collecting remeasurement data, the case management organization can compare the two (baseline and remeasurement data) to assess the impact the case management intervention had on the process or system. Once measured, the outcomes may demonstrate that case management interventions caused improvement, deterioration, or had no effect. In the Evaluation stage, the organization must decide the reasons for the change (or lack of change), and what to do next.

A basic principle in outcomes management is that *uniform collection of data is critical.* The same quality indicators and data abstraction tools must be used for measuring baseline data and remeasurement data, whether the data compare the same organization over two time periods, or comparing several organizations. This can be difficult, especially with the variation in case management practice patterns and a lack of common information systems. To vary from the details of the study will yield results that cannot be compared; therefore, the data collection methods must take these challenges into consideration.

V. Evaluation

Evaluating what was done well, or what could be improved, is a critical stage of an improvement project. CQI studies have demonstrated that many organizations neglect the evaluation stage. To measure a process, and not evaluate the process for potential improvement, is an incomplete project. To evaluate a process for opportunities for improvement, and then do nothing, is a serious waste of effort and resources.

By evaluating the reasons behind poor outcomes, sometimes organizations may find other hidden opportunities for improving processes. Earlier in the section, such factors as variation, validity, reliability, and interrater reliability were discussed as having an important impact on the data collection results. However, during evaluation, investigate further for less obvious reasons for poor compliance. For example, information in the medical records may simply be inaccurate: wrong procedural codes used, wrong primary or secondary diagnosis coded, wrong information documented on a patient's chart, information documented on the wrong chart, or any type of documentation error.

Another common occurrence in data collection is that abstractors may not find the necessary data in the chart. This could be because of incomplete or inaccurate documentation, or because abstractors had not been provided with the necessary portion of the patients' medical records. When abstracting data on mammography, one insurance company appeared to have low mammography rates. The medical records used for data abstraction came from PCPs' offices. However, a new benefit rule allowed women to self-refer to OB/GYN physicians, where a large number of mammography reports were found. After review of both the PCP and OB/GYN medical records, the mammography compliance rate significantly improved. Another opportunity for improvement was also discovered: that of increasing the rates that OB/GYN reports reach the patient's record in their PCP's office.

A second example of the abstractors lacking proper documentation occurred when the data collection included a quality indicator monitoring smoking cessation advice in acute myocardial infarction patients in the hospital setting. Although this may be discussed during the admission, it was rarely documented in the main patient record, lowering compliance rates in many hospitals. However, most hospitals had documented the smoking cessation advice in the cardiac rehabilitation portion of the patient's medical record; this portion of the chart did not get copied, and therefore the abstractors could not show compliance in this quality indicator.

This problem could be overcome in several ways. Next time the project was being remeasured, the organization could plan, in advance, what section of the patient's medical record would yield the information being collected. Or the organization could have quality improvement personnel or cardiac case managers modify or develop a discharge checksheet that would include all quality indicators being measured. This is especially useful advice with the many national HCFA (Health Care Financing Administration) projects commencing in 1999; know the quality indicators that will be measured, and take appropriate measures to assure your organization receives optimal credit for its performance.

The evaluation stage of an improvement project is actually another "planning and assessment" phase and includes several important considerations:

1. *Evaluation of the impact of case management interventions.* This is accomplished though assessing and analyzing the remeasurement data. Compare the baseline data with the remeasurement data. Next, study the results of the current project with the intent of discovering methods to improve current processes.

2. *An assessment of lessons learned.* Ask yourself, "If your organization was going to do another outcomes project, what would you do differently this time?" What aspects of the project would you keep? What were barriers encountered? Can the barriers be overcome? How? Do the quality indicators need to be modified? In a CQI environment, the lessons learned in the course of any project can be applied to improve the planning and implementation of subsequent projects involving the same or similar objective, populations, or interventions.

3. *Plan methods to improve processes based on lessons learned.* This may encompass either significant changes, or small but essential changes in a process. In essence, this is recycling the improvement process, and is discussed in detail in the section on the PDCA Cycle.

4. *Plan for sustaining improvement.* This is an important component of the improvement process. Often, improvement occurs when attention is brought to a process. This attention can be the result of a national project requiring good compliance rates, an imminent accreditation survey, or an adverse occurrence that needed immediate attention. However, once the pressure is off, it is not uncommon for the improvement gains to go down the slippery slope of deterioration.

Maintaining the improvements achieved involves careful consideration of all systems impacted by the change. Case managers are familiar with patient compliance issues; what is the best method to keep patients independent and compliant in their treatment? The same issues need consideration in improvement projects. The checksheets and new behaviors will be replaced with other, more pressing issues unless a collaborative plan is organized. When the JCAHO or HEDIS accreditation is over, or the HCFA improvement project has completed the remeasurement phase and your organization has done well, or the fear of making headlines for poor care has passed, what can be done to build capacity, or independence, in those who changed behavior to improve performance? Those who planned the improvement project in the first place also must plan for exiting the project, comfortable that the birds they are pushing out of the nest can fly.

5. *Dissemination of the results and future plans of the project.* The organization has already drafted a communication strategy during the initial planning stage. Now it is time to share the results with others. Administration will want to know what has been accomplished with the resources that were used. Internal and external customers that are impacted will also be interested in the results. Consider publishing an article on the project; include lessons learned so others may build on your knowledge base and not have to "re-invent the wheel."

   When several similar groups have all participated in an improvement project, a particularly convincing method of disseminating data is called "*comparative feedback.*" Some experts believe that *measurement without comparison is meaningless.* "Comparative feedback" is the ticket that enables any collaborator who participated in the improvement project to compare his or her data with those of another collaborator, on any (or all) quality indicators measured. One large insurance plan, realizing that physicians are a competitive group, routinely collects data on their physicians and sends them letters such as, "Dear Dr. Jones, Your diabetic patients have an average HbA1c of 9.5. Your peers average 8.0." There are no instructions given; only the data information. But these letters have impacted the care to diabetic patients.

   After the data are analyzed, a table can be developed, listing all those who participated in the project: case management organizations, providers, facilities, or any comparable group of collaborators. Instead of actual names of organizations or facilities, use letters or numbers as a code to ensure confidentiality among the group. Next, list the quality indicators that were measured for each collaborator. (See sample Comparative Feedback Tables on Pneumonia [Table 5–1] and Diabetes [Table 5–2].) This is a proven powerful tool, because the comparison displays how well one group is performing in contrast to their peers.

TABLE 5-1 Pneumonia Project Comparative Data: Percentage of Quality Indicators and Mean Antibiotic Time by Hospital at Baseline

HOSPITAL	ANTIBIOTIC RECEIVED WITHIN 4 HOURS OF PRESENTATION*	MEAN TIME TO 1ST ANTIBIOTIC	SPUTUM GRAM STAIN PERFORMED	SPUTUM CULTURE PERFORMED	BLOOD CULTURE PERFORMED	PNEUMOCOCCAL VACCINE DOCUMENTED	INFLUENZA VACCINE DOCUMENTED
A	48.2	5.7	51.2	51.2	79.1	2.3	0.0†
B	43.9	6.9	40.5	40.5	59.5	2.4	9.5
C	29.6	11.2	48.8	46.5	62.8	4.6	4.6
D	52.2	8.0	59.6	59.6	68.1	8.5	4.3
E	37.1	6.6	60.5	60.5	65.1	9.3	4.6
F	51.2	8.3	51.0	51.0	71.4	44.9†	51.0†
G	35.8	8.8	55.1	53.1	75.5	4.1	4.1
H	46.8	5.1	48.9	48.9	78.7	6.4	4.3
I	52.0	7.0	39.6	41.2	66.7	4.2	0.0†
Total	43.0	7.5	50.6	50.4	69.8	9.9	9.5
Benchmark	72.1	4.0	51.6	71.1	70.3	60.0	60.0

*Eleven cases were excluded because of missing admission, emergency room, or antibiotic administration time.
†Significantly different from aggregate at baseline.

120

REVIEW OF BASIC OUTCOMES MANAGEMENT PRINCIPLES

- *Outcomes* are simply results, or endpoints; a *process* is the intervention taken to achieve the outcome; *accountability* is being responsible.
- Outcomes must be measurable, credible, and feasible.
- Collect data on large numbers to be statistically significant. This is one reason to combine strategies as a case management group. Smaller numbers may reflect rare outcomes, rather than common outcomes.
- Collect data using a uniform method. Use the same data collection tools. Assure that the data collection is performed accurately and consistently.
- Clearly define what is being measured. Assure that all those who contribute to the database are using the same *operational definition*. For example, the definition of a patient's condition, or level of medical complexity, must be consistent when collecting data. This is another priority for case managers to define as a group. For example: What characteristics constitute a low-/moderate-/high-priority congestive heart failure case?
- Risk adjustment and risk factors must be addressed consistently and in relationship to the outcomes being measured; risk factors for congestive heart failure are different from risk factors for a mortality outcome measurement.
- Start small. New outcome programs should choose one or two outcomes to measure.
- Start with something objective and well-defined; the more concrete the outcome (*i.e.,* laboratory results, number of case management encounters, number of patients on a case management roster), the easier it is to prove. Cost savings are easier to prove than quality of life changes.
- Sophisticated information systems can ease the burden of data collection. However, when comparing your case management outcomes with others, unless the same system is used, the comparison may be inaccurate.
- When possible, identify resources that are already "tried and true"—for example, when available, use indicators that are already written, validated, and found reliable, rather than starting from scratch. If it is necessary to tweak the indicator to match your organization's requirements, have an expert determine whether the "tweaking" will change the validity or reliability of the instrument.
- By reducing unintended variation, resources are more effectively managed, and quality can be improved.
- As in case management, outcomes management can be fun.

TABLE 5-2 Diabetes Project Comparative Data

QUALITY INDICATOR	1996 MEDICARE B/R	1996 MEDICAID BASELINE	1998 BENCH-MARKS	COLLAB-ORATOR A*	COLLAB-ORATOR B*
Process Quality Indicators					
Blood pressure quarterly	42/41	41.0	**64.0**	34.50	32.11
Hemoglobin A1c (HbA1c) twice a year	33/47	31.0	**59.0**	56.88	59.06
Foot examination twice a year	17/27	32.0	**53.0**	50.47	25.03
Retinal examination yearly	51/54	59.0		39.26	25.37
Lipid profile annually	51/47	35.0	**60.0**	60.58	59.91
Proteinuria dipstick annually	57/64	65.0		47.57	37.71
All process indicators				48.15	38.75
Diabetes Education Quality Indicators					
Diet	48/62	74.0		65.68	69.29
Exercise	18/43	83.0	**53.0**	55.28	35.77
Medication	35/66	42.0		77.40	81.80
Self-monitoring blood glucose	18/55	58.0	**72.0**	72.38	81.65
All education indicators				67.68	65.05
Outcome Quality Indicators					
ACE inhibitor if hypertensive	35/53	56.0	**57.0**	68.85	64.00
ACE inhibitor if proteinuria	35/58	47.0		72.00	68.23
Treatment if hyperlipemic	16/43	65.0	**52.0**	62.54	53.38
Ophthalmologic referral if abnormal retinal examination	73/99	95.0		100.00	100.00
Microalbuminuria strip testing if routine dipstick negative				16.56	59.33
All follow-up indicators				61.90	63.40
Measurement Quality Indicator					
HbA1c < 8.0			**71.37**	79.55	72.19
All 16 Indicators				**58.26**	**52.57**

NOTE. All values are in percentages.

(continued)

CAUTIONS AND CONCLUSIONS

Case managers have practiced the skill of "maintaining balance" in so many ways that not becoming overly absorbed by outcomes management should be a "given." In an effort to show both sides, this section ends with some cautions about outcomes management. Outcomes management topics such as the dark side of risk adjustment, stress on providers, using an evolving terminology, and use of large databases are discussed.

COLLAB-ORATOR C*	COLLAB-ORATOR D*	COLLAB-ORATOR E*	COLLAB-ORATOR F*	COLLAB-ORATOR G*	COLLAB-ORATOR H*	AGGREGATE DATA COLLAB-ORATOR A–H
27.07	35.48	45.00	28.87	35.91	52.49	34.03
55.19	42.61	35.00	34.75	56.46	54.22	47.65
35.07	22.46	23.50	15.58	25.73	32.08	32.12
21.35	27.35	25.63	18.10	42.99	55.39	35.51
42.85	44.98	28.00	46.11	64.64	51.75	46.19
43.29	44.98	45.00	31.61	62.00	46.54	45.64
37.99	35.14	32.36	29.67	47.11	45.25	43.03
53.98	48.43	44.50	43.49	53.33	52.73	52.07
49.90	41.61	27.50	33.57	46.78	45.78	43.05
72.04	72.95	86.93	77.02	82.44	74.37	76.12
68.64	48.69	55.50	55.26	62.56	72.90	64.60
58.14	53.92	55.82	48.83	64.53	62.19	57.56
56.87	47.22	54.96	46.62	45.24	63.79	56.42
57.46	52.19	53.63	43.74	48.15	73.19	57.03
55.65	52.75	52.85	46.22	44.86	41.19	52.08
86.71	95.88	94.00	100.00	94.83	100.00	95.84
37.46	5.31	22.68	5.12	33.59	19.52	20.09
53.81	46.09	51.88	42.50	46.94	51.18	53.86
87.52	59.81	53.03	72.05	65.55	78.63	73.73
49.78	**44.20**	**43.00**	**39.07**	**54.57**	**54.76**	**48.71**

An Overabundance of Risk Adjustment

When the results are in, some insurers may decide that certain outcomes are not worthwhile and refuse to pay for them. Risk adjustment plays an important role here; it may be statistically proven that the odds of some patients to benefit from a procedure, surgery, or service is poor. "The negative effect of controlling for these factors through a risk-adjustment model might be to reduce a plan's incentives to target treatment to populations that might require more expensive or complex interventions" (McGlynn & Asch, 1998, p.6). For example, if return to work is predicted to be unlikely, why pay for rehabilitation? Or would insurers refuse to pay for substance abuse services if research shows this group has a poor chance to sustain benefits achieved in rehabilitation? This must be carefully watched with the new payment systems in skilled nursing facilities and home health agencies as well. Will certain "risk-adjusted" patients be denied admission? In some post-acute levels of care, it could turn out that the healthiest and sickest may be most acceptable; the healthiest, because care can be provided within the financial limits allowed; and the sickest, because financial incentives allow extra dollars for the "outliers." The middle-risk patients could actually be considered the fiscally undesirable ones.

Provider Stress

Studies that measure outcomes have created additional stress on providers. Not only are providers operating under increasing levels of financial risk, but they are often having to please multiple health plans and regulatory agencies. Rather than using a single set of disease guidelines or looking at a common set of quality indicators, they are often required to adapt patient care to multiple taskmasters. HbA1c levels must be drawn annually for one requirement; they must be addressed two or four times annually to satisfy other requirements. This also happens at the insurance company level. A study recommends mammograms every 2 years; another project recommends mammograms every year; this is further complicated by the fact that each may have different age ranges or insurance coverage requirements included in the measures. And the need to obtain rapid answers puts additional pressures on many organizations. Accreditation requirements, national projects with tight timeframes, and limited staff resources all pool to create a dilemma. Do organizations conduct studies with sound methodology, or do they work rapidly, under pressure to quickly change processes in the hopes it will change outcomes?

Evolving Terminology

Terminology in the outcomes management field is still poorly defined. Words such as *performance outcomes, performance measures, clinical indicators, quality indicators, outcome measures,* or *outcome indicators* are still used interchangeably. Even "quality" means different things to different people. In CQI, a basic principle states that *operational definitions* must be clear. Poorly defined operational definitions is one of the major barriers to success. This tenet has proved true in the health care field, when recurring problems occur because of poor definitions; consider definitions such as "medically necessary," "homebound," or "preventive treatment." With the ongoing acceptance of the CQI philosophy, it is hoped that clear operational definitions will be treated as a priority in health care and outcomes management.

Large Database Cautions

The use of large databases poses many reservations, from confidentiality to lack of accurate data. One concern for case managers is that human individuality can be lost. *As patient advocates, case managers may find new challenges, knowing that within any large population's data are individuals who can beat the odds.* This may be our most important asset that case managers bring to the outcomes table: the role of patient advocate. Just as case management's "bottom line" is the patient, so must be the efforts of outcomes management. Strive to improve the quality of life in our patients, first, and work to allay costs as a secondary incentive. It has been said many times that quality care is cost-effective care. Like case management, outcomes management is a dynamic process. Be clear on goals and objectives; obtain reliable data to make accurate conclusions; and use the information to continuously improve case management services and processes.

PART II: REFERENCES, RESOURCES, AND BIBLIOGRAPHY

Agency for Health Care Policy and Research (AHCPR). (1995). *Using clinical practice guidelines to evaluate quality of care: Vol. 1. Issues.* AHCPR Pub. No. 95-0045. Rockville, MD: Author.

Agency for Health Care Policy and Research (AHCPR). (1995). *Using clinical practice guidelines to evaluate quality of care: Vol. 2. Methods.* AHCPR Pub. No. 95-0046. Rockville, MD: AHCPR.

American College of Emergency Physicians (ACEP). (1998). Quality of care and the outcomes management movement. Retrieved 1997 from the World Wide Web: http://www.acep.org/POLICY/QUALCARE.HTM.

Barry, M. (1996). Searching for the definition of outcomes in subacute care. *Continuing Care, 15*(9), 14–17.

Bayer Quality Network. (1997). *Sharing success in CQI, 1*(4), 1–15.

Blackwell, S. (1997). Measuring clinical outcomes spells success. *Continuing Care, 1*(16), 18–23.

Braunling-McMorrow, D., & Fralish, K. (1995). Theoretical, ethical, and practical issues in outcomes assessment of acquired brain injury rehabilitation. *The Journal of Care Management, 1*(1), 56–63.

Camp, R., & Tweet, A. (1994). Benchmarking applied to health care. *Journal of Quality Improvement, 5*(20), 229–238.

Campbell, A. (1994). Benchmarking: a performance intervention tool. *Journal of Quality Improvement, 5*(20), 225–228.

Case Management Society of America (CMSA). (1998). Center for case management accountability (CCMA). Retrieved 1998 from the World Wide Web: www.cmsa.org.

Carneal, G. (1998). In search of quality and customer service in managed care. *Continuing Care, 17*(9), 20, 34–35.

Center for Health Systems Research and Analysis (CHSRA). (1998). Methodological issues in using QIs. Retrieved 1998 from the World Wide Web: hsra.wisc.edu.

Center for Health Systems Research and Analysis. (1998). Quality indicators versus quality measures. Retrieved 1998 from www.chsra.wisc.edu.

COR Healthcare Resources (1997). Medical management network: Strategic tools for implementing evidence-based care. *5*(9), 1–18.

Davies, A., Doyle, M., Lansky, D., Rutt, W., Stevic, M., & Doyle, J. (1994). Outcomes assessment in clinical settings: A consensus statement on principles and best practices in project management. *Joint Commission Journal of Quality Improvement, 20*(6).

Ellwood, P. (1988). Shattuck Lecture. Outcomes management: A technology of patient experience. *New England Journal of Medicine, 318*:1549–1556.

Epstein, R. & Sherwood, L. (1994). From outcomes research to disease management: A guide for the perplexed. *Annals of Internal Medicine, 124*(9), 832–837.

Goldfield, N., Pine, M., & Pine, J. (1993). *Measuring and managing health care quality: Procedures, techniques, and protocols.* Gaithersburg: Aspen Publishers.

Gosfield, A. (1997). Guidelines in case management. *The Case Manager, 8*(3), 103–108.

Hughes, D. (1997). *Decision support systems and their impact on the performance improvement function.* National Association for Healthcare Quality; Special Report from the 22nd Annual Educational Conference, September 1997, pp. 8–9.

Issel, L. (1997). Measuring comprehensive case management interventions: development of a tool. *Nursing Case Management, 4*(2), 132–138.

Joint Commission on Accreditation of Healthcare Organizations (JCAHO). (1989, November). Characteristics of clinical indicators. *QRB,* pp. 330–339.

Joint Commission on Accreditation of Healthcare Organizations (JCAHO). (1998). Nation's three leading health care quality oversight bodies to coordinate measurement activities. Retrieved 1998 from the World Wide Web: http://www.jcaho.org/news/nb137.htm.

Jennings, B., & Staggers, N. (1997). The hazards in outcomes management. *The Journal of Outcomes Management, 1*(4), 18–23.

Kiefe, C., Thomas, Woolley, T., Allison, J., Box, J., & Craig, A. (1994). Determining benchmarks: A data-driven search for the best achievable performance. *Clinical Performance and Quality Health Care, 4*(2), 190–194.

Kiefe, C., Weissman, N., Farmer, R., Weaver, M., Allison, J., & Williams, O. (1998, October). Measuring quality by achievable benchmarks of care (ABC). *UQHC, 14*(5).

Kopin, L. (1997). An integral part of comprehensive cardiac care. *Case Review, 3*(3), 30–32.

Kongstvedt, P.R. (1993). *The Managed Health Care Handbook.* Gaithersburg, MD: Aspen Publishers.

Kozma, C. (1997). Process versus outcomes: What is acceptable evidence of success in developing disease state management programs? *Medical Interface, 10*(1), 75–76.

Kozma, C. (1996). Evaluating disease state management interventions. *Medical Interface, 9*(6), 110–111.

Lamb, G., Donaldson, N., & Kellogg, J. (1998). *Case management: A guide to strategic evaluation.* St. Louis: Mosby.

Mateo, M., Matzke, K., & Newton, C. (1998). Designing measurements to assess case management outcomes. *Nursing Case Management, 1*(3), 2–6.

McGlynn, E., & Asch, S. (1998). Developing a clinical performance measure. *American Journal of Preventive Medicine, 14*(3), 14–21.

McLaughlin, C., & Kaluzny, A. (1994). *Continuous quality improvement in health care.* Gaithersburg, MD: Aspen Publishers.

Med Group. (1997, Fall). Outcomes assessment easier said than done. *Respiratory Review, 14,* p. 1.

Rieve, J. (1997a). Benchmarking and using outcomes data. *The Case Manager, 4*(8), 55–61.

Rieve, J. (1997b). Outcomes: the quality connection. *The Case Manager, 5*(8), 44–47.

Rieve, J. (1997c). Quality management tools: part I. *The Case Manager, 6*(8), 38–41.

Rieve, J. (1997d). Quality management tools: part II. *The Case Manager, 1*(9), 22–24.

Rosenstein, A. (1997, Nov/Dec). Outcomes management: Opportunities and objectives. *Health Care Innovations, 1997.*

Schecter, S. (1995, April/May/June). Case management outcomes: Report on the case management outcomes workshop. *The Case Manager,* pp. 48–52.

Sierra Health Foundation. (1998). *The managed health care improvement task force report.* Sacramento: Sierra Health Foundation.

Spath, P. (1997, May). Revamp data sources for measuring performance. *Hospital Peer Review,* pp. 67–70.

Sousa, J. (1997). Patient satisfaction and outcomes. *Case Review, 3*(2), 57–59.

Stewart, M. (1995). Development of disease-specific outcomes instruments. Retrieved 1998 from the World Wide Web: http://utsph.sph.uth.tmc.edu/www/utsph/CS/hmwk4.htm.

Todd, W., & Nash, D., Eds. (1997). *Disease management: A systems approach to improving patient outcomes.* Chicago: American Hospital Publishing, Inc.

Williams, D. (1998). Demonstrating the benefits of case management. *Nursing Case Management, 4*(3), 139.

Wojner, A. (1997). From case management to outcomes management. *The Case Manager 2*(8), 77–82.

Resources

Note: Entire books have been written on Internet resources for healthcare. They may be useful for outcomes research. This is a small, but important, sample of literature.

- Some Evidenced-Based Sources of Indicators:
  — CONQUEST—sponsored by AHCPR
  — Cochrane Collaboration
  — NIH Consensus Conferences
  — Computerized Databases
    – MEDLAR
    – Physician Data Query
    – American College of Physicians
  — USPSTF
  — Professional Association Guidelines

- Clinical outcomes Research Center—to expand the academic field of outcomes research through national activities. www.hsr.umn.edu/corc.html

- Medical Outcomes Trust
  SF-36 copyright held by Medical Outcomes Trust
  (617) 426-4046
  www.outcomestrust.org

- Health Institute at the New England Medical Center (SF 36)
  http://www.sf-36.com
  Contains on-line health status information

- NCQA Guidelines
  http://www.ncqa.org

- AHCPR
  http://www.ahcpr.gov

PART II: STUDY QUESTIONS

1. How will the additional responsibilities of being an "outcomes manager" affect your job description?
2. List important reasons for adding this role to your job description.
3. Prioritize six quality indicators that relate to the disease management diagnoses determined during study questions in Part I (two for each diagnosis).
4. Are any of the quality indicators process indicators? Are any of the type quality indicators–outcome indicators? Include both types of quality indicators in your list.
5. Develop the quality indicators in numerator/denominator format.
6. Plan and design a quality improvement project, using the steps in the text. Use the quality indicators as measures of success.
7. Do the quality improvement project in your organization on a small scale.

Continuous Quality Improvement (CQI) and Case Management

"It isn't that they can't see the solution.

It is that they can't see the problem."

G. K. CHESTERTON

PART III: IMPORTANT TERMS AND CONCEPTS

Bar Chart
Brainstorming
Cause-and-Effect Diagram
CASE© PDCA
Common Cause
Consensus
Continuous Quality Improvement
    (CQI)
Control Chart
CQI Tools for Process Improvement
Data Box
Defining Stage
Deming's "Fourteen Points"
Discussion Stages
Edward Deming
Exploratory Stage
Facilitator
Fishbone Diagram
Flowchart
Force Field Analysis
Ishikawa Diagram
Joseph Juran
"Just in Time (JIT)" Training
Lower Control Limits (LCL)
Multidisciplinary Patient Care Team
Multivoting
Negative Correlation
Nominal Group Technique
Outlier
Pareto Diagram

PDCA Cycle
Performance Improvement Team
Pie Chart
Positive Correlation
Problem Statement
Process Flow Diagrams
Process Improvement Team (PIT)
Project Team
Quality Action Team (QAT)
Quality Advisor
Quality Council
Quality Improvement Projects
Quality Improvement Team (QIT)
Root Cause Analysis
Run Chart
Scatter Diagram
Sentinel Event
Special Cause
Stages of Team Development
Statistical Process Control Chart (SPCC)
Steering Teams
Shewhart Cycle
Stephen Covey
Trend Chart
Upper Control Limits (UCL)
Variation

CHAPTER 6

Overview of Continuous Quality Improvement (CQI)

INTRODUCTION TO CONTINUOUS QUALITY IMPROVEMENT (CQI)

Case managers have always played a prominent role in reducing health care costs. Now that the relationship between cost and quality of care is being closely examined, case managers—if they are to retain their credibility—must meet the challenge of participating in the Quality Revolution. This mandates understanding the relationship between continuous quality improvement (CQI) tools and techniques, outcomes, and processes. Case managers have been instrumental in the creation and utilization of critical/clinical pathways, protocols, guidelines, and other interventions to improve health care quality. The next step, as leaders, is to self-evaluate our profession using statistically valid methods. CQI tools and techniques are used to analyze and assess the impact of case and disease management processes, pathways, and protocols; this is how we can "prove our worth" in a language business people and CEOs understand.

In the Outcomes Management chapters, quality improvement projects were discussed, and their processes of development and performance were detailed. The CQI chapters contribute adjunctive tools to aid the case manager in evaluating, organizing, and presenting the outcomes. For example, in the chapter on Quality Improvement Projects, several pages were dedicated to the planning and assessment required before starting a project. In CQI fashion, an acronym, **CASE PDCA,** has been provided as a tool to build the quality improvement process. The "CASE" portion will walk the case manager through the extensive planning phase, using a familiar word as a reminder system.

Continuous Quality Improvement (CQI) is a cyclical process, thus the word *continuous.* And the foundational problem-solving method, the PDCA Cycle, is also cyclical. CQI is a process that continuously and cyclically seeks to improve performance to enhance quality, efficiency, and efficacy. Case management is, itself, a continuous process. Except in managing conditions such as high-risk pregnancy (assuming mother and baby are doing well), and especially with the "through the continuum" trend, the nature of case management is ongoing. It is even more important to have the mindset of continuous quality improvement.

CQI applies tools of process improvement and believes that if you can measure it, you can improve it. Several CQI tools and techniques will be addressed. Some present with very statistical components. The goal of this section is not to teach statistics or construction of the more advanced tools; in fact, it is recommended that a statistician or data analyst be included in any CQI team that requires more than elementary mathematics. The intent of this chapter is to aid case managers in statistical thinking, so they can participate in analyzing the processes of our profession. Donald M. Berwick, M.D., President and CEO of the Institute for Healthcare Improvement, states that, "Many clinicians and other health care leaders underestimate the great contributions that better statistical thinking could make toward reducing costs and improving outcomes." Dr. Berwick is a leader in the heath care quality improvement movement and does not believe in timidity; rather, boldness creates change. Case managers have always been bold and are major change agents; a little statistical thinking will not slow us down.

Some types of charts are easy to learn and can be valuable to case managers in many ways, such as flowcharts. Others, such as Pareto diagrams and statistical process control charts (SPCC), are more complex. Not every case manager will need to create them; but case management will benefit from accurate analysis and interpretation of them. One type of simple SPCC is an invaluable patient teaching tool for some case management applications.

Tools for process improvement are much like computer software in that, if they are not used immediately or frequently, they will be lost somewhere in the gray matter. A CQI concept called "just in time (JIT)" training has proved to be a very effective approach to using the CQI tools. In essence, "just in time" education is given to the teams when they can immediately apply it. For example, if hospital case managers need to evaluate their process for handing-off patients to home health, health maintenance organization (HMO), or skilled nursing facility (SNF) case managers, a process flowchart may be the perfect tool for this, and the perfect time to learn how to use and appreciate this tool.

The CQI Gurus

DR. W. EDWARDS DEMING

Many books and articles have been written by and about the people who laid the foundation for CQI. This overview discusses a few of the pioneers. Perhaps of all the CQI gurus that are credited with moving the quality improvement revolution to where it is today, Dr. W. Edwards Deming is the most well known. In the mid-1900s, Dr. Deming could not acquire buy-in for his ideas in Detroit. However, someone heard his "message" and assigned him to rebuild the Japanese economy after World War II. It may well be that he is responsible for changing the perception of "it is disposable because it is made in Japan," to "the merchandise is of excellent quality because it is made in Japan." Deming's "Fourteen Points" are considered the basis for the transformation of industry. Some of them seem so fundamental today, but were eye-opening (and criticized) several decades ago. Many are meaningful in the organizations where case managers are employed. They include such Deming pearls of wisdom as (Gibbons, 1994):

- Stress the importance of continuous and well-informed on-the-job training; also encourage education and self-improvement for everyone. "What an organization needs is not just good people; it needs people that are improving with education" (Deming quote).
- Drive out fear from the workplace because "no one can put in his/her best performance unless he/she feels secure" (Deming quote).
- Cease dependence on mass inspection. In other words, once a product is poorly made or a service is poorly rendered, it is too late to do anything about its quality. Rather, change the process and do it correctly the first time. Quality does not come from inspection but from improvement of processes. Inspection is used for the purpose of monitoring quality services, not to find the "bad apple."
- Improve constantly and forever the system of production and service. Improvement is a never-ending process, not a one-time event. This is the basis of the CQI philosophy.
- Institute leadership. "The job of management is not supervision, but leadership" (Deming quote). There is a fine line, and a deep distinction, between supervision and leadership. (See Stephan Covey—CQI Guru)
- Remove barriers to pride of workmanship. Most people want to do a good job. Barriers may include lack of data, poor training, poor supplies, managers who do not care, ignoring suggestions and personal problems, and poor communication. All of these can lead to loss of motivation.
- Take action to accomplish the transformation. Teamwork is the key. Deming recommends the Shewhart Cycle (see PDCA) to guide improvement. Deming also believes the key to quality is the use of statistical data and analysis for decisions, rather than relying on hunches or experience alone.

DR. JOSEPH M. JURAN

Dr. Joseph M. Juran is also known for his work in Japan after World War II. Like Deming, much of his work was ignored in the West until after the dramatic improvements made by the Japanese were apparent. He founded the Juran Institute, where his quality philosophy is taught today. In organizations that are using CQI philosophies, many of Juran's ideas are a part of the organizational culture: quality councils, the team concept, estimating measures of performance, providing recognition to employees/teams through a reward system, and most of all, Juran's "Ten-Step Quality Improvement Process," which is used by major health care organizations (Gibbons, 1994):

1. Build awareness of the need and opportunity for improvement.
2. Set goals for improvement.
3. Organize to reach the goals (*e.g.*, establish a quality council, identify problems, select processes that need improvement, appoint teams, train facilitators and team members).
4. Provide training throughout the organization.
5. Carry out projects to solve problems.
6. Report progress.
7. Give recognition.
8. Communicate results.
9. Keep score.
10. Maintain momentum by making annual improvement part of the regular systems and processes of the company.

DR. STEPHEN R. COVEY

Dr. Stephen R. Covey is a contemporary expert in quality and leadership and is the founder of the Covey Leadership Center. He believes that systems must be managed according to universal principles; these are natural laws that cannot be broken. He also believes that managers manage things; leaders lead people. His books discuss principles of leadership. Two books by Covey that are highly recommended (and from which most of this overview is taken) are:

- *The Seven Habits of Highly Effective People*
- *First Things First*

Not too many years ago, while on the plane home from one of the Case Management Society of America's annual conferences, I realized how quickly case management has evolved. As case management matures, we are no longer merely case managers; we are case leaders. Leadership techniques are necessary in all essential case management and administrative job functions. Leadership skills critical to the health and well-being of case managers are discussed in *The Seven Habits of Highly Effective People:*

Habit #1. Be proactive. Case management is a proactive process. Habit #1 talks about proactivity as it applies to one's personal relationship with events. It means being responsible for one's decisions and actions. A proactive person acts rather than is acted on. Highly proactive people recognize that they are responsible for their actions. Broken down, the word *responsibility* equals "response" and "ability," or the ability to choose responses. Their behavior is a function of their decisions, and they do not blame circumstances, conditions, or conditioning for their behavior. However, it is not unusual for case managers to work with family members or coworkers who are reactive, the opposite of proactive. A nonproactive person reacts with blame and fault finding. Highly effective case managers do not react to reactive people.

Habit #2. Begin with the end in mind. To do this, one must have a clear understanding of the desired direction and destination. Covey believes all things are created twice: first is the mental creation, then the physical creation (much like a blueprint precedes the actual building). The alternative is to climb the "ladder of success (or life)" only to realize that, after all the work, you do not like the wall it is leaning against.

Habit #2 has far-reaching ramifications in the area of outcomes management. First, the case manager must know what is to be measured (the endpoint); then the method to measure and evaluate that endpoint can be strategically determined. One of the best, and possibly the earliest, CQI gurus was the Cheshire Cat in "Alice in Wonderland." When Alice asked him which way she ought to go, he replied with, "If you don't know where you're going, any road will take you there!" Highly effective case managers know where they are going; they begin with the end in mind; then the roadmap can be constructed.

Habit #3. Put first things first. Essentially, first things are those that are deemed most important. Goethe said, "Things which matter most must never be at the mercy of things which matter least." Putting "first things first" involves organizing and managing time and events according to one's personal priorities; ask what is truly important at any given time. Case managers must sometimes make critical choices that change their priorities suddenly and dramatically; however, by putting "first things first," Covey believes that there will be less crisis. Covey states that people spend their time doing one of four activities: those that are impor-

tant; those that are not important; those that are urgent; and those that
are not urgent.

I. Urgent/Important—These are important, crisis tasks that must be
attended to. They are necessary and must be managed.

II. Not Urgent/Important—Covey states that as one spends more time in
this quadrant of planning and clarifying, less time will be spent in
the urgent/crisis quadrant. This is the quadrant of leadership and
quality. Focusing one's time in this quadrant will eventually lead to a
state of fewer crises. This need not take a lot time; often highly effective case managers plan and clarify throughout the day, tweaking priorities so they can go home at a reasonable hour.

III. Urgent/Not Important—This quadrant can be reduced with good
planning. These tasks are often deceptive (unnecessary interruptions,
for example) and often can be avoided.

IV. Not Urgent/Not Important—This quadrant can be eliminated almost
entirely. It is a quadrant generally of waste and should be avoided.

The goal of habit #3 is to decrease urgency and crises. Urgency, or a
style of management known as "crisis management," is addictive. Many
people who are locked into this way of management like it because it
makes them feel as though are accomplishing something. Emotionally,
this makes them feel worthwhile; physically, they are addicted to the
adrenaline "rush" put out by the adrenal glands when a person is in a
constant state of stress. A survey that tested how addictive the participants were to "crises" was given to dozens of people in 1997. It was
interesting to note that most of those addicted were nurses no longer
practicing in a patient care environment; and the ones with the highest
scores were either intensive care unit (ICU) or emergency department
dropouts (or graduates, depending how they looked at it). The results of
the survey made them jokingly refer to themselves as "recovering RNs."
However, none had practiced in acute care for many years. Habits die
hard.

Habit #4. Think Win–Win. Covey believes in an "abundance" mentality.
Any interaction where there is a Win–Lose, or Lose–Lose, attitude
denotes a "scarcity" mentality. Win–Win sees life as a cooperative (not
competitive) arena where mutually beneficial solutions are sought out.
There is a four-step process to seeking Win–Win solutions. Highly
effective case managers use these problem-solving techniques frequently:

1. See the problem from the other point of view. Really seek to understand (habit #5) and to give expression to the needs and concerns of
the other party.

2. Identify the key issues and concerns (not positions) involved.

3. Determine what results would constitute a fully acceptable solution.

4. Identify possible new options to achieve those results.

Habit #5. Seek first to understand, then to be understood. Typically, most people seek first to be understood, then, maybe, to understand. Communication is the most important skill in life, and certainly in case management. But many have not understood the difference between "hearing" and "listening." Without the ability to listen, one cannot understand another human being. Furthermore, people usually listen, not with intent to understand, but with intent to reply. They are either speaking, or preparing to speak, filtering what they are hearing through their own paradigms, and listening within their own frame of reference. But without truly understanding another's point of view, no real teamwork or problem solving can be accomplished. Highly effective case managers have exceptional listening skills.

Habit #6. Synergize. The basis for synergy is valuing people's differences. Here, the whole is greater than the sum of its parts. This is more evolved than compromising, where both parties give up a part of themselves to make peace. Sometimes a third solution can be found that is better than the two original ones. Highly effective case managers use creative thinking to find synergistic solutions to seemingly impossible problems.

Habit #7. Sharpen the saw. There is a story about a strapping young man who wanted to be a lumberjack. On his 18th birthday, he set out to get a job in the logging industry. Being young, strong, and healthy, he quickly got his wish. He was given his axe and set out to work. On the first day, he singlehandedly felled 12 trees. The boss was very pleased and commended him on his energy and strength. On the second day, the young man seemed to work just as diligently but cut down only 10 trees. On the third day, he cut 7, and on the fourth day, still trying very hard, only 3 trees came down. By the fifth day, with all the effort he could muster, no trees were cut.

The boy went to his boss, feeling terrible, and explained he had not cut one tree today. The boss asked why. "I am working as hard as I can. I'm really trying, sir," was the reply. Then the boss asked, "Have you taken the time to sharpen your axe?" The boy had not. He had been working so hard he did not take the time to work smart (Powell, 1996).

Sharpening your saw, axe, or your skills saves in time and effort. Time is a limited commodity, and case managers usually have a lot to do within their allotted timeframe. The time spent sharpening the saw—learning new skills—will be rewarded in multiples in reduced stress and frustration. Sometimes people are so busy cutting trees that they forget to sharpen the axe. Highly effective case managers take time to be sharp on all levels: physically, emotionally, spiritually, and mentally.

CHAPTER 7

Tools for
Process Improvement

INTRODUCTION

Measuring and assessing outcomes is no longer an option in today's health care market; it is mandatory for many accreditation requirements, which in turn are often mandatory for "winning" contracts. It has been said that one cannot improve what cannot be measured. An organization must know how to systematically assess, measure, and evaluate their processes to improve the outcomes, that is, the results of those processes. Continuous quality improvement (CQI) methods and tools provide the foundation for this work. It is important to use the correct CQI tool for the job; just as a crowbar should not be used to take apart a computer (although we may want to do this at times), a bar chart will not elicit the information needed when we want to take apart and examine a process.

First, decide what needs improving.
Second, decide what is the current process versus the best process.
Third, make changes in the direction of the improvement.

CQI is that simple. The complexity comes in knowing how to elicit the correct answers using the right tools. Sometimes that tool may be in the form of a question. Three fundamental questions should be asked before starting any improvement process (Langley, Gerald, Nolan, & Nolan, 1992):

1. *What are we trying to accomplish?*
   What is the aim of this improvement effort? This resonates with Covey's habit #2 (Chapter 6): *Begin with the end in mind.* Does the case management organization or department want to improve the way they are doing a process; increase their capture of a disease-specific population; find out why clinical pathways are not being adhered to?
2. *How will we know that a change is an improvement?*
   To answer this question, one must have a working knowledge of the total situation. Not unlike a patient's case, the whole universe of the current process must be understood, including who are the customers and what would constitute improvement in their eyes; how does the process work, and what are

the current outcomes of the process? Then the organization must have a way to measure the impact of any change initiated. Outcomes measures before a change (at baseline), and after a change, provide the answer to this question.

3. *What changes can we make that will result in improvement?*
   Data are needed to answer this question to:
   - Increase knowledge to develop a change
   - Develop and test a change
   - Implement the change (Langley et al., 1992)

On a more statistical note, Walter Shewhart, the creator of the PDCA Cycle, believed that *statistical process control charts,* described later in this chapter, help organizations to understand variation; and understanding variation in a process is the key to answering this question.

There are dozens of CQI tools in the literature. Each tool has a unique application, and some are more statistically complex than others. The *CQI Tools for Process Improvement* that will be examined in this chapter include:

Flowcharts
Run (trend) charts
Statistical process control charts (SPCC); a.k.a. control charts
Pie charts
Bar charts
Pareto charts
Cause-and-effect diagrams (fishbone or Ishikawa diagram)
Scatter diagrams

It is evident from Table 7-1, *CQI Tools and Techniques,* that each CQI tool and technique is useful for many important improvement process functions. The information provided in this text will give the reader a template to work with. Like case management, CQI techniques must be used to fully appreciate their value.

FLOWCHARTS

Flowcharts, also called **process flow diagrams,** are pictorial representations of the steps in a process. Although each team member may be fully knowledgeable about his or her segment of the work being done, they may not be clear about the complete process or system. Flowcharts take complicated routines, jobs, and events and display them so that they can be analyzed by individuals inside and outside that area of expertise.

Case management work is made up of processes within processes. Most often, quality failures are due not to faulty people but to the result of a faulty process.

TABLE 7-1 CQI Tools and Techniques

THE CHART	PRIMARY FUNCTION	USE TO:
Flowcharts	Displays the process	• Increase understanding of problems • Analyze processes • Identify gaps between current and desired situation • Identify opportunities to improve • Plan for change
Run charts	Displays data trends over time	• Increase understanding of problems • Identify gaps between current and desired situation • Identify opportunities to improve • Analyze processes
Control charts	Determines stability of data trends over time	• Increase understanding of problems • Identify gaps between current and desired situation • Monitor process performance • Identify opportunities to improve • Analyze processes • Evaluate tasks
Pie charts	Displays the percentage each variable contributes to the whole	• Increase understanding of problems • Identify gaps between current and desired situation • Identify variables affecting process • Identify opportunities to improve
Bar charts	Compares categories of data at one point in time	• Increase understanding of problems • Identify variables affecting process • Identify opportunities to improve
Pareto charts	Determines the most frequent causes of a problem (*i.e.*, the most important problems of a process)	• Increase understanding of problems • Identify and list problems • Indicate reasons likely to yield the most improvement • Separate the "vital few from the trivial many" • Identify variables affecting process • Identify opportunities to improve • Analyze processes • Evaluate tasks
Cause and effect	Displays multiple causes of a problem	• Increase understanding of problems • Identify and list problems • Identify root causes • Identify variables affecting process • Identify opportunities to improve • Analyze processes • Plan for change
Scatter diagram	Displays the relationship between two variables	• Increase understanding of problems • Identify opportunities to improve • Analyze processes • Plan for change • Evaluate tasks

Joseph Juran believed that 85% of the problems are process problems; 15% are proficiency problems. In *The Team Handbook* (Scholtes, Joiner, & Streibel, 1996), there is a picture of a hen laying eggs from a high platform. The worker's job is to grab a Band-Aid from the Band-Aid dispenser, place it on the cracked egg after it breaks (from hitting the table), and put the egg in the egg carton. He is doing a great job and has not missed a Band-Aid on a single egg. But there is a problem with the process! How often do case managers feel frustrated, not by the job we are doing, but by the processes in which we find ourselves?

A process, when it is at its finest, runs smoothly and has no unnecessary, redundant, or misplaced steps. Donald Berwick, M.D., states that "Every system is perfectly designed to get exactly the results it gets . . . a good outcome is the result of a good process." If a different result (outcome) is desired, a new process must be identified. Crude or erratic processes will lead to poor outcomes; sensible, dependable processes will lead to good, consistent outcomes. Enter flowcharts—the queen of evaluating processes. Flowcharts can be used:

1. To outline the sequence of events and their relationship to one another in a process
2. To identify redundant steps, loopholes that are potential sources of trouble, unnecessary complexity, and inefficiency in a process. A handy acronym (source unknown) is that flowcharts can be used to identify CRUD:
   Complexity
   Redundancy
   Unnecessary steps
   Delays
3. To create a common understanding of the flow of a process among various members of the multidisciplinary team. Furthermore, this CQI tool works well when there are inconsistencies in such activities as handing off patients among various levels of care, or between external and internal case managers.
4. As a training tool to train new case managers in various case management processes such as utilization review, discharge planning, assessment, use of clinical tools, or facility-specific processes
5. As an effective method of educating others about a process and where the opportunities for improvement may be. It is a good way to expose problems. Flowcharts also serve as an excellent method to write or recheck policies and procedures. Case management departments may choose to:
   a. Draw a flowchart of what steps the process actually follows.
   b. Draw a flowchart of what steps the process should follow if everything is correct and accurate. Use guidelines such as the *Case Management Standards* or your facilities' policies and procedures as a template.

c. Compare the two charts to find where they are different; this is usually where opportunities for improvement can be found.

The Flowchart Symbols and Definitions

Flowcharts use a series of symbols to represent actions and decision points. There are many available symbols, but few are essential for most basic flow-charting purposes. Using the correct symbols when producing a flowchart is important. A well-dressed flowchart is easy to read; the eye can go straight to the significant decision points and decide what to do and whether the answer is "yes" or "no." It also demonstrates that the facility/agency is knowledgeable about some CQI tools. Most processes can be flowed with the following few symbols:

BEGINNING AND END ⬭

This symbol can be an oval or elliptic shape and is used to show the beginning and end of a process. The ovals should reflect the boundaries of the process. When it is used to show the last step of a process, some choose to put the word "END" inside. This removes any doubt that this is the conclusion of the process.

PROCESS ACTION ☐

A process action is represented by a rectangle or box and is the most commonly used symbol in flowcharting. Include a brief description of the step or activity inside the rectangle. Only one arrow should emerge from a process or activity rectangle. If two flow lines are needed, a decision diamond (below) is more appropriate.

DECISION ◇

A decision is represented by the diamond shape. The decision point has one entry and two exits. State the decision in the form of a question that can be answered with "Yes" or "No." Each decision should have a "yes" path and a "no" path. Although not a rule, if you show all "yes" choices branching down, and "no" choices branching to the left, it is easier to follow; at the least, be consistent.

BREAK/CONTINUED SYMBOL Ⓐ

This symbol is used when part of the flow is continued in another area or page. "A,B,C . . ." or "1,2,3 . . ." can be used inside the circle; again, be consistent in the way the break is marked.

CONNECTORS ←⌐ → ←

Connectors are lines with arrows on the end showing the direction of the flow. Always have your arrows flowing in the same direction when you join lines. Flow is like a river; it only moves in one direction.

There are several types of flowcharts, such as *top-down flowcharts* or *responsibility flowcharts*. Several of the excellent books on Quality Improvement and CQI tools go into detail about the many types (see Resources and References at the end of this section). A case manager will also hear about "high-level flowcharts" and "low-level flowcharts." A high-level flowchart is a basic flowchart with an general overview of all the steps. It does not include detailed processes (see Figure 7-1, High-Level Flowchart Showing DME Order). A low-level flowchart is more detailed and will include more steps. These may have a medium amount of detail or may include precise details of the process. These flows can be one, two, or a dozen pages long, depending on the process being evaluated and pictured (see Figure 7-2, Low Level Flowchart Showing DME Order). These definitions may be initially confusing for case managers, because they are the opposite of how we describe rehabilitation patients: for example, in rehabilitation, a high-level patient is one who can follow or perform more details; a high-level flowchart is one that has few details.

Steps to Create a Flowchart

1. *Decide what needs to be flowcharted.* Brainstorm processes that are not working as smoothly as the case managers would like. Prioritize a process to focus on. It is best if the first attempt at changing a process is one that will have

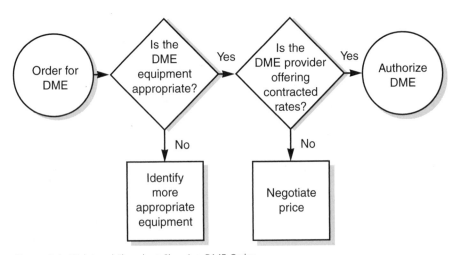

Figure 7-1. High-Level Flowchart Showing DME Order.

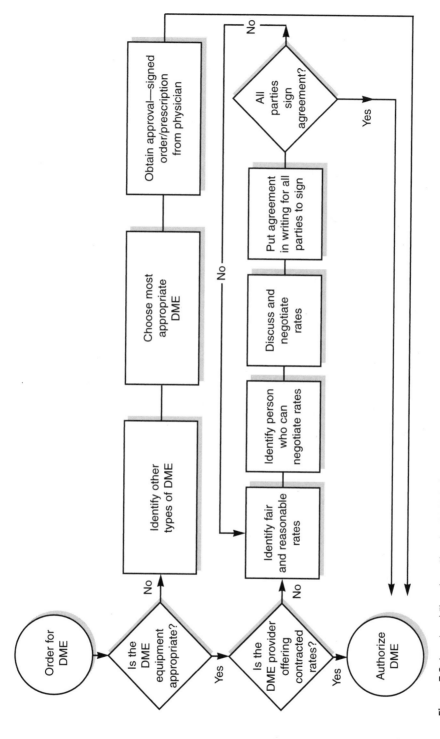

Figure 7-2. Low-Level Flowchart Showing DME Order.

145

the greatest impact with the least amount of changes and disruption to the existing system. This priority is not always easy to find, but initial successes in the CQI effort are imperative.

2. *Assemble a team that is knowledgeable about the process.* This team may or may not consist only of case managers. If the process to be evaluated needs a representative from respiratory, dietary, pharmacy, radiology, utilization management, finances, a specific level of care (acute, post acute, hospice), or an HMO (to name a few possibilities), include them on the initial team. However, do not allow the team to consist of more than six to seven members. The core people should have the most to gain by improving the process; others can be invited to meetings as consultants on an "as-needed" basis. (See Chapter 9 on Teams)

3. *Team members should agree to the level of detail they must show on the flowchart* to clearly understand the process and identify problem areas. The team may want to start with a high-level flowchart (basic flowchart), then add details later or only where it is needed. However, be consistent in the level of detail shown.

Do not try to flow too much. If you want to flow a huge process, do it at a very high level. Complicated processes are just a collection of smaller processes. If you need to show how the process fits into the whole, create a separate high-level diagram to demonstrate its place in the whole system. In the example of the low-level DME flowchart, note that more details and decision points could have been added.

Clearly define the first and last steps in the process. These two steps are also known as *boundaries*. Boundaries can be moving targets: what is the beginning/input to a case manager (*e.g.,* the referral to case management by the utilization review department) may be the endpoint/outcome for another staff member (*e.g.,* once the utilization manager refers a patient to a case manager, he or she is no longer involved in the case).

4. *List the steps that are involved in the process.* The steps may already be in narrative form in written policies and procedures, or in the heads of managers or employees. Brainstorm a list of all major activities and decisions. Ask, "what happens next?" Use large sticky notes on which to write the steps; this will make number 5 (below) easier.

If you are flowing an existing process, *show how it is currently being done.* If you interview employees to get information, make sure they are telling you how it is being done (rather than how it *should* be done—which is their first inclination!). This is necessary to see where the problems are in the process. Then, produce an ideal flowchart of the process. Compare and contrast the *current process* with the *ideal process* to identify discrepancies and opportunities for improvements.

5. *Sequence the steps.* Move the sticky notes around.

6. *Create a graphic diagram of the process using the correct flowchart symbols and add the arrows.* A lot of symbols can be used in a flowchart; but sometimes it is cleaner and clearer to keep it simple. Flowchart decision diamonds have only two answers; "Yes" and "No" are the most common. If it cannot be answered with "Yes" or "No," the process may not have been broken down far enough.

    Everything goes toward the END. Flowcharts have a single beginning and a single end (which may be pointed to from several directions). Create a single "END" symbol and point to it; it creates finality and clarity to the reader. If a process loops backwards, this may be a clue for an opportunity for improvement.

7. *If needed, break down the activities to show their complexity.* However, do not become so detailed in your process flow diagraming that you lose sight of the scope of the original problem. If the flowcharting is taking a long time, step back and ensure that you are still addressing the case management issue. Good flow charts are understandable, readable, and usable, and are meant to clarify, educate, and provoke thought. Hopefully, they are not as confusing as the process itself! Create a flowchart and use wording that is clear and understood by anyone.

8. *Title the diagram.* Place a date on the flowchart.

9. *Test the process.*
    - Is this process being run the way is should be?
    - Is the staff following the process as charted?
    - Are there obvious complexities or redundancies that can be reduced or eliminated? Check for CRUD.

GRAPHS AND LINE CHARTS

Many of the CQI tools for process improvement are in the form of bar graphs and line charts. In their simplest form, they are the same as taught in junior high school math classes. The more advanced CQI tools borrow components from the basic graphs and charts and add their own level of complexity. To be useful, it is important for the graphs and charts to include three pieces of information:

1. *A Descriptive Title:* This title should be a meaningful description of what the graph or chart is about, even if it is long. The purpose of a graph or chart is to show a picture of a situation. The title may be the first item looked at and should say that this graph has an important message to convey. For exam-

ple, a graph may be named "Average Number of Case Management Hours Per Congestive Heart Failure Patient: May–September 1999."

2. *A Data Box:* A box labeled "Data Collected" should answer "when, where, and by whom." For the above graph, "when" is May through September 1999; "where" would be the facility or company where the data was collected; "by whom" may be case managers or other personnel.

Data Collected:
Date:
By:
At:

3. *The Population Used to Create the Graph:* A population can be any patient population such as asthmatics younger than age 18 years, diabetics who received angiotensin-converting enzyme inhibitors, acute myocardial infarction patients who received thrombolytics within 1 hour of admission, or any group being studied. A population also can be a number of surveys, occurrences such as intravenous lines that infiltrated, or situations such as waiting times for a primary care provider appointment in an HMO. Three symbols one might see on a graph include:

$\overline{X}$ = this is the symbol for average and should be placed on any line that represents an average of the data

N = This symbol is used when the total population was included in the project. If all congestive heart failure patients in an HMO were included, N would be used to describe the population.

n = This symbol is used when a sample (or portion) of the total population was used. Rather than all the congestive heart failure patients in an HMO, this symbol might represent when a random sample of congestive heart failure patients were chosen.

RUN (TREND) CHARTS

A *run chart*, also referred to as a *trend chart*, is a basic line graph that displays similar data over time. Run charts are easy to create and interpret. They monitor processes or occurrences to identify trends. The time component may be in minutes, hours, days, weeks, months, or years. Most nurses have used run charts for trending patient temperatures. The vertical axis (the y-axis) displays the variable that is being measured; in this example it is the patient's temperature either in Centigrade or Fahrenheit. The horizontal axis (the x-axis) displays the time units; hospital temperatures may be taken every 4 hours, and home health temperature may be charted every 3 days. Run charts present a good visual representation of such case management issues as utilization management data, infection rates, or patient satisfaction scores. (Figure 7-3 gives an example of a run chart.)

Steps to Create and Interpret Run (Trend) Charts

1. Draw and label:
   The y-axis (vertical). For total hip replacement patients, this axis could indicate length of stay.
   The x-axis (horizontal). For total hip replacement patients, this axis could indicate the number of patients for each length of stay.
2. Draw the average, mean, or median line. This line may indicate the benchmark to target. For human temperatures, this would be placed at the 98.6°F line. For length of stay for total hip replacement patients, this may be 3.5 days.
3. Plot the data on the chart.
4. Connect the dots with a line.
5. If a more complex run chart is being used with more than one line, use different colors, thickness, or textures and create a "key" to explain what each line represents. Dotted lines are often reserved for future projections of the data.
6. Look for trends in the data points. In general, if at least 20 data points were used, then six changes in the same direction are considered significant; if fewer than 20 data points were used, five changes in the same direction are considered significant, or a trend. The reasons for the data changes may be clear, or they may take further investigation. The data may need to be gathered differently: by hour instead of day; by day instead of week.

   In the temperature example, temperature spikes may occur at certain times in the day, or after a specific medication or dietary meal. Individual patients may require investigation into other activities in their medical records.

   When further evaluated, the length of stay for total hip replacement patients that are over the targeted benchmark may be traced back to a specific physician. To find this out, the patients would need to be tracked individually by physician.

   Conversely, the longer length of stay may be due to the day of the week the surgery was performed; do Wednesday and Thursday surgeries cause

longer length of stays because of lack of discharge planning or physical therapy assistance on the weekends? Those with longer length of stays may
require a chart indicating the day of the week the surgeries were performed.

Once the cause of the trend is noted, and an action plan is in place, it is
a good idea to periodically check the process through another run chart exercise. A spot check of the trends can show whether the revised process is still
working.

Run charts are a simple method of data collection. A disadvantage is that
they have a limited application. However, they can be used as a stepping stone.
The run chart example below displays an average length of stay (LOS) by
month for total hip replacement patients. The LOS decreased over the months.
But what else happened? Did the patients do as well with the shorter LOS? An
interesting adjunctive study would be to survey the patients during the same
months, with a patient survey such as the SF 36/SF 12. Did the LOS affect the
patient's perception of their postoperative functionality?

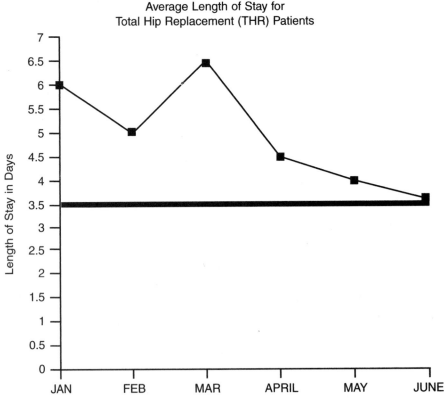

Figure 7-3. Example of a Run (Trend) Chart.

CONTROL CHARTS (STATISTICAL PROCESS CONTROL CHARTS [SPCC])

A *control chart*, also known as a *statistical quality control chart* or *statistical process control chart (SPCC)*, is similar to a run chart in that it shows trends of data over time. In addition, control charts exhibit *control limits* known as *upper control limits* (UCL) and *lower control limits* (LCL). These control limits define the acceptable range of the data being monitored, and are statistically determined by allowing the process to run untouched and then analyzing the results using a mathematical formula. There are several types of complex control charts, but for our purposes, we will discuss them at their most basic level. The hope is that case managers will see the value of this remarkable CQI tool. Control charts can be used to examine variation over time and can be used as a vital teaching tool for some important case management applications. Deming called control charts a "gift" from Dr. Walter A. Shewhart, whose purpose is to "to stop people from chasing down causes."

Understanding *variation* is germane to the appreciation of control charts. A variation is simply a change in the data. The old quality assurance "variance criteria" looks at variation in a negative light, but actually it is a natural occurrence that exists in all processes. Body temperature varies according to foods eaten, infection present, activity performed, or a variety of other common factors. Many of the temperature variances are not only acceptable, but needed for a healthy and balanced system. (See Box 7-1 for examples of variation.)

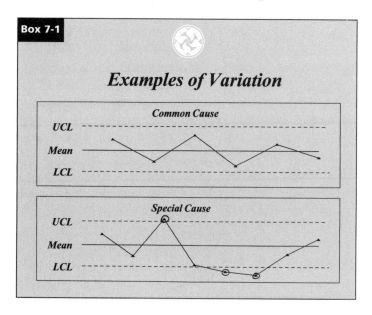

Box 7-1

Examples of Variation

However, when variances get "out of control" or are far from the mean (the average), this may signal an opportunity to improve the process. For example, if a patient's temperature is unstable, or out of control, a medical practitioner would examine the cause for the variation; if the temperature is varying around the normal temperature of 98.6°F, then it would not be a cause for major examination. The same is true for all processes. It is critical to know whether a variation is from a stable *common cause* or from an unstable *special cause* (see Box 7-2).

Box 7-2

COMPARISON OF COMMON CAUSE AND SPECIAL CAUSE

COMMON CAUSES	SPECIAL CAUSES
1. Also known as a random or unassignable cause of variation	1. Also known as a nonrandom or assignable cause of variation (*i.e.*, variation in the process is assignable to a special cause)
2. **In a Control Chart:** Shown within the upper and lower control limits	2. **In a Control Chart:** Shown outside of the upper and lower control limits
3. All processes have common cause variation; they are routine, expected, and are produced by variables of the process itself	3. Are activated by irregular or unnatural causes that are not a part of the system or process (*i.e.*, happens when there is a change in the system or process)
4. Reasons for common causes are sometimes harder to detect because they are an integrated part of the process	4. Easier to detect than common causes because they are due to an unusual event
5. a. Results from many small causes or minor variations in the process, and in time, may affect everyone in the system and all outcomes of the process	5. a. Results from unexpected and specific circumstances

(continued)

Box 7-2 (Continued)

COMPARISON OF COMMON CAUSE AND SPECIAL CAUSE

COMMON CAUSES	SPECIAL CAUSES
b. Fundamental changes to the system are usually needed to affect an improvement	b. Easier to eliminate than common causes (ex: scheduling problem because MRI machine broke)
6. Results in a *stable* process; therefore, the variation is predictable	6. Results in an *unstable* process; therefore, the variation is not predictable
7. Are said to be "in statistical control"	7. Are said to be "out of statistical control"
8. Improvement to a process or system can be obtained by understanding what the common causes are	8. Improvement to a process or system can be obtained by understanding what the special causes are

- *Common causes* hover in the mid-range between the UCL and LCL; they are considered an inherent part of the system and are predictable and in control; improvement to processes can be gained by understanding common causes, although they are often harder to detect than special causes. Common cause process outcomes may not be "good" or meet customer needs, and it may be possible that the UCL and LCL need to be recalculated. For example, if the UCL allows a 25% infection rate, there is cause for reconsideration of the UCL; perhaps initial thresholds should have been more realistic. But some control chart experts caution not to recalculate the control limits unless the actual process has been changed and to use new data after the change has occurred.

- *Special causes* fall outside of the UCL and LCL; they are considered unpredictable and out of control. Improvement to the process can be obtained by understanding special causes, and they are often easier to expose or eliminate than a common cause: for example, schedules may be delayed because of machine malfunctions; transfers may be delayed because of difficulty obtaining insurance authorization. One method used to get to the root of the special cause is to ask "why" several times (See Root Cause Analysis, Chapter 9). Suppose a large teaching hospital sees a significant increase in medication errors in June and July. A few rounds of "why" may easily determine that June and July invites the influx of new interns, residents, and RNs, and seasoned staff goes on vacation. This does not always mean, however, that a special cause is to be avoided; sometimes a special cause produces a positive impact on the system and should be built into the process! (See Figure 7-4, the flowchart "Variation Analysis—Common and Special Causes.")

Deming once said, "If I had to reduce my message for management to just a few words, I'd say it all had to do with reducing variation." Variation is treated differently depending on whether it is due to a common cause or to a special cause. And control charts are the CQI tool to expose the difference.

A control chart is a powerful CQI tool for monitoring and maintaining processes. The organization can see whether it is making changes, and whether the changes are moving in the desired direction. The trends, or patterns, on control charts can also help predict how a process might act in the future through the discovery of special cause variation. There are approximately seven types of statistically elaborate control charts, and it is recommended that the books listed in the resources at the end of this section be used for further investigation. However, the following information on control charts can be used as a practical application for case managers.

One application that has proved effective is for the purpose of patient self-monitoring. Dr. Larry Staker, Director of Clinical Practice Improvement at Intermountain Health Care, presented a study in which diabetics were taught how to monitor and chart their blood sugars using a control chart. Figure 7-5 ("Patient Diabetic Control Chart") shows an approximate version of what the patients were given. The UCL and LCL were set at the accepted range for a healthy blood sugar. Blood sugars outside of that range needed attention. In the manufacturing industries, control charts are often called "stop and go" charts because they add red, green, and sometimes yellow to the chart, as in a traffic light. Color coding the acceptable range as green and the nonacceptable ranges as red may be effective for some patients.

In Dr. Staker's study, the value of self-monitoring proved to be what case managers always suspected; it was discovered that blood sugars in their diabetic patients were more "in control" when patients were able to visually see the blood sugar trends. Figure 7-6 ("Diabetic Control Sheets") displays the trends of blood sugars **before** and **after** the patients were taught to use the control chart (two charts).

Control charts of this type can be used for many other case management teaching or monitoring activities. Every disease management program has a patient education component. The control limits that are set on each chart will

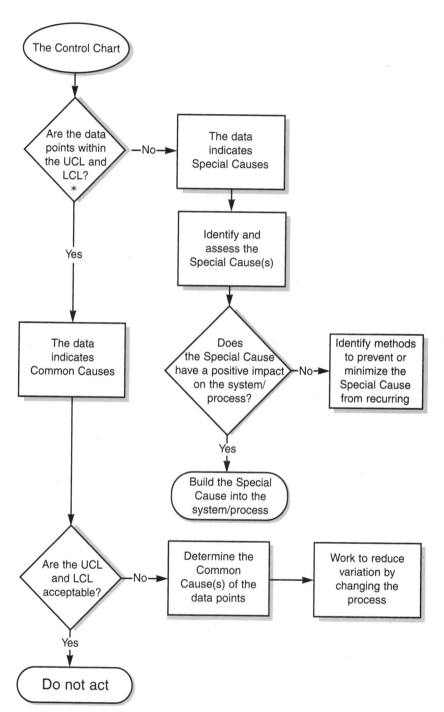

Figure 7-4. Variation Analysis—Common and Special Causes.
*UCL, upper control limits; LCL, lower control limits.

155

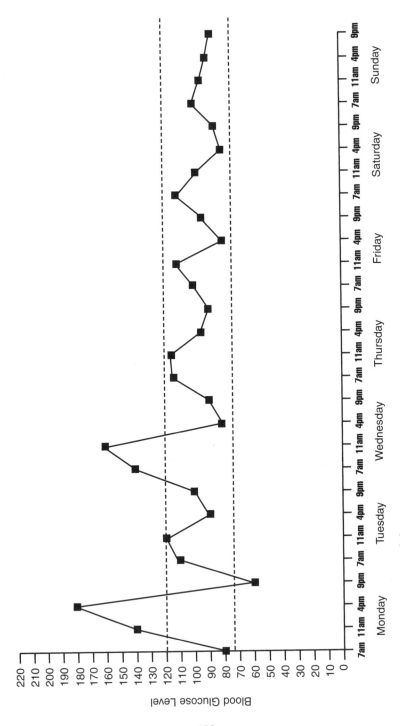

Figure 7-5. Patient diabetic control chart.

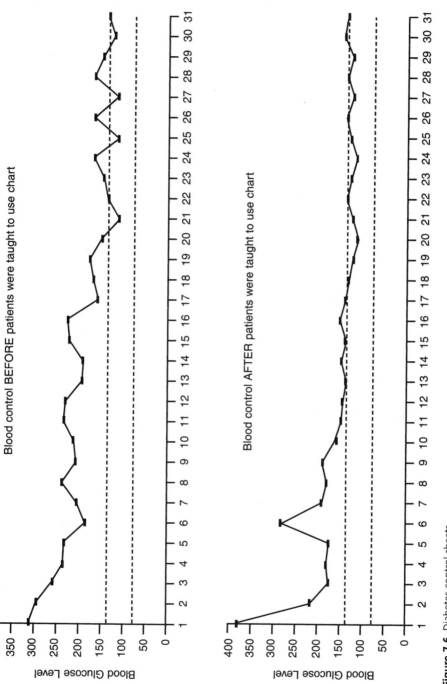

Figure 7-6. Diabetes control sheets.

depend on the patient's needs (such as weight ranges) and acceptable limits according to medical practice (such as blood sugar ranges). This tool is ideal for many applications, a few of which are listed:

- Diabetes patients—blood sugar monitoring and education
- Congestive heart failure—weight monitoring and education*
- Renal patients—weight monitoring and education *
- Coumadin patients—monitoring INR levels
- Asthma patients—monitoring Peak Flow Meter results
- Pain management—chart pain levels and pain medication administration

Steps to Create and Interpret Control Charts

1. Draw and label the x-axis (horizontal), which is the time sequence (hours, days, months). In Figure 7-5, the "Patient Diabetic Control Chart" example, the time sequence is 7 AM, 11 AM, 4 PM, and 9 PM for 1 week.
2. Draw and label the y-axis (vertical), which shows the data that will be trended.
   Data generally falls into two categories:
   a. Data that can be measured: lengths, temperature, volume, pressure, blood sugar, weights, blood pressure
   b. Data that can be counted: missed or canceled physician appointments, units of physical/speech/occupational therapy, number of home health visits
   On the "Patient Diabetic Control Chart" example, the blood glucose level, in 10-unit increments, forms the vertical axis.
3. Draw the center line, which is the arithmetic mean or average. This line is usually solid and indicates the benchmark to target. In the diabetic example, no median line is differentiated.
4. Calculate and plot upper and lower control limits according to the appropriate statistical formula (see books in the resource section) or use a computer program. Use dotted or dashed lines. The UCL and LCL are usually based on 2 to 3 standard deviations from the mean. Benchmarks or clinically accepted ranges also can be used. In the diabetic example, the acceptable blood sugar range is the standard accepted by every clinical facility (between 70 and 120).
5. Plot the data on the chart. Most of the time it is recommended that raw numbers are not used when plotting the data points; percentages and data

---

*The control chart for renal and congestive heart failure patients would require a chart tailored for the patient's specific weight prescription.

obtained with indicators created with a numerator/denominator will yield comparable numbers. If hospitals in one state compared their medication errors for the month of September as raw numbers, then the lowest number "wins." But what if hospital A had 15 medication errors and a census of 1,000 and hospital B had 25 medication errors with a census of 3,000 in the same timeframe? Rather, the data should be plotted using a numerator/denominator format:

the number of medication errors / 1,000 patients

It levels the playing field. Although hospital A has fewer medication errors for the month, using a numerator and denominator exposes that hospital B actually has fewer medication errors per 1,000 patients. On the "Patient Diabetic Control Chart" example, blood sugars for 1 week are plotted; but blood sugars are comparable, stable numbers for everyone and can be used accurately in control charts. (See chapters on Outcomes Management for more on numerator/denominator construction of indicators).

6. Connect the dots with a line.
7. To really see a trend, it is best to have at least 20 data points to look at. Then, look for variation; examine which points indicate common causes or special causes. Ascertain reasons for the special cause variations. When the blood sugar went "out of control," was the patient eating improperly, did he have an infection, was he under stress, or did he miss an insulin dose?

PIE CHARTS

Pie charts are used to display the percentage that a category contributes to the total of all categories. For example, if a case management agency or department wanted to see "at a glance" where their case management referrals are coming from, they may collect data on all referrals (the whole pie). The various referral sources would become the different slices of the pie.

Steps to Create a Pie Chart

1. Divide all the data into categories and collect the data. In this case, referral sources may include:
   - The social worker
   - The primary care physician
   - The employer (in a self-funded situation)
   - Other case managers (from the HMO, home health agency, SNF)
   - Patient or family member

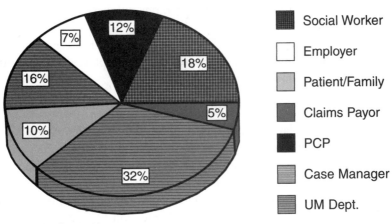

Figure 7-7. Example of a Pie Chart.

- Utilization management department
- Claims payor
2. Calculate the percentage of the whole that each referral source represents:
   - The social worker (18%)
   - The primary care physician (12%)
   - The employer (in a self-funded situation) (7%)
   - Other case managers (from the HMO, home health agency, SNF) (16%)
   - Patient or family member (10%)
   - Utilization management department (32%)
   - Claims payor (5%)
3. It is easiest to use a software program to draw pie charts. Assign each referral source to the whole pie. Label each slice of the pie and include its percentage to the whole. Provide a meaningful title.
4. If there are several small categories, assign one slice as "other"; however, the "other" category should always be the smallest slice. (Figure 7-7 gives an example of a pie chart.)

BAR CHARTS

A bar chart, at its simplest level, is used to compare data at one point in time. From the pictorial diagram, data analysis efforts can be enhanced. If a case management agency or department would like to see reasons for case management closure, a simple bar chart, as described in the steps below, would suffice.

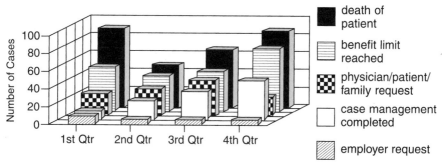

Figure 7-8. Example of a Bar Chart.

Bar charts can be more detailed with clusters of the categories shown over several quarters. Histograms and Pareto charts are more advanced forms of bar charts.

Steps to Create a Bar Chart

1. Divide the horizontal axis into categories for the bars. If the bar chart will display "Reasons for Case Management Closure," the categories may include:
   - Death of patient
   - Benefit limit reached/lost eligibility
   - Physician request
   - Patient/family request
   - Case management completed
   - Employer (self-funded group) request
2. Divide the vertical axis into segments. In this example, the segments would be numbers.

Note: If the bar chart is used to compare the categories in various quarters, all case management closure reasons will be displayed in bar form for *each* quarter. See Figure 7-8 for an example.

PARETO CHARTS

In health care, it is estimated that 20% of the patients account for approximately 80% of the health care dollars. It was Dr. Joseph Juran who coined the famous 80/20 rule, when he observed through testing that 80% of the problems typically are caused by 20% of the contributing factors. The *Pareto chart* can show this visually; it consists of a series of bars (as in a bar graph) that are displayed from tallest (most frequent contributing factor) to smallest (least frequent contributing factor); it also has a line graph component that displays a cumulative percentage. The Pareto chart is useful to create a clear description of the situation, to gain consensus on which direction to pursue, and to establish an action plan for either further data collection or improvement strategies (Schroeder, 1994).

The *Pareto Principle* separates "the vital few from the trivial many" (Vilfredo Pareto); it states that, whenever a quality problem has multiple causes, a relative few of those causes account for most of the incidents (McLaughlin & Kaluzny, 1994). The Pareto chart displays the frequency and relative importance of the causes, thereby seeing "at a glance" which account for the bulk of the problem. Rarely can problems be solved all at once, especially when there are multiple factors causing the difficulty. With a Pareto chart, the team can focus on problems that have the greatest potential for improvement. However, to complicate things, this does not mean that working on the cause with the greatest frequency is the always wisest choice. The team must take into consideration what effect the change will have on the whole, and whether the change is worth the effort in time and expenses relative to the potential gain.

Steps to Create a Pareto Chart

I. *Identify a problem that your case management department/organization wants to understand more fully.*

Pareto charts can be used to help identify which case management interventions are most costly/least costly, what problems account for the most dissatisfaction (of patients, payors, employers, case managers, providers), or why patients are falling through the cracks (in which referrals were made too late, or not at all). For example, a Pareto chart can identify which of the "vital few" types of case management referrals are getting overlooked most often. What would have been the reason for the case management referral, had it been referred to at an appropriate time? After displaying the missed reasons for case management referrals, the improvement team can work on methods to stop these important cases from falling through the cracks. After the reasons are sorted out, the team may want to apply a *Root Cause Analysis,* to find out why these cases are getting overlooked. (See Root Cause Analysis in the chapter on teams.)

There are multiple reasons that a case management referral may be triggered. At any time, these same patients may go without case management because of an oversight in the case management process. Some potential reasons are:

- Psychosocial issues
  — Suspected or actual child or adult abuse
  — Crime victim
  — Homelessness
  — Inadequate social, financial, or insurance support
  — High-risk behaviors
  — Drug-seeking behaviors
  — Language, cultural issues or barriers
  — Home environment, safety issues
  — Mental health issues
  — Suicidal (actual or potential)
  — Potential risk management/litigation issue
  — Unable to return to previous living environment
  — Unable to meet previous caregiver responsibilities
- Clinical conditions
  — Terminal condition
  — High risk procedure planned
  — Catastrophic illness/event
  — High-risk, high-dollar diagnosis
  — Chronic disease state with comorbidities
  — Readmission within 15 days (or 1 month)
  — Multiple admissions

II. *Develop a list of possible categories that may explain the reason for the problem chosen in step I.* This list can be generated through a brainstorming session or through a cause-and-effect diagram (see Brainstorming and Cause-and-Effect Diagram).

Rules:
1. Categories must be defined so that they are clearly distinct entities.
2. Have at least 30 data points if four to six categories are chosen.
   Have at least 60 data points if 7 to 10 categories are chosen.
   Have at least 100 data points if 11 or more categories are chosen (Executive Learning, 1997).

For the example Pareto chart (see Figure 7–9), three psychosocial issues and three clinical conditions were chosen:

1. Inadequate financial/insurance support
2. Mental health issues
3. Unable to return to previous living environment
4. High-risk procedure planned (e.g., brain surgery)
5. Chronic disease state with comorbidities
6. Multiple admissions

TABLE 7-2 A Table Used to Create a Pareto Chart

CATEGORY	FREQUENCY	PERCENTAGE OF TOTAL	CUMULATIVE PERCENTAGE
1. Inadequate financial/insurance support	15	50%	50%
2. Multiple admissions	10	34%	84%
3. Unable to return to previous living environment	2	7%	91%
4. High-risk procedure planned (e.g., brain surgery)	1	3%	94%
5. Chronic disease state with comorbidities	1	3%	97%
6. Mental health issues	1	3%	100%
Grand total	**30**	**100%**	**100%**

III. *Collect the data on the list in step II.* Identify how often each occurred. A simple check sheet can be used for this step.

IV. *Rank order the data in descending order.* Lump minor categories together and label them "other"; this category should not constitute more than 20% of the total (Executive Learning, 1997).

V. *Calculate the percentage of the total for each category; also calculate the cumulative percentage for each category with all previous categories* (Executive Learning, 1997).

VI. *Draw a table* (Table 7-2 is an example) and include the information above:
- In the first column, list the categories in the order of most frequent to least frequent.
- In the second column, list the frequency that the categories occur.
- In the third column, list the percentage of total for each category.
- In the fourth column, list the cumulative percentage (Executive Learning, 1997).

VII. *Construct the Pareto chart.* Draw the axes:
- a. The x-axis (horizontal) will display the list from step II. Label the categories from largest to smallest, left to right.
- b. The left-side y-axis (vertical) will display the units of measurement being compared; draw the total number at the top.
- c. The right-side y-axis (vertical) will display the cumulative percentages from 0% to 100%, with 100% directly opposite the total number (top).

VIII. *Draw the bars of the Pareto chart with the height being the unit of measurement.*
- Bars should be equal width.

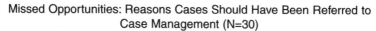

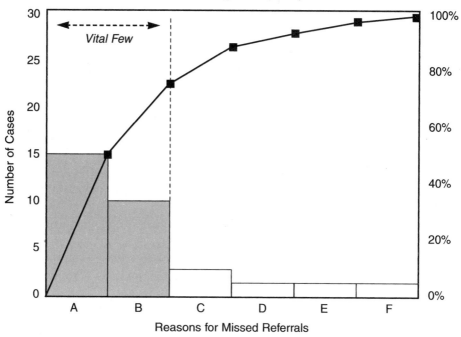

A. Inadequate financial/
   insurance support
B. Multiple admissions
C. Unable to return to
   previous living environment

D. High-risk procedure planned
   (brain surgery)
E. Chronic disease state with
   comorbidities
F. Mental health issues

Figure 7-9. Example of a Pareto Chart.

- The bars should touch each other.
- The right-sided bar should touch the right axis; the left-sided bar should touch the left axis.

Note: If the bars on the chart are flat, consider examining the data from a different perspective (Executive Learning, 1997).

IX. *Draw a line graph that will depict the cumulative percentages above the bars.*

X. *Label the Pareto chart with title, source of data, date, who collected the data, and any other pertinent information.*

CAUSE-AND-EFFECT DIAGRAMS
(FISHBONE OR ISHIKAWA DIAGRAM)

Cause-and-Effect Diagrams are used to explore all the factors that influence a process or situation. Before a team can "fix" a problem, they must first identify and understand the multiple causes for the problem. These diagrams are used in conjunction with a brainstorming session, where the team will look at all the "causes" that can be attributed to the "effect" being evaluated. Cause-and-effect diagrams are also known as the *Ishikawa diagram*, after its originator, Kaoru Ishikawa, or as a "*fishbone*" diagram because of its shape.

In Ishikawa's book, *Guide to Quality Control*, he summarizes the advantages of cause-and-effect diagrams:

- The creation of the diagram itself is educational and gets important players speaking to each other about the problem process.
- It helps focus the discussion; irrelevant discussion and complaints are reduced.
- It is an active process with a goal: to uncover the root cause of a problem.
- Data usually must be collected with this tool. This increases objectivity and reduces personal opinion.
- It demonstrates the level of the staff's understanding of the process. The more complex the diagram is, the more the workers know about the process.
- It can be used for a large variety of problems.

Steps to Create Cause-and-Effect Diagrams

1. *Define the Effect:* Clearly define the outcome, end result, or problem; write this out in a *problem statement*. This is the "effect" that is occurring. It is important that everyone agree on the problem statement. Place the problem statement in the middle, right-hand side of the paper inside of a box.
2. *Draw the Diagram:* Draw a horizontal line from the "problem box" toward the left of the paper. Place an arrow, pointing toward the problem box (See Figure 7-10).
3. *Develop the Categories:* Determine and define the major categories of causes that will be investigated. These branch off the main horizontal line, and describe the system or process under examination. The main categories require some flexibility. These categories may be specifically customized to the issue; they may be more general, like those used in the mechanical industry; or they can be a combination of both.

   Industry has devised several possibilities for these branches, or fishbones. Some examples of industrial categories are materials, procedures/methods,

A. General Cause-and-Effect Diagram

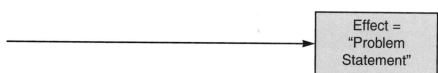

Effect =
"Problem
Statement"

B. Potential Causes for Poor Mammogram Rates in Medicare Women

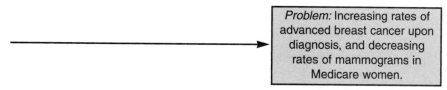

Problem: Increasing rates of advanced breast cancer upon diagnosis, and decreasing rates of mammograms in Medicare women.

Figure 7-10. A. General Cause-and-Effect Diagram. **B.** Case management/disease management Cause-and-Effect Diagram.

equipment/machines, environment, money, and people. Easy reminder lists have been made:

The 5 Ps are used for administrative purposes: People, Provisions, Policies, Procedures, Place

The 5 Ms are used in the manufacturing industry: Manpower, Materials, Machines, Methods, Measurements

Some of these categories will "fit" case management cause-and-effect requirements by customizing the definitions. For example, the "People" category in industry may include buyers, manufacturers, salespeople, etc.; in case management, this category may include caregivers, patients, other case managers, providers, physicians, claims payors, home health agencies, or pharmacists. Machinery in the trucking industry will be different from the high-tech patient care equipment in a hospital. In this step, always keep the categories general. Each problem statement may require a different set of categories. In the case management/disease management example of a cause-and-effect diagram, the categories are specifically tailored to the problem statement. There is not a set number or type of categories; rather, use what "fits" the issue (See Figure 7-11).

4. *Determine the Causes:* It is not always easy to define categories before defining the causes; some recommend first searching for causes, then placing them in appropriate categories. Even if this sequence is chosen, step 4 should undergo another round of brainstorming to assure that all causes have been identified. Note that the team will start with general areas of "cause" and then get more specific through brainstorming each category.

A. General Cause-and-Effect Diagram

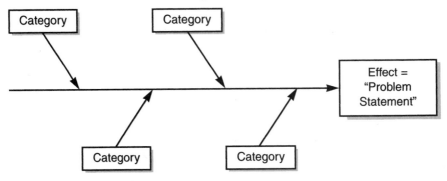

B. Potential Causes for Poor Mammogram Rates in Medicare Women

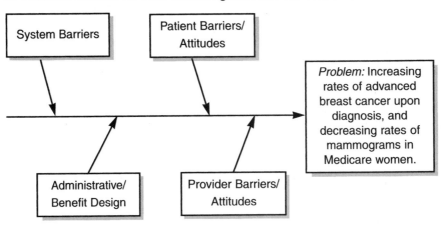

Figure 7-11. A. General Cause-and-Effect Diagram. **B.** Case management/disease management Cause-and-Effect Diagram.

These causes will branch out from the "categories" and be placed parallel to the main horizontal line placed in step 2. If there are any subcauses, these can branch out further from the "fishbones."

Develop the "causes" by repeatedly asking the question, "Why?" or more specifically, "Why is this occurring?" This step is similar to the *root cause analysis* technique discussed in Chapter 9. The team must continue this process until a useful level of detail has been reached. This occurs when the root cause is specific enough to be measured. Only when it is measurable can the team plan action (Executive Learning, 1997). If the root cause is controlled by more than one level of management removed from the group that is exploring the problem, it may not be one that the group can impact. Change the team members, use other staff closer to the problem as "consultants," or develop a subgroup to explore the problem.

It is important to list only causes; steer clear of listing anything that resembles symptoms or solutions (Figure 7-12).

5. *Evaluate the Fishbone:* When a root cause reappears in more than one major category, it is a significant problem and would benefit from an intense evaluation. Some improvement options will stand out as obvious choices. Others may be classified as easily remedied or already remedied. Circle the most likely root cause(s) within each category that the team will focus on.

6. *Prioritize the Categories:* Redraw the "fish" with the most likely root causes toward the head.

7. *Cause-and-effect diagrams are not an end in themselves; they will only identify the problem.* Use other CQI methods to move the process and solve the problem. In the case management/disease management example, the causes have been identified for potential reasons why mammogram rates are low; this, in turn, may be the reason for advanced breast cancer on diagnosis. However, the "causes" for the problem are not yet solved; and a whole lot of work may be required once "Pandora's Box" has been opened.

A. General Cause-and-Effect Diagram

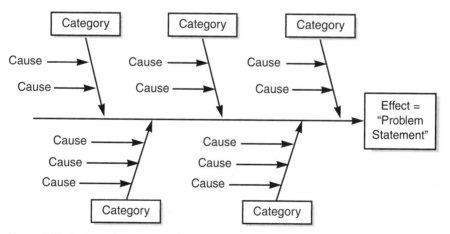

Figure 7-12. A. General Cause-and-Effect Diagram *(continued).*

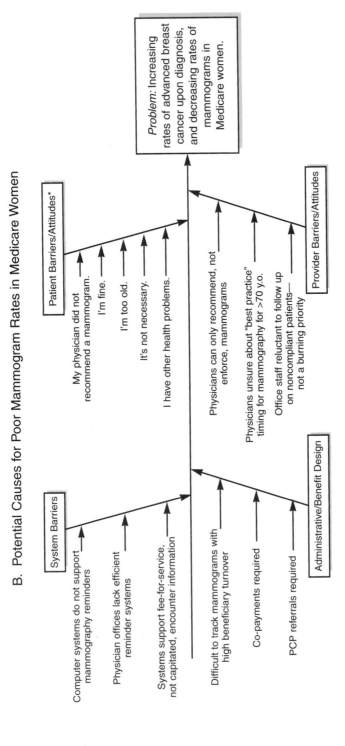

B. Potential Causes for Poor Mammogram Rates in Medicare Women

System Barriers

Computer systems do not support mammography reminders

Physician offices lack efficient reminder systems

Systems support fee-for-service, not capitated, encounter information

Difficult to track mammograms with high beneficiary turnover

Co-payments required

PCP referrals required

Administrative/Benefit Design

Patient Barriers/Attitudes*

My physician did not recommend a mammogram.

I'm fine.

I'm too old.

It's not necessary.

I have other health problems.

Physicians can only recommend, not enforce, mammograms

Physicians unsure about "best practice" timing for mammography for >70 y.o.

Office staff reluctant to follow up on noncompliant patients— not a burning priority

Provider Barriers/Attitudes

Problem: Increasing rates of advanced breast cancer upon diagnosis, and decreasing rates of mammograms in Medicare women.

* Attitudes about mammograms from an actual Arizona Insurance survey

Figure 7-12 (Continued). B. Case management/disease management Cause-and-Effect Diagram.

SCATTER DIAGRAMS (SCATTERGRAMS)

Scatter diagrams display the relationship, or correlation, between two variables; they are useful because they display all the data as a whole, rather than individually. Anytime two case management variables intersect, a scattergram is the tool-of-choice to see whether a relationship exists between them. It is a good idea to at least suspect that the two variables affect each other.

Often, scatter diagrams pair a process variable with a quality issue, although that is not the only practical application.

- On one axis, measure case managers' caseloads.
  On the other axis, measure case manager satisfaction with the job.
- On one axis, measure case managers' caseloads.
  On the other axis, measure the patient's satisfaction with case management.
- On one axis, measure the number of case management encounters with the patient.
  On the other axis, measure patient satisfaction with case management.
- On one axis, measure a (process), such as education, coordination, or providers, etc.
  On the other axis, measure patient SF-12 scores.

Or explore the relationship between a case manager's caseload to see whether it affects length of stay:

- On one axis, measure case managers' caseloads.
  On the other axis, measure length of stay.

Interpretation of Scatter Diagrams

Once several data points between two variables have been plotted, a pattern emerges. Depending on the "scatter" of the points, the two variables may have a positive correlation, a negative correlation, or no correlation. In general:

- *Positive correlation:* The points run in a linear fashion from the lower left corner to the upper right corner. "Higher" scores of one variable correlate with "lower" scores of the other variable. Improving one variable will likely improve the other variable (Schroeder, 1994). See Figure 7–13E.
- *Negative correlation:* The points run in a linear fashion from the upper left corner to the lower right corner. "Higher" scores of one variable correlate with "lower" scores of the other variable. Increasing one variable will likely decrease the other variable (Schroeder, 1994). See Figure 7–13F.
- *No correlation:* The points are scattered all over the plot with no obvious pattern. There is no definite relationship between the two variables. See Figure 7–13C.

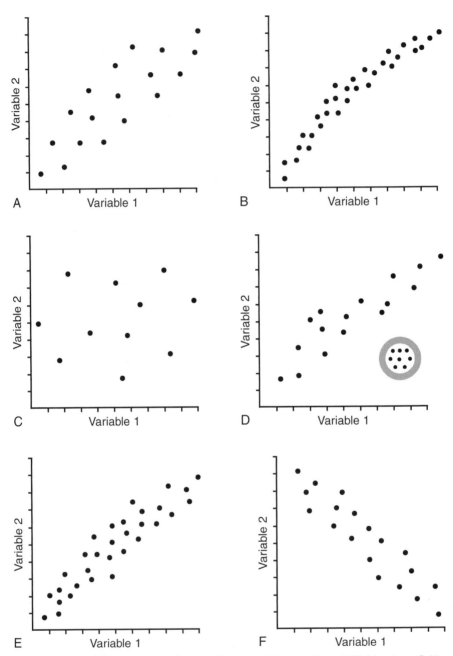

Figure 7-13. The different patterns of scatter diagrams. **A.** Loose pattern. **B.** Tight pattern. **C.** No correlation. **D.** Outliers. **E.** Positive correlation. **F.** Negative correlation.

- If, in a positive or negative plot structure, there is a group of points in one quadrant, this group is known as "outliers" and may represent "special causes" (Executive Learning, 1997). (See control charts, this chapter, for "special causes"). See Figure 7–13D.
- If the pattern in the positive or negative correlation scatter diagram is "tight," the factors being studied are probably responsible for most of the variation; if the pattern is "loose," there may be other factors affecting the data. See Figure 7–13A and B.

Steps to Create Scatter Diagrams

1. Clearly define the two variables that will be measured and plotted; these two variables should be suspected of having a logical relationship (Executive Learning, 1997).
2. Collect the data; at least 25 pairs of data for the two variables are recommended.
3. Draw and label the axes. The x-axis (horizontal) will display one variable: the y-axis (vertical) will display the other variable.
4. Plot the paired sets of data by marking a dot at the intersection of their values.
5. Label the scatter diagram with title, source of data, date, who collected the data, and any other pertinent information.

This chapter has identified some of the most useful CQI tools for process improvement that can be applied in case management practice. Chapter 8 will discuss the continuous quality improvement process and the PDCA method of problem-solving. Chapter 9 will examine important concepts when case managers work in improvement teams, including decision-making techniques.

The Continuous Quality Improvement (CQI) Process

THE PDCA CYCLE

Problem-Solving Methods

Problem-solving models, or strategies, abound at this time. It is good that they do. In this fast-changing world, they provide a way for us to organize our thinking. When a problem appears or persists, specific information must be attained to evaluate what is currently happening; then specific actions must be taken to remedy the situation. If the situation is not improving to the degree the team planned, it is not uncommon for the team to flounder, and ask, "Where do we go from here?" With problem-solving methodologies, the team has a roadmap for success.

One problem-solving model that is tried-and-true is the *Shewhart Cycle*—or the *PDCA Cycle*. It is named after its originator, Dr. Walter A. Shewhart, who developed the *Theory of Statistical Quality Control* and created the cycle while working at Bell Telephone Laboratories in the 1920s. Dr. Deming continued to advocate its use decades later, and "PDCA" remains the cornerstone of CQI problem-solving methodologies.

PDCA stands for Plan-Do-Check-Act. Deming made one small change. He changed the "Check" word to "Study," because he believed that merely checking one's progress was not enough; one must study the results carefully. "Check" and "Study" are often seen interchangeably. According to Dr. Deming, the PDC(S)A Cycle stands for (Scholtes et al., 1996):

PLAN a change or a test aimed at improvement.
DO the change; carry it out (preferably on a small scale).
STUDY the results. What was learned?
ACT. Depending on what was learned in the STUDY Phase:

1. Adopt the change
2. Abandon the change

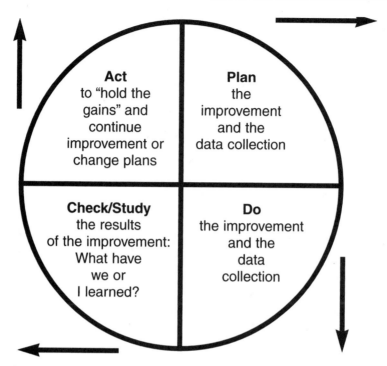

Figure 8-1. The PDCA cycle.

3. Run through the cycle again, possibly under different environmental conditions

The PDCA Cycle is at the heart of continuous quality improvement (CQI), because it uses a cycle to identify problems, causes, and solutions, and then evaluates if those solutions were effective. It is said (source unknown) that *anything that can be done, can be done better.* Therefore, continuously repeating the cycle over again can further improve the process. Brian Joiner, one of the authors of *The Team Handbook,* once said, "The basic notion of PDCA is so simple that when I first heard it I felt I understood it in five minutes. Now, more than a decade later, I think I might understand it some day. . . but I have come to realize that PDCA is the essence of managerial work: making sure the job gets done today and developing better ways to do it tomorrow" (Joiner, 1994, pp. 44, 46).

UNDERSTANDING THE RELATIONSHIP BETWEEN QUALITY IMPROVEMENT PROJECTS AND THE PDCA CYCLE

In Chapter 5, the planning and sequencing of quality improvement projects was discussed in detail. The five essential steps in a quality improvement project include:

1. Baseline measurement
2. Initiation of case management interventions
3. Early interim measurement to assess success of interventions
4. Remeasurement
5. Evaluation

However, before any measurement, an intensive planning and assessment phase must clarify exactly what the problem is and the potential interventions that may bring about an improvement. That PLANNING step corresponds to the "P" phase of the PDCA cycle. Chapter 5 detailed important questions and considerations that must be clarified before "baseline measurement."

Therefore, the "P" phase will determine:

- What the organization will measure; what is important to the organization
- An acceptable budget
- What/Who is the target population of the measurement
- Clarification of case management goals and objectives
- Which specific quality indicators will give measurable, objective data
- How the data will be selected, collected, and measured, including the data collection methods and designs, the data sources, and how data analysis will take place
- What the known risks are of applying/withholding the intervention(s) chosen
- The communication strategy
- And, perhaps most importantly, the feasibility of the interventions selected

In the "DO" stage of the PDCA Cycle, the quality improvement project begins in earnest. Baseline data are measured, and the case management interventions are initiated. Some CQI experts believe that the whole PDCA cycle should be done initially on a small scale. This allows small-scale changes if problems arise, rather than major overhauls. This concept will become especially apparent during the DO stage.

The "CHECK" phase of the PDCA Cycle involves the evaluation of the progress of the quality improvement project. The quality improvement project step of "early interim measurement to assess success of interventions" is a good method to check the progress. On a small scale, use the quality indicators decided on in the planning stage as a measure to compare the baseline measurement and the interim measurement. Check and study:

- Whether there is improvement, deterioration, or no change from the baseline measurement
- The impact of case management interventions
- Any lessons learned

The fourth stage of the PDCA Cycle is the "ACT" phase. At this time, the quality improvement team has a small interim measure. The ACTION planned will depend on what was confirmed from the CHECK/STUDY phase. Did the case management interventions result in improvement, deterioration of the process, or no change? What could be done differently? What were the lessons learned? The evaluation of the results of the interim measurement should be done before the actual "remeasurement" of data. This will allow time to change courses, if necessary, so that a better remeasurement can be realized.

Finally, the *remeasurement of the data* is done; it is then compared with the baseline data and the interim measurement data. When the results of the remeasurement data show that the case management interventions were not as successful as hoped for, cycle back to the PLANNING step of Evaluation, to determine whether small (or large) changes in the interventions may produce better results. *This cycling back to the PLANNING step can occur in either the "CHECK" stage or the "ACT" stage.* Lastly, ACT to sustain the improvement, and disseminate the results, conclusions, and recommendations of the project to administration and others who would benefit by the information.

The remaining chapter will detail the PDCA Cycle, with a "case management twist."

Plan DCA CYCLE

Plan a Change or a Test Aimed at Improvement, Plan the Data Collection

The planning phase of the PDCA Cycle is perhaps the most important of all aspects of the cycle; it is certainly the most intensive. In the Assessment Stage in case management, the assessment is the critical link between the patient and the case management plan. The planning phase of the PDCA Cycle is the critical link between the project and the success of the improvement effort. This phase is actually one of assessment and planning. One CQI tenet is that is it wise to spend 80% of the project's time in the "planning" part of the cycle and 20% in the "doing" part of the cycle. The oriental countries recognized this fact (probably from the influence of the two Americans, Juran and Deming) and therefore spent much less time in the "fixing" phase. It may well be that many other countries, and certainly individual organizations, reverse these percentages.

A great deal of effort is required in the planning phase. The organization must determine goals and methods of reaching these goals. An action plan must be prepared that addresses *key quality indicators* or *key performance indicators*. These indicators will target:

- **What** will be done; which improvements will need to be made; identification of aspects of the improvement that will have the greatest impact on customer needs

The **Planning Phase** also will determine:

- **Who** will be responsible for each action. Assure that the "owner" of the process is involved. Empower the team and help to remove barriers.
- Set the timelines: **When** will the tasks be done?
- **Where** will the tasks be accomplished?
- **How** will the tasks be accomplished? How will the data collection be accomplished? How shall we measure to answer our questions—to confirm or reject our prediction?

Because of its complexity, the **Planning Phase** will be broken down into four components by applying the acronym **CASE**. Like utilization management modalities, this acronym is a "tool, not a rule" to be used as a road map and a reminder system to aid the case manager or project manager in remembering all aspects of the planning process. Note that in Display 8-1, The Case Management Continuous Quality Improvement Process, CASE is embedded within the "P" Phase of the PDCA Cycle.

Clarify case management opportunities for improvement
Assess the initial data
Strategize the target interventions for improvement
Evaluate the feasibility and plan the pilot test

The Case Management Continuous Quality Improvement Process chart displays this case management PDCA Cycle. It also suggests various tools for

DISPLAY 8-1 **The Case Management Continuous Quality Improvement Process**

Plan the improvement and the data collection

  Clarify case management opportunities for improvement

  Assess the data

  Strategize the target interventions for improvement

  Evaluate for feasibility and plan the pilot test

Useful Tools and Techniques in the Plan Phase

Force field analysis
Pareto chart
Brainstorming
Flowcharts
Check sheets
Control charts
Nominal group technique/ Multivoting
Cause-and-effect diagram
Run charts

Do the improvement and the data collection on a small scale

Useful Tools and Techniques in the Do Phase

Check sheets	Surveys
Run charts	Control charts
Flowcharts	Pareto charts
Scatter diagram	Histograms
Cause-and-effect diagrams	

Check the results of the pilot project

Useful Tools and Techniques in the Check Phase

Control charts	Run charts
Histograms	Pareto charts
Cause-and-effect diagram	

Act to continue improving the process

Useful Tools and Techniques in the Act Phase

Flowcharts	Check sheets
Control charts	Pareto charts
Brainstorming	
Cause-and-effect diagrams	
Nominal group technique/multivoting	

CASE © PDCA is an acronym that can be used by case managers to assess, plan, test, evaluate, and put into action efforts of quality improvement. The acronym CASE is actually embedded in the "Planning" phase of the PDCA cycle.

process improvement and decision-making techniques that may clarify issues as they come up in each phase. The tools for process improvement are discussed in detail in Chapter 7; the problem-solving, decision-making techniques are discussed in Chapter 9.

Clarify Case Management Opportunities for Improvement ASE

During the "C" planning phase, improvement opportunities are revealed by looking at processes, services, and aspects of case management performance. The problem is often the part of the process that creates a "bottleneck." The team that is to prioritize the selection of the process or condition to be measured and improved may want to start by brainstorming possible areas to examine. Opportunities for improvement can be identified from many sources. Customer feedback is often the noisiest, and a case manager's "customers" may include patients, physicians, various levels of care/facilities, and other case managers. Claims data, utilization management, or case management performance data may also point an improvement team in a specific direction. Policy and Procedures may be old or invalid and need updating. Rarely is there a lack of improvement opportunities; more often, there is lack of time and personnel to improve all of the areas selected. Some important processes, services, and aspects of case management performance that may be examined as potential areas to improve include:

1. *The Case Management Process—Evaluation of Performance*
   The Case Management process is followed appropriately and completely according to the needs of the patient/family/multidisciplinary team. Investigate the following processes/case management tasks:
   a. Case screening, referral, and selection
   b. Assessment (of all medical, psychosocial, financial issues)/problem identification
   c. Coordination and development of the treatment and discharge plans
   d. Implementation of the plans
   e. Continuous monitoring, assessment, evaluation of case status, plans, outcomes
   f. Evaluation of outcomes
   g. Follow-ups throughout the continuum as needed
2. *Confidentiality*
   a. Patient information is kept confidential in accordance with policies and applicable laws
   b. Patient information is limited and shared solely on an "as needed" basis
3. *Use of: CMSA (Case Management Society of America) "Standards of Practice for Case Management" and CCMC (Commission for Case Manager Certification) "Code of Professional Conduct for Case Managers"*
   a. Case Managers are knowledgeable about above Standards/Code.
   b. Case Managers will work within the established Standards/Code.

4. *Case Management Orientation/Training*—Is the training:
   a. Thorough and accurate
   b. Appropriate to the type of case management performed
   c. Ongoing and continuous
   d. Clinically accurate for the type of cases being case-managed
5. *Performance Evaluations of Case Managers*
6. *Case Management Reports*—Examine the reports for:
   a. Timeliness/regular updates
   b. Accuracy
   c. Completeness
7. *Understanding of Insurance Types/Issues as They Relate to Case Management*
8. *Conducts Case Management Activities Ethically;* Guided by *CMSA Statement Regarding Ethical Case Management Practice*
9. *Practices Case Management in Accordance with Applicable Laws*
10. *Resource Utilization*—appraise for:
    a. Appropriateness
    b. Integrated with factors relating to quality, safety, efficiency, and cost-effectiveness of whole case
    c. That case managers are knowledgeable about various utilization management modalities
    d. Negotiation attempts for more extensive services than Plan allows are done appropriately, professionally, and proper people are notified

After a list of potential improvement candidates has been generated, the next step is to prioritize the list to the critical few that need immediate attention. "Think 20/80." What 20% of the work is creating 80% of the problems (Executive Learning, 1997)? Prioritizing of selections is important. Today's resources are limited; therefore, it is critical that the team's time and energy are spent on something that can be impacted on (*i.e.,* that is feasible). Along the same vein, choose something that is meaningful; the people involved must desire a change in the process or condition and believe that their efforts to change will be worthwhile.

After it is clear what the process will be that needs improvement, the next step will be to evaluate the team. Does it include everyone that is needed to identify the steps in the process? Select multidisciplinary members who have a good understanding of the process being evaluated. The team also may need a data analyst or statistician (at least as a resource for the team). Team selection is important because teams will be responsible for:

- Designing the scope of project
- Identifying the problem(s)

THE THREE "Ms" FOR PRIORITY SELECTION
MUST BE CONSIDERED:

1. **Is it Meaningful?**
   If it is not a priority to the team, the change may not come to completion.
2. **Is it Measurable?**
   If it can't be measured, how will you know the change is an improvement?
3. **Is it Manageable?**
   The change must be feasible.

- Developing solutions
- Implementing solutions

Collect information to clarify *current knowledge of the process.* It is recommended that a problem statement be put in writing. This is to assure that everyone on the team understands clearly and precisely the problem and the target improvement. It should describe the condition/process as it currently exists (see section on flow charts as an excellent tool for this process), including identification of standards, suppliers, and customer requirements and expectations. Next, compare current processes and the results of those processes with requirements and expectations. Look for any problems or opportunities for improvement in the chosen condition/process.

TIPS FOR THE "C" PLANNING PHASE

- Be diligent about COMMUNICATIONS to everyone involved—from those on high to those who will be affected by the change. When the team has a *short* timeline with which to do the job, the team may ask for *written* input from the actual workers in the process about what they perceive the problems and potential solutions are.
- Pick a project for change that is not already in the middle of a revision.
- Set timelines and time limits for everyone.
- Gain support from top management—they can help remove barriers or **be** the barrier. Another essential team member is a "champion" who is respected (such as a physician).

- BUDGETS! Secure support and resource commitment. Improvement teams are valuable; over the long term, CQI efforts will save money and improve quality. However, they can be expensive. Allocation of resources must be considered. For example:

	the time spent (hours × number of meetings + individual work)
×	the number of people
×	the salaries
=	$$$ spent for meetings, work time plus miscellaneous charges (supplies, overtime, etc.)

C Assess the Initial (Baseline) Data SE

The definition of *data* is simply facts or figures from which conclusions can be drawn (Webster's). Assessing data may be the most intimidating part of CQI for case managers, yet it is essential to understand and measure outcomes. To show improvement, it is imperative to be able to analyze the problem or opportunity for improvement from data; this is how we will know that the action or intervention caused a change in the outcomes. That does not mean case managers must be statisticians; statisticians or data analysts can be "borrowed" or used as consultants. These resource people can help define the correct data to collect to elicit the information desired and therefore not waste time and resources collecting unnecessary data.

After the team has done the "C" planning phase of clarifying which opportunity for improvement to target, baseline data must be gathered. The baseline data will be compared with the data after implementation of the chosen intervention to improve the process. In the simplest of terms, an entire quality improvement project can be broken down into three steps (see Outcomes Management chapters for more on Improvement Project steps):

1. Gather baseline data and measure them.
2. Do the intervention/action.
3. Remeasure and evaluate changes in the outcomes.

The data in step 1 (baseline data) and step 3 (data from remeasurement after a new intervention has started) will be compared. The expectation is that the intervention conducted in step 2 will cause the remeasurement data to demonstrate that improvement has occurred.

Here the team must decide *what* to measure to evaluate the process chosen, and *how to* measure it. This may include identifying a sample size to study and the correct methodology with which to study the process. Identify a list of influential factors or *root causes* of the problem. An excellent tool for evaluating this process is the *cause-and-effect diagram* described in Chapter 7. Assure that a clear data collection plan is developed and adhered to. "Just in time" training may be needed about a variety of topics: understanding the "how" and "why" of data collecting, reading control charts, etc.

An important recommendation for this phase of data collection and assessment involves the importance of *operational definitions*. An operational definition "is a description in quantifiable terms of what to measure and steps to follow to measure it consistently. . .operational definitions are the most frequent reason for poor data collection and problems in getting meaningful information from the data collected" (Executive Learning, 1997). For example, if timeliness is a measure that the team deems to be important, then the team will have to operationally define what the customer views as timeliness. Without that fact, the target to work toward is nebulous.

Remember, this is *baseline* data you will be collecting. And *any method used for baseline data collection also must be used for remeasurement data collection.* To change the collection methods will skew the results. *Run charts* and *control charts* are often used to measure and compare health care data. "It is critical that performance indicator information be placed onto a run chart or control chart so that the picture of the process performance is created. A single point of data in a report does not show how the process is performing over a period of time" (Executive Learning, 1997). When the remeasurement data run chart or control chart is created, it can easily be compared with the chart made at baseline (done in this step); this before-and-after "picture" will be worth a thousand words to the business side of the health care world. An example of this type of data is in the section on control charts (Chapter 7). The "Diabetic Control Sheet" demonstrates a comparison of "before-and-after" the patients were taught to monitor and chart their own blood sugars. The blood sugars were more "in control" after the patients were taught to use the control chart. The "after" blood sugar chart is generated in the *Check Phase* of the PDCA Cycle.

C A Strategize the Target Interventions for Improvement E

In the "S" planning phase, the team will develop strategies and a plan for implementation that enhances a vision of a more ideal condition. As in the "C" planning phase, it is time to generate another rich selection of options; however, rather than determining processes to improve, the team will determine which intervention(s) may be the key to improvement (See section on

Interventions in Chapter 5). At this time, the team must answer three questions:

1. *Which interventions are going to be conducted?* To answer that question, generate a list of promising solutions; decide on which processes to change; use benchmark data or other available indicators/data whenever possible; review the literature; and look at improvements others have made from other comparable departments, facilities, or agencies.

    An intervention also can be the elimination of a step or steps in a process. Consider the flowchart exercise where the team develops one flowchart showing exactly how a process occurs; a second flowchart indicates the ideal method of the same process. Perhaps several redundant steps were identified. Then the team must ask, "if this step was missed would anyone be hurt by it?" Consider how one change will affect other people, processes, and systems as a whole.

2. *How much improvement is the team going to strive for?* If the intervention can be plotted in numeric terms, set a numeric target for improvement that is significantly beyond the current performance. As Dr. Berwick says, "don't be timid"! Team goals may include improvement of customer satisfaction by 20%; reduction of timeframes by 50%; or improvement of productivity by 35%.

3. *How will the team know that an improvement has occurred?* It is essential to use the planning phase to determine ahead of time how the team will assess progress.

Nothing is more wasteful than to plan a change, make the change, and be unable to tell whether it had any significant effect. . . Before making a change, write down the expected benefits and how you will know whether they have been achieved. As you carry out the plan, capture notes on key events, anything related to what does or does not go according to plan. Then force yourself to study the results. It will be a humbling exercise! Document the lessons learned and take action. Keep it up. The next experience will also be disappointing, but less so. Momentum will build as you continue to turn the PDCA wheel. (Joiner, 1994, p. 50)

TIPS FOR THE "S" PLANNING PHASE

- Consider the three "Ms" for priority selection. The intervention must be meaningful, measurable, and manageable.
- "Think 20/80." What 20% of the work is creating 80% of the problems (Executive Learning, 1997)? What few changes will give us the greatest gain?

- Be diligent about communications to everyone.
- Set timelines and time limits for everyone.
- Obtain support from top management.
- Secure support and resource (budget) commitment.

Lastly, remember to "connect the dots." Confirm that this step relates to the original selection for improvement in the "C" planning phase.

CAS Evaluate for Feasibility and Plan the Pilot Test

In the "E" planning phase, the team must accomplish two tasks:

1. *Plan the pilot test that will establish the new process.* Essentially, the team will create an implementation plan including a decision about which tasks are to be accomplished and which processes need to be implemented. It is also useful to identify and plan for resistance to change; it is almost inevitable. The planning team may even decide to establish an implementation team specific for the "Do" phase of the PDCA Cycle, when the implementation will actually be accomplished. Specific tasks to be determined include:
   - How the pilot test will be run on a "small, manageable scale," and the combinations and number of proposed changes to run
   - How to sequence the steps
   - The timeline for each step, including how to schedule the interventions
   - The use of "varying conditions" (different days of week, times of day, departments) to test the efficacy of the interventions in several ways
   - What remeasurement data will be collected (who, where, how, when)
   - If training is required for data collection, and how data collection will be abstracted and monitored
2. *Determine whether the plan is feasible.* This is critical and feasibility means that the plan is capable of being accomplished. To determine whether the plan is feasible, the team must determine potential barriers to improvement. These barriers may be in the form of people, resistance to change, lack of resources (personnel or financial), tight timeframes—the list can be very long (see barriers to change in Disease Management chapters). However, it is better to know hurdles the teams must overcome *beforehand*; the team can then plan for them. No project plan can be labeled a feasible plan unless this exercise in exorcizing the barriers is accomplished.

It is essential that communication to everyone who may be impacted is continuous and clear. Here is where leadership support is essential—they are the ones who can remove barriers to change, or be the barrier to change!

PDoCA CYCLE

Do the Experiment

Begin the pilot improvement and the data collection on a limited scale. Education and training of all key people is done in this stage. This will include training those who are collecting the data and those who are performing the process. Data collection training will include testing for *interrelater reliability* during the training sessions. Education for those performing the process being evaluated will be specific to the details of the *quality indicators* used (see Chapter 4 for a discussion on quality indicators).

Implement the planned work; however, testing the process improvement on a small scale will conserve resources. If the test is "off the mark," problems can be identified early, and changes in the improvement plan can be implemented quickly and with less interruption to the areas being tested.

TIPS

1. A process is best understood by seeing it at the best of times and the worst of times; therefore, collect data and test improvement on the extremes of a process. This may necessitate testing a process at different times of the day, different days of the week, different levels of care, or in different departments/units.
2. Collect data that is limited and concise.
3. Post-intervention (remeasurement) data must match the pre-intervention (baseline) data collected to be able to make direct comparisons and see the true effects of the improvement effort.
4. Take care that, while improving one aspect of the process, another aspect of the process does not deteriorate.

PD CHECKA CYCLE

Check/Study the Results of the Pilot Project. What Was Learned?

Of all the steps in the PDCA cycle, the *Check phase* is the most important for rapid learning; "without it, improvement is nearly impossible" (Joiner, 1994, p. 47). Many organizations perform the *planning step* and the *doing step* consistently. However, the *checking step* is often done haphazardly. Here is where the lessons are learned, and "failures" are recycled into successful new insights. Sometimes this phase uncovers concerns that the organization would just as soon leave unexposed; but those are the issues that need to be revealed and changed. If there were negative outcomes, what was learned? Were they expected or unanticipated? Would staff training or educational efforts improve the process? Are more resources needed? Are more resources feasible?

Analyze the remeasurement data for results. Again, a key point to remember about remeasurement is that the data must be measured in the same way, using the same tools for remeasurement as was used in gathering baseline data. This allows an accurate and honest comparison and evaluation. Look at trends and patterns. Assess what factors most influence the problem/opportunity for improvement. Compare baseline data with the target benchmarks and your personal target improvement (established in the "S" planning phase); the difference between the remeasurement data and the desired benchmark data becomes the "gap in performance." Reducing or eliminating this gap is the goal of improvement efforts (Executive Learning, 1997). Then decide which change, or combination of changes, will produce the most improvement in the process.

Once the results of the pilot test have been thoroughly evaluated, one of three PDCA actions can become the next step:

1. If the pilot test was effective, move to the ACT phase.
2. If the pilot test was somewhat ineffective yet showed promise, begin the PLAN phase again (recycle PDCA), possibly under different environmental conditions. Running through the PDCA cycle will also continuously improve the process. Add a new monitoring component for measuring improvement. Examine what was learned during this cycle and improve on it as the pilot is recycled with a new change.
3. If the pilot test was ineffective or caused deterioration of the process, abandon the intervention. However, valuable lessons can be learned from "failed" experiments; therefore, this, too, becomes an opportunity for improvement.

PDCAct CYCLE

Act to Continuously Improve the Process

The team has selected the intervention(s) with the most positive impact on the indicator and little or no ill effects on the rest of the process. It is time to adopt the intervention. Take appropriate action based on the findings in the "Check" Phase. This may mean:

- Putting the pilot into "policy and procedure"
- Changing current flowcharts
- Train the staff

The ACT phase is about putting into practice the lessons learned from the whole quality improvement project. As needed, return and plan to repeat the PDCA Cycle again.

Act to "Hold the Gains"

"Holding the gains" is a CQI term for doing what is needed to sustain whatever improvement has been accomplished. This is essential. Many case managers have seen successful changes in their organizations falter after time. This can occur for several reasons. Perhaps the "champion" or "owner" of the project became involved in other activities or left the organization; or the reminder systems that were once used are now forgotten (and so is the improved process the reminder system was created for); or "more important" matters take priority. There is no lack of "reasons."

Many important improvement projects have been created to satisfy accreditation requirements or to gain an understanding of outcomes. These projects take a great deal of time, resources, and effort. It is unsettling to see an important critical area of patient improvement deteriorate after the JCAHO or NCQA team has left the building. But it happens. CQI teams disband, and the organization moves on to the next big adventure—too much to do and too little time and resources to do it.

The idea of "building capacity" in an organization is critical; this means that the organization will be independent, capable, and competent in the area recently improved—without the project team's constant supervision. Teams must move on; priorities do change; the same people cannot sustain the same project forever. The solution lies in teaching others to carry on important aspects of the new process. This is not unlike teaching a new diabetic or asthmatic how to sustain their health independently. More research is needed in this arena of "building capacity" both for sustaining improvement and in patient teaching. What factors lead to capacity building? What obstacles are encountered? How can these obstacles be overcome? Without it, the improvement project is a temporary expenditure of effort with temporary results. Case managers are well aware that education alone does not always change behavior. Education can result in short-term behavioral changes, to do well in the accreditation effort, or the remeasurement of a patient care indicator, or even to gain approval from a case manager or supervisor. Long-term behavioral changes are needed, as is an understanding on how to successfully promote and sustain these behaviors.

Disease management programs can benefit from being run through the PDCA Cycle on occasion. But can the PDCA Cycle be used for actual patient case management? In some ways this cycle resembles the case management process:

1. Case selection
2. Assessment/problem identification
3. Development and coordination of the case plan
4. Implementation of the plan
5. Evaluation and follow-up

PLANNING includes case selection, assessment, problem identification, and the development and coordination of the patient's individual case plan. DO corresponds to the case management implementation of the plan. CHECK is the constant monitoring, reassessment, and evaluation of the plan. ACT is the case management interventions and follow-up that occurs each time a case manager rechecks and recalibrates the patient's progress.

Case Managers Working in Project Teams

TEAMS AND TEAM MEETINGS

> A **team** is a group of people who have come together for a spe-
> cific purpose; ideally, teams are empowered to assess problems,
> initiate changes, and evaluate the impact of those changes.

Case managers are accustomed to working in teams. In fact, it is this aspect of
case management that offers one of our most valuable assets. In addition to
coordinating the care of multiple providers and systems, the case management
multidisciplinary team approach provides organizations with an important
function that is required for accreditations. Many of the techniques in this
chapter will be useful for all team encounters; some will be most useful when
working in improvement teams. Case managers well acquainted with multidisciplinary team work will find the continuous quality improvement (CQI) type
of team rewarding. However, there are fundamental differences between a *multidisciplinary patient care team* and a *CQI cross-functional team.*

Patient care teams may be planned for weekly or biweekly meetings. The
agenda and purpose is focused around patient care. Sometimes, patient care
conferences are impromptu, almost emergent, in their timing. Often, the team
members depend on which patient(s) need attention, and what the underlying
problems may be; this necessitates a constant changing of important team players. For example, if Mrs. Smith is having a sudden change of mental status, the
multidisciplinary team would consist of different members than for Mr. Jones,
who was recently a pedestrian in an automobile altercation.

A CQI team, however, most often has a set schedule, a specific goal or goals,
an assigned group of team members (with occasional experts called in) that will
change only infrequently, and has the initial luxury of a meeting or two to
get to know the team members and establish meeting guidelines. The cross-

functional team members can include almost anyone, depending on the reason for the initiation of the team: physicians, case managers, biostatisticians, computer programers, data analysts, administrators, financial personnel, etc. The team members are chosen for their ability to contribute to the problem needing to be solved.

The CQI cross-functional teams are Joint Commission on Accreditation of Healthcare Organizations (JCAHO) and National Committee for Quality Assurance (NCQA) mandated for regulatory requirements. They are also hailed as a "breakthrough in organization" by CQI guru Joseph Juran. It is this type of team that is discussed in the following pages. If a CQI team is organized with care and consideration, the experience can be productive and gratifying. Simple, basic, yet important team tips that follow can make the difference between a constructive use of time and a frustrated waste of everyone's time and resources.

Types of Teams

There are several types of CQI teams. Two of the most important for case management applications are the *steering teams or councils* and *improvement teams.* Typically, these teams are not permanent. Once the improvement is completed, they are disbanded (unless another round of continuous improvement will commence). The major function of a steering team/council is to coordinate and support improvement in the organization. This team plans, organizes, and facilitates other teams. Quality Councils are a type of steering team; they assess the organization and initiate and "steer" improvement teams in the right direction.

Improvement teams exist to improve processes, products, services, morale, etc. Common names of improvement teams include process improvement teams (PIT), quality improvement teams (QIT), quality action teams (QAT), or performance improvement teams. These teams identify causes of problems using process improvement tools, plan process improvement, monitor the effectiveness of the action plan, maintain new standards, and identify opportunities for further improvement.

Understanding Stages of Team Development

Teams go through fairly predictable stages before reaching maturity and synergy. Understanding these stages as normal may keep groups from overreacting or setting unrealistic expectations too soon in the team process. Initial team meetings are essential for both learning about the process being studied and learning about the team members. The first few meetings set the tone for the team and will take the team through the "norming" and "storming" stages discussed below. In time-sensitive meetings such as impromptu patient care meetings, these steps are neither practical nor advised. However, when a team will be together for several weeks or months, the first few meetings should "set the stage." These meetings provide time to define specific goals:

TEAM BUILDING GOALS

- Getting to know team members' skills, backgrounds, and styles
- Learning to work together as a team
- Reviewing roles and expectations
- Working out decision-making issues
- Setting meeting ground rules

PROJECT GOALS

- Understanding and agreeing on the scope of the project
- Examining and evaluating available resources
- Developing a work plan
- Reviewing the organization's and team's mission statements

EDUCATIONAL GOALS

- If the team is expected to use tools and methods that are unfamiliar to them, provide educational resources. "Just in time" training should be considered. For example, if the team requires knowledge about flowcharts, Pareto diagrams, or building consensus, bring in experts to teach the team these skills *when* they are needed.

After the first few meetings, much of the groundwork has been laid, and the work can begin in earnest. These are the "norming" and "performing" stages. The team's work should settle into a routine of reviewing progress of the project, discussing and deciding what the next steps might be, providing new or revised project plans, and planning "between meeting" assignments.

One team, perhaps the best and most productive I have ever been on, consisted of long-term, stable employees who had always worked well together. It came as a surprise when, at about the third meeting as a Quality Council team, irritation set in and tempers flared. The team was well versed in team dynamics; so when one member came up with the enlightened reason ("we are in the `storming' stage"), the team relaxed and got down to business. The four stages are:

1. Forming
2. Storming
3. Norming
4. Performing

During the *forming* stage, there are feelings of excitement, anticipation, optimism, and pride in being chosen for the team. However, there also may be some suspicion, fear, and anxiety about the team's responsibility, and perhaps a little resentment about the additional time demands. Team members may struggle to discover acceptable group behavior or may have difficulty in identifying relevant problems. Complaints about the organization's barriers to the task may be a common cry. Case managers who are responsible for leading the group can help move the team past this stage by helping team members get to know each other, provide a clear direction and purpose, suggest goals, involve all members in developing plans and clarifying roles, provide information the team will need to get started, and set a motivational climate.

During the *storming* stage, the members may feel resistance to anything new, different, or uncomfortable. There may be defensiveness, competition, resentment of authority, tension, or jealousy. Team members may display arguing, even when there is apparent agreement; they may be defensive, establish unrealistic goals, be concerned about excessive work, and create discord and a perceived "pecking order." Case managers who are responsible for leading the group can help move the team past this stage by helping team members resolve issues of power and authority, create a climate of change, encourage creativity and nonjudgmental participation, help to obtain resources, manage conflicts, adapt the leadership role to allow the team to become more independent, and encourage team members to take on more responsibility.

During the *norming* stage, team members are able to get down to work. There is more excitement, optimism, relief, acceptance, trust, and a healthy ability to express criticism in a constructive manner. Team members will confide more in each other, and they will discuss team dynamics honestly. There is more of a team spirit and a strong sense of common goals. This is a time to relook at team ground rules (the "norms") and tweak them. There is an underlying relief that things seem to be working out. Case managers who are responsible for leading the group can assist by helping team members fully use skills, knowledge, and experience, encourage collaboration and respect for fellow team members, review progress constantly, assist in correcting mistakes, push people out of their comfort zones, and reward successes as they occur.

During the *performing* stage, the atmosphere is one of enthusiasm, comfort with group processes, learning to accept personal differences, and understanding of individual strengths and weaknesses. There is satisfaction with the team's progress. The team will be more cohesive, more work gets done during this stage, and there is an ability to prevent, or work through, group problems. Case managers who are responsible for leading the group can assist by updating the team's methods to encourage cooperation and problem solving, help the team to understand and manage "change," monitor work progress, and delegate more decision-making and problem-solving to the team.

Team Roles and Responsibilities

Suppose a health maintenance organization's (HMO) upper management team (we will call them a Quality Council) decides that an improvement team should be initiated; they would like to address a new disease management program and use case management as a pivotal intervention. Deciding who should be on the team is one of the most important steps in initiating a successful project. The Quality Council may choose a primary member to get the team started: one who has a good working knowledge of the process that is to be created or improved. That person will then have to ask defining questions for selection of the other team members:

- Who has the organizational influence to move mountains? (You will want that person on your team!)
- Who must be represented for their "perspective" of the whole project?
- Who are impacted by the process being studied or the potential new process?
- Who can contribute to an understanding of the process (financial, clinical, information systems)?
- Who has special skills that can be used in the improvement process?

Teams that are too large (more than about eight members) often have problems. It is difficult to get schedules merged for meeting times; there are often too many varied perspectives to come to a consensus; and it is expensive in salary and time resources. Another idea is to have a small core of improvement team members; then have expert guests who have specialized knowledge of the topic invited as a resource.

Once a team is in place, roles within the team must be clearly defined for a smooth-functioning unit. Just as *Job Descriptions* are necessary in an organization, they are also essential in a team setting. The following represent the main roles to consider in team meetings:

The *Quality Advisor* is often a member of the Quality Council. This person acts as a team advisor or consultant and has expertise in the quality improvement process. The goal of the quality advisor is to move the team to one of self-sufficiency in working together as a group and in use of the process improvement tools; as self-sufficiency increases, involvement of the Quality Advisor decreases. The Quality Advisor

- Is a process improvement expert
- Does not need to be knowledgeable about the process being evaluated. Often, by being a nonexpert in the process that requires improvement, the quality advisor also serves as a clear voice-of-reason if disagreements mount.
- Provides "just in time" training. The Quality Advisor is more focused on process than outcome (for example, focuses on how decisions are made rather than what decisions are reached).
- Is not responsible for running meetings or handling administrative details
- Assists with the team's learning process by helping with tools and acting as a resource
- Assists the Team Leader in assigning and structuring tasks and individual assignments
- Works with the Team Leader between meetings to plan meetings and revise plans in response to team member suggestions
- Tracks the team progress and works with the Team Leader and management to implement the new process
- Helps the team to construct pictures from the data to make it clear to people outside the team
- Helps the team to decide which data to collect and what would be most useful
- Helps the team to prepare for presentations
- Is an advisor and mentor; continually develops personal skills in facilitating, group processes, and training
- Breaks down barriers to success

The *Team Leader* is often recognized as the "facilitator" of the work process being evaluated. Team Leaders coordinate and direct the work of the team. They often facilitate the team meetings and are also team members who contribute ideas, help to interpret data, and participate in all team decisions. The meeting's facilitator role is sometimes rotated; this is a good idea when organizations are teaching CQI principles, because it gives experience to a wide range of employees. However, in some circles, rotating the facilitator role causes a lack of continuity and consistency. Facilitators responsibilities include

- Managing and coordinating team activities; keeps the team on schedule
- Keeps communication channels open

- Is the "content" expert, having a functional knowledge of the process
- Is a "change agent" to influence other workers
- Calls the meetings and leads the team meeting according to the agenda (may be responsible for writing the agenda)
- Leads the team through the improvement process
- Helps the team use the quality tools and techniques
- Communicates with the Quality Advisor and other pertinent people before and after team meetings to minimize risk and surprises
- Leads the team through the stages of team growth/development
- Establishes an environment that encourages individual participation and growth
- Delegates administrative duties for the team
- Reports/presents progress to the Quality Council or others who "need to know"
- Implements approved recommendations
- Recognizes team members' contributions

Quality improvement teams are made up of *Team Members*. Team Members should consider their participation as a priority responsibility, rather than an intrusion on their "real jobs." They are the functional core of any team. A Team Member:

- Must have a fundamental knowledge of the process being evaluated/implemented
- Contributes as fully as possible to the project, sharing their knowledge and expertise, and participates in and attends all meetings and discussions
- Develops and implements improvement plans
- Carries out assigned tasks between meetings
- Communicates a positive picture of the team's progress, successes, and "lessons learned" to co-workers
- Learns appropriate quality improvement tools
- Analyzes the process, applying appropriate quality improvement tools (*e.g.,* flowcharts, charts, and diagrams)
- Is a "team player" (listens, communicates, participates, is enthusiastic, cooperative, hard-working, dedicated, punctual, customer-oriented, and has a sense of humor)
- Is receptive to change

The *Recorder* is the eyes and ears of the team process. The Recorder is responsible for the meeting minutes, which are the historical reference for the team. This position may be assigned permanently, for a set period, or may be rotated. The recorder:

- Records the team's mission as defined by the consensus process
- Summarizes and records the work and decisions of the team
- Composes the minutes of each meeting and distributes them to the team and Quality Advisor

The *Scribe* may be assigned permanently, for a set period, or may be rotated. The Scribe should write large enough for the team to see clearly, write legibly, check with the team for accuracy, and not worry about spelling. The Scribe:

- Keeps ideas "visible" during the meetings (*e.g.,* on flipcharts)
- Organizes the team's key ideas, questions, agreements, etc.
- Gives the flipcharts to the Recorder at the end of the meeting to include in the minutes

The *Timekeeper* may be assigned permanently, for a set period, or may be rotated. It is the team's responsibility to manage time, but the timekeeper assists the team in this function. The Timekeeper:

- Keeps the team on track according to the time set on the agenda
- Calls out the time remaining on each agenda item at intervals determined by the team

Characteristics of Effective Teams

Teams increase the probability of successfully discovering and implementing a solution to a problem; the sum total knowledge of a group is greater than that of a single individual. However, poorly run teams can result in a waste of time, expense, and frustration for all involved. Productive teams will have many of the following characteristics, although it may take some time (and a few norming and storming meetings) to reach this level of maturity.

- Team members are clear about the team's mission and goals.
- Team members have clearly defined roles and responsibilities.
- Communication is direct, succinct, and there is free expression; criticism is constructive.
- Team members actively listen to each other; input from all members is valued.
- Only one person speaks at a time; interruptions are minimal.
- All team members participate in discussions in balanced doses.

- A cooperative, friendly, supportive climate exists; members seem to enjoy each other.
- Team members are committed and complete assignments; they work toward a common goal.
- Team members use an agenda; the agenda is mostly adhered to.
- The team has well-defined decision-making procedures that are understood by members.
- The team agrees to and adheres to a set of "team ground rules."
- Good minutes are kept so that past decisions are easily found.
- Periodically, the team stops to assess its own performance.
- Team members share knowledge for the benefit of the project.
- Team members use a scientific approach to drawing conclusions about causes/solutions.
- Members feel free to express disagreement during discussions; conflicts are worked out.
- Team members make every attempt to attend meetings; it is a priority for them.
- Team decisions reflect a consensus; this is facilitated by the team leader.
- The work of the team is accepted and used; management supports the team's recommendations or changes.
- The whole team is given credit and recognized for accomplishments; success is shared.

Characteristics of Effective Team Meetings

USE OF GROUND RULES

Ground rules are explicit agreements about how a team will work together, define roles and responsibilities, and apply general courtesies. These will become the "norms" for the group, and the group is encouraged to intervene if these rules are consistently broken. It is highly recommended that ground rules be discussed and agreed to early in the "forming" developmental stages of the team. In fact, this is an excellent avenue to help the group understand each other and learn what is important to the group. An example of a ground rule may be that the group decides to start and end on time (as Parkinson's Law states that work expands to fill the available time). Other examples are in Box 9-1. They may be used as a template, or the team may prefer to use the following list and start their ground rules from scratch. The important point is that consensus should be reached on each rule. General areas for the team to discuss and make ground rules for include:

Box 9-1

EXAMPLE RULES FOR EFFECTIVE MEETINGS

Planning and Conducting Meetings

1. Arrive on time.
2. Start on time.
3. End on time.
4. Have an agenda.
   - The development of the agenda is the responsibility of the facilitator.
   - Agenda items from team members must be in the facilitator's "In Box" by _____ days before the meeting.
   - Distribute the agenda before the meeting (preferably 24–72 hours before the meeting.)

   The standardized agenda should include:
   a. Topics for discussion and a facilitator for each topic
   b. Time estimates for each topic
   c. Attachments for each topic, if applicable
   d. Old business/new business
   e. Action plans
   f. Five minutes at the end of the meeting to summarize
5. Facilitator responsibilities are rotated. If the facilitator cannot attend the meeting, she/he is to ask the next assigned facilitator to take over. If that is not possible, another facilitator may be requested.
6. Notify the facilitator/team leader if you cannot attend. No substitutes are to be sent in your absence.
7. Assign a Timekeeper to keep the meeting topics within allotted timeframes.
8. Assign a recorder to take notes.
9. At the conclusion of the meeting, take time to summarize decisions reached, including action plans and timeframes. This will allow everyone to leave the meeting with a clear direction.

Participation Etiquette

10. "Seek first to understand, then to be understood."
11. Be loyal to those present and absent.
12. Keep confidential discussions confidential.
13. Stay within the topic. Do not digress from the agenda unless the consensus agrees to do so. Watch "hidden agendas."
14. Be courteous: avoid nonconstructive criticism; speak one at a time; do not interrupt. It is alright to disagree; it is not alright to be disagreeable.

(continued)

Box 9-1 *(Continued)*

15. Use the "100 Mile" rule: No one should be called from a meeting unless it is so important that the disruption would occur even if the meeting was 100 miles away from the meeting.
16. Be prepared.
17. Everyone participates.
18. Discussions will be candid and open; creativity is encouraged.
19. Votes are based on a quorum of at least _____.
20. Meetings will not be canceled unless there is a consensus of agreement.
21. Follow-up on your commitments; display integrity.
22. Have fun! (and refreshments are nice.)

- Attendance at meetings
- Assignments and between-meeting work (preparation)
- Responsibilities for record keeping, logistics, communication
- Conflict management
- Decision-making
- Promptness to meetings
- Participation
- Interruptions (phone calls, beepers, etc.)
- Rotation of roles and chores
- Fun, humor, celebration
- Confidentiality
- Basic communication courtesies

USE OF AGENDAS

Agendas provide structure to a meeting. Some teams prefer to write the next agenda at the conclusion of the current meeting. This works well, because the ideas are fresh and everyone can agree on priorities as a team. Some teams allow time between meetings to "add" to the agenda. This is useful when important items come up unexpectedly; but assessment and caution are advised because:

- The agenda item was not agreed to by the whole team.
- When new, unexpected agenda items arise every week, it could sway the team into tangents; adhere to the original focus of the team whenever possible.

MEETING CHECKLIST

Preparation for a meeting:
- ☐ Decide on purpose/meeting objectives
- ☐ Notify participants
- ☐ Prepare and distribute agenda in advance of the meeting
- ☐ Book meeting room for correct date/time
- ☐ Set up meeting room (chairs, tables, equipment, materials, etc.)
- ☐ Team Leader/Facilitator is identified

During the meeting:
- ☐ Start on time
- ☐ Use printed agenda
- ☐ Introduction of the Team Leader/Facilitator, members
- ☐ Assign roles (Timekeeper, Scribe)
- ☐ Review, change, order the objectives on the agenda
- ☐ Manage time—ensure time limits are clear
- ☐ Ensure the group keeps objectives in focus
- ☐ Use of meeting etiquette/ground rules

Ending the meeting:
- ☐ Summarize decisions and important points
- ☐ Assign between meeting responsibilities
- ☐ Set next meeting (date, time, place)
- ☐ Evaluate the meeting
- ☐ End on time
- ☐ Clean the room after the meeting

After the Meeting:
- ☐ Prepare the minutes and distribute
- ☐ Follow up on assignments—support team as needed
- ☐ Go to "Preparation for a Meeting"

FILL KEY MEETING ROLES

Each team should decide which positions will be permanent, semipermanent, or rotated for each meeting. If the position is rotated (perhaps a timekeeper or scribe), address this at the beginning of each meeting, or have a rotational schedule. Facilitators are key to the meeting process. Team Leaders or Quality Advisors may fill this role, but the team also may choose to rotate the facilitator role to allow everyone to gain valuable experience.

TAKE MINUTES

Minutes are the major communication avenue for the team and are a record of the team's progress; they are essential to reconstruct past decisions and help absent team members stay current on the decisions of the team.

ADHERE TO THE "100 MILE RULE"

No one should be called from a meeting unless it is so important that the disruption would occur even if the meeting was 100 miles away from the workplace.

SUMMARIZE THE MEETING AT THE END

At the conclusion of the meeting, allow time to summarize decisions reached, including action plans and timeframes. This will enable everyone to leave the meeting with a clear direction.

DRAFT THE NEXT MEETING AGENDA

Some teams prefer to draft the next agenda at this time. Include time and place of the next meeting.

COMPUTE COST OF THE MEETING

Periodically, compute costs of the overhead, personnel salaries, materials, etc. Use this information to ensure that meetings are not a waste of time and resources. I was recently in a 2-day meeting where over 100 people, including a team of "experts," were expected to plan the foundation for an important project. The team was flown in from over five states and stayed in a comfortable hotel for 2 nights. The room was filled with physicians and PhDs. By the second day (when the team was somewhere between the forming and norming stages—partly due to the size), I tried to compute the cost per hour. Although there was no way I would really know the figure, I am sure it was quite impressive. And I wondered whether there was, perhaps, a better way to establish the project parameters.

PROJECT CLOSURE

Know when to say goodbye. All projects, and most teams, will reach a natural endpoint. The following are clues to a project's closure:

1. When the purpose of the project has been finished
2. When the work plan has been completed
3. When the indicators of improvement show progress, and further progress will clearly require a new, intensive effort
4. When there is agreement that this is the wrong team to do the project (*e.g.*, investigation has shown that the real problem is different from what was first thought, and a different team would better handle it)

DECISION-MAKING TECHNIQUES FOR PROCESS IMPROVEMENT

Decision-making steps in case management patient care conferences most often consist of gathering the clinical, financial, social, and insurance benefit information, adding in some creativity, and coming to a consensus on a patient care plan. It is not that techniques such as brainstorming or nominal group technique are never appropriate; however, the mood and time constraints of patient care conferences do not usually align with these techniques. In other types of meetings, the following are the tools for collaborative progress. Use them for getting to the core of problems and generating feasible ideas.

- Brainstorming
- Multivoting
- Nominal group technique
- Force field analysis
- Root cause analysis
- Consensus

There are basically two discussion stages involved in all decision-making techniques:

Stage 1: The *exploratory stage* is when the group is generating a rich pool of ideas, options, and perspectives. Brainstorming is a common method for this stage.

Stage 2: The *defining stage* is when the multiple choices must be whittled down to a necessary few, or one. During this stage, the choices are evaluated, sorted, and selected. Multivoting is a common method for this stage.

The decision-making techniques defined may initially feel awkward. But with practice, these techniques will flow in meetings at just the right time, and case managers will be acknowledged as brilliant meeting facilitators.

Brainstorming

Brainstorming is an easy way to generate a wide variety of ideas from all participants in a short amount of time. Anytime there is dissension among the case management ranks, brainstorming can be used to calm the storm. For example, if there is a major dispute about "handing-off" patients (and this could be within a hospital setting, or throughout a continuum), invite all the players into one arena. *Focus on processes, not people;* this is critical. And use brainstorming to simply list all of the possible processes that could be contributing to the problem.

GUIDELINES FOR BRAINSTORMING

1. Identify a facilitator and scribe.
2. Start by reviewing the topic. Make sure everyone understands the issue(s).
3. Explain the **RULES.** Some brainstorming rules include the following:
   a. Decide whether the brainstorming session will be a *round-robin* or *popcorn* style. Round-robin is where the team goes around the group and everyone says one idea until all finally "pass." Popcorn is where anyone can call out an idea, in no order, until all ideas are out.
   b. There is only one idea stated at a time.
   c. No criticism allowed; not even a groan or grimace!
   d. No idea is too "far out."
   e. It is alright to "hitchhike" (to build on the ideas of others).
   f. Anyone can "pass."
   g. There is no discussion during the brainstorm session.
   h. Each person takes a turn.
4. Give everyone a minute or two of "thinking time."
5. When the ideas start to flow, do not hold back.
6. Write the ideas where everyone can see them.
7. Brainstorm until the group "Brainstems"! End the session when everyone "passes."
8. Review or clarify the ideas as needed.
9. Rank/vote on the ideas (see other Decision-Making Techniques).

One variation on brainstorming is "paperstorming," in which the ideas are committed to paper or e-mail. This saves time and can be more private, although it does not allow for "hitchhiking," which is a powerful method of squeezing out more ideas.

Multivoting

Multivoting is designed to reduce a list of more than 10 ideas to a manageable number with limited discussion and difficulty. This is accomplished through a series of votes; each vote will cut the list more. Multivoting often follows a brainstorming session. If, for example, the brainstorming session above resulted in a list of 22 possible reasons for confusion and patients falling through the cracks during "hand-offs," then multivoting can limit the number to a manageable few.

Note that this is still a consensus of everyone's opinions. If there is time (a sparse commodity), the more scientific method would be collecting actual data about the problem, and perhaps using the brainstorming list as a data collection tool. Then, "Pareto" the results; put them on a Pareto chart to actually see which of the brainstormed problems rank as most common (See Pareto Charts, Chapter 7). Another method to really understand the process is to flowchart the way the process actually works, then flowchart the ideal process, and lastly, compare the two flowcharts (See Flowcharts in Chapter 7).

STEPS IN MULTIVOTING

1. Generate a list of items (this was done in a brainstorming session); number each item.
2. Combine similar items if the group agrees they are the same idea.
3. Agree on the number of ideas for which each member will vote. A general guideline is 25% to 33% of the ideas listed.
4. Have all members choose several items they would like to discuss or address by writing down the numbers of these items on a sheet of paper.
5. Tally the votes by asking for a show of hands for each item on the list that was voted on. Record and add the votes on a flipchart.
6. Decide which ideas should receive further consideration. Eliminate those items with the fewest votes. If any member feels very strongly about an idea, the team may decide to keep that item on the list. The size of the group affects the results. A rule of thumb:
   5 or fewer members—cross off items with only 1 or 2 votes
   6 to 15 members—eliminate anything with 3 or fewer votes
   >15 members—eliminate items with 4 or fewer votes

7. Repeat steps 3 through 6 on the remaining list of choices. Continue this until only a few items remain.

Nominal Group Technique

Nominal Group Technique (NGT) is a structured method of generating a list and then narrowing it down. The first phase is silent brainstorming (paper-storming). The second phase is voting to reduce the list. There is a relatively low level of interaction of the group members during phase 1; therefore, it is good for highly controversial issues. Again, this eliminates the often productive technique of "hitchhiking."

NOMINAL GROUP TECHNIQUE—PART ONE: A FORMALIZED BRAINSTORM

1. Clarify the objective of the NGT. The Team Leader/Facilitator may want to write the objective or question down so the members can refer back to it. Going back to the brainstorming problem, the leader may write: List all possible reasons why "handing-off" patients is not a smooth process; focus on processes, not people.
2. Generate ideas. It is important to have team members write down their list in silence. Eliminate distractions and allow adequate time for members to generate as many ideas as possible. Members should sit quietly until all are finished.
3. Go around the table and call out ideas in round-robin fashion with each member giving one idea at a time. Continue until all ideas are spoken. No discussion, criticisms, or compliments are allowed. List the items on a flipchart. (Or turn in papers to be put on the flipchart.)
4. Clarify and discuss the ideas. Have all flipcharts displayed at once. If anyone has questions, the initiator of the idea should answer, but others also may join in to help define and clarify the items. Condense the list as appropriate by combining similar items if the group agrees that they are the same idea.

NOMINAL GROUP TECHNIQUE—PART TWO: MAKING THE SELECTION

1. If there are more than 50 items, use multivoting to reduce the list to 50 items.
2. Give the team members 3 × 5 cards. Give four cards to each member for up to 20 items on the list; six cards for 20 to 35 items; eight cards for 35 to 50 items.

3. Each team member writes their preferred items on the cards; then they rank them, giving the highest score to their most important choice. (Here you rank your selection.)
4. The votes are tallied on the flipchart. The item that ends up with the highest point total is the group's selection.
5. If the members agree on the highest scored items, then the group can decide what are the next steps in the process. If the members do not agree, the team can investigate other items with high scores.

Force Field Analysis

A *force field analysis* can be considered one of the tools for process improvement; however, it is also useful in the decision-making process. After the team has developed a control chart and has decided on what the variances are, a force field analysis is a method to find out what forces are causing problems in the process. This tool is based on the speculation that all events are the result of *driving forces* (forces that push for change), and *restraining forces* (forces that restrict change). These forces impact case management's ability to change a process. In this CQI section, the focus is on processes and process improvement; however, as case managers, we also may find an invaluable use for this tool in such areas as defining reasons for patient noncompliance (of course this would take patient/family cooperation).

When a force field analysis is used in a CQI team meeting, the team may want to build on, and strengthen, driving forces; the team may want to address, and decrease, restraining forces. Anytime the case management department is in the midst of change and there is disagreement and conflict, this is a practical tool to sort out what is really bothering people. Use brainstorming techniques during analysis of the forces that are affecting change (See Box 9-2 for an example of a force field analysis).

STEPS TO CREATE A FORCE FIELD ANALYSIS

1. Accurately define the issue or circumstance. In this tool's example, the development of an outcomes management program is the focus.
2. Create two lists: one is for the *driving forces,* the other is for the *restraining forces.*
3. Brainstorm for possibilities in each list. Adhere to the brainstorming rules above; this exercise (especially when developing the "restraining forces" list), can bring out organizational problems.
4. Use the knowledge gained to promote effective strategies for change.

Box 9-2

SAMPLE FORCE FIELD ANALYSIS: DEVELOPMENT OF A CASE MANAGEMENT/OUTCOMES MANAGEMENT PROGRAM

Restraining Forces

- Fear of statistics
- Lack of outcomes management experience
- Lack of experience with CQI tools for process improvement
- Lack of time
- Shortage of case management staff to develop and perform outcomes projects
- Lack of resource people for projects
- Lack of administrative support
- Comfort with `the way things are'

Driving Forces

- To prove the value of case management
- To standardize case management processes
- To use the outcomes as a marketing tool for case managers when payors require hard data to justify the cost of case management
- To track costs and predict future costs
- To demonstrate the contribution of case management in accreditation efforts
- To demonstrate which case management interventions provide the best outcome in a specific population
- To identify opportunities for improvement
- To measure case manager performance
- To identify problems, which leads to improved case management services
- To develop a large database of results
- To predict needed skills for professional development
- To identify gaps in services which may lead to poorer quality and increased costs

Root Cause Analysis

A *root cause analysis* is another tool for process improvement. After a control chart (see Chapter 7) has demonstrated what the variances are, a root cause analysis is an investigative method to get to the root, or cause, of a problem. In many ways, this technique holds the key to successful change efforts. Improvement requires change; however, the change made must correspond to the true cause (or root) of the problem. A root cause analysis uncovers the bottlenecks that impede the free flow of a process; this bottleneck is often the cause of poor performance.

This tool is required for some accreditation applications. Effective April 1, 1998, The JCAHO Board of Commissioners significantly revised its sentinel event policy. Hospitals believed that the way the JCAHO policy on sentinel events was written could further expose them to malpractice suits; now, those that self-report sentinel events are not placed on the "accreditation watch" list. JCAHO defines a *sentinel event* as an unexpected occurrence that involves death or serious physical or psychological injury. Sentinel events are reportable to JCAHO on a voluntary basis; however, it is expected that the facility will maintain records that a root cause analysis and an action plan was completed within 30 days. Failure to perform an adequate root cause analysis will result in an accreditation status change, ranging from accreditation watch to loss of Joint Commission accreditation (NAHQ, 1998).

Whether the incident is reported to JCAHO or not, a root cause analysis, and an effort to improve the situation, shows good faith and is good practice. Case managers will find it an easy and useful scrutinizing method when patients fall through the cracks, when hand-off methods to other case managers cause friction, and for a variety of other case management aches and pains.

HOW TO PERFORM A ROOT CAUSE ANALYSIS

The simplest method to get to the underlying cause of the problem is by merely asking the team, **"Why?"** Some CQI experts say that a series of "five whys" will usually suffice. If the "root" does not appear to be uncovered, ask a few more "whys," or see whether any of the answers lead the team down the wrong path (with half-truths or hidden agendas). This approach uses the distinguished case management skill of intense assessment. Ultimately, the exercise should identify changes needed to improve processes or systems, to decrease the likelihood that the event will recur in the future.

Consider the following case management event:

Issue: As ordered, a home health nurse obtained blood work on a complex, but nondiabetic case management patient. The laboratory called and recommended the patient go to the emergency department (ED), because her blood sugar was 650. They also faxed the laboratory results to the ED. The outcome was that the patient spent 36 hours in acute care for severe **hypoglycemia.**

1. Why?
   Because her blood sugar decreased into the 20s after being placed on an insulin drip
2. Why?
   Because she did not have a blood sugar of 650
3. Why?
   Because the laboratory made an error, and the ED acted on the faxed orders
4. Why?
   Because the staff did not question whether the laboratory results were correct before starting an insulin drip
5. Why?
   Because:
   - The staff requires training in "critical thinking." This was a nondiabetic patient; the results should have been confirmed.
   - The ED had a critical shortage of professional staff.
   - There was no formal hospital policy requiring finger sticks to be performed before starting insulin drips on all nondiabetic patients.
   - **Note:** The laboratory would also benefit from a root cause analysis.
   - **Plan:** Institute a policy requiring that all patients (especially those not known to have a history of diabetes) have a finger stick to confirm external laboratory results.

The actual root cause analysis is the bulk of the work when a sentinel event occurs. After the "five whys," ascertain whether the big picture has been evaluated. JCAHO's Root-Cause Analysis Model includes other components to examine.

- Examine why the occurrence happened and what systems affect those processes.
- Discover the details of the occurrence. Examine all departments and service lines that played a role.
- Find the proximate causes of the occurrence.
- Identify a strategy to minimize the risk of another similar event from occurring.
- Initiate risk reduction strategies.

Consensus

Misunderstandings about what consensus is and is not are common. Consensus is a decision in which all the team members find a common ground that is acceptable enough for everyone to support the decision. The key word is "support." In other words, no member actively opposes it. The members believe the decision was reached fairly and openly and represents the best solution at the time.

Consensus is not a unanimous vote that represents everyone's first choice. Nor is consensus a majority vote, in which only the majority get something they are happy with, and the minority get something they do not want at all. It does not mean that everyone is totally satisfied. Consensus does not represent a compromise; a creative solution can still be achieved with consensus. And lastly, consensus is not a "don't rock the boat" mentality; creativity cannot be achieved with "group think."

CONSENSUS GUIDELINES

1. Allow time. Consensus takes time for a full and thorough discussion of the issues.
2. Encourage all members to actively participate. Periodically, have each member state their current view of the issue. Encourage everyone to share information.
3. Creativity and open-mindedness are important. Skills in communication, listening, conflict resolution, and facilitation are essential.
4. Listen carefully. Investigate the meaning behind what the members are saying. Listen for **content** and **intent** (which may be different).
5. Look for a win–win solution. Search for ways to meet the goals of all members.
6. Seek out differences of opinion; this is often where the best solutions are hidden.
7. Avoid changing your mind only to avoid conflict. Do not agree too quickly. Do not bargain or trade support.
8. Do not vote.
9. Avoid arguing blindly for your own point of view. Try to incorporate criticism of your ideas into your proposals.
10. Those with more authority in the group should state their views late in the discussion, after others have had a chance to be heard. The more meek members of the team may find it difficult to state a difference of opinion from the one senior management expressed.
11. After consensus has been reached, check to ensure that everyone understands why the decision was made. Recheck for support.

See Box 9-3 for a summary of decision-making techniques.

Box 9-3

DECISION-MAKING TECHNIQUES FOR
PROCESS IMPROVEMENT

The Chart	Primary Function	Use To:
Brainstorming	Generates multiple ideas in a short time	• Increase understanding of problems • Identify and list problems • Clarify customer (internal or external) expectations • Consider multiple solutions • Identify root causes • Identify variables affecting process • Identify opportunities to improve • Analyze processes • Plan for change • Evaluate tasks
Multivoting	Narrows long lists of ideas, variables, etc.	• Increase understanding/ priorities of problems • Evaluate tasks
Nominal Group Technique	Generates multiple ideas, then narrows and prioritizes the list	• Increase understanding of problems • Identify and list problems • Consider multiple solutions • Identify root causes • Identify variables affecting process • Identify opportunities to improve • Analyze processes • Plan for change

(continued)

Box 9-3 (*Continued*)

The Chart	Primary Function	Use To:
Force Field Analysis	Depicts driving and restraining forces that impact a proposed change	• Increase understanding of problems • Identify and list problems • Identify variables affecting process • Analyze processes • Plan for change
Root Cause Analysis	Identifies the root cause of a problem	• Increase understanding of problems • Identify and list problems • Identify root causes • Identify variables affecting process • Identify opportunities to improve • Plan for change
Consensus	Generates agreement among members	• Increase understanding of problems • Plan for change • Evaluate tasks

CQI CONCLUSION

The tools, techniques, and principles of CQI may appear awkward; it is not something taught in the professions in which most case managers have their license. There are many reasons why this knowledge is important to case management; two of the most important are:

1. Outcomes management is not a passing trend in health care, and it requires strategic planning and objective data. The tools and techniques of CQI are the road map that is used for outcomes management projects. Case managers are intimately involved in all phases of patient health and outcomes; we will be increasingly responsible for demonstrating positive outcomes, both on a patient level and as a profession.

2. CQI principles promote leadership abilities. Case managers are the "movers and shakers" of health care. Our next stage of evolution is one of management and leadership on a larger scale than we have addressed previously. The leadership principles that Dr. Stephen Covey and others promote are ethically based. This can only strengthen and enlighten us further, as case managers continue to be placed in positions and roles that require ethically balanced decisions.

PART III: RESOURCES AND REFERENCES

Brassard, M., & Ritter, D. (1994). *Memory jogger II.* Goal/QPC-Methuen: Joiner Associates.

Covey, S. (1994). *First things first.* New York: Simon & Schuster.

Covey, S. (1992). *Princple-centered leadership.* New York: Simon & Schuster.

Covey, S. (1989). *Seven habits of highly effective people.* New York: Simon & Schuster.

Deming, E. (1986). *Out of the crisis.* Cambridge, MA: MIT Center for Advanced Engineering Study.

Executive Learning. (1997). FAST PDCA—Leaders Guide. Brentwood: Executive Learning, Inc.

Executive Learning. (1997). *Handbook for improvement: A reference guide for tools and concepts* (2nd ed.). Brentwood: Executive Learning, Inc.

Fisher, R., & Ury. (1991). *Getting to yes: negotiating agreement without giving in.* New York: Viking Press.

Gibbons, S. (1994, Oct/Nov). Three paths, one journey. *Journal for Quality and Participation,* pp. 36–45.

Ishikawa, K. (1990). *Introduction to quality control.* Tokyo: 3A Corporation.

Joiner, B. (1994). *Fourth generation management: The new business consciousness.* New York: McGraw-Hill.

Juran, J. (1989). *Juran on leadership for quality: An executive handbook.* New York: The Free Press (Macmillan, Inc.).

Langley, G.J., Nolan, K.M., & Nolan, K. (1992). *The foundation of improvement.* Silver Spring, MD: API Publishing.

McLaughlin, C., & Kaluzny, A. (1994). *Continuous quality improvement in health care: Theory, implementation, and applications.* Gaithersburg, MD: Aspen.

National Association for Health care Quality (NAHQ). (1997). NAHQ guide to quality management (7th ed.). Glenview: NAHQ.

National Association for Health care Quality (NAHQ). 1998. *NAHQ guide to quality management* (8th ed.). Glenview, IL: NAHQ.

Powell, S.K. (1996). *Nursing case management: A practical guide to success in managed care.* Philadelphia: Lippincott, Williams, and Wilkins.

Scholtes, P., Joiner, B., & Streibel, B. (1996). The team handbook (2nd ed.). Madison, WI: Joiner Associates.

Schroeder, P. (1994). *Improving quality and performance: Concepts, programs, and techniques.* St. Louis: Mosby-Year Book.

Senge, P. (1990). *The fifth discipline.* New York: Doubleday/Currency.

Temme, J. (1996). *Team power.* Mission: Skillpath Publications.

1. Choose one of the quality points from the CQI Gurus. Apply it to your organization. How can your organization be improved using this idea?
2. Apply appropriate tools for process improvement to evaluate various aspects of your organization. You may choose to use the issue determined in question number one.
   - Flowcharts
   - Run (trend) charts
   - Statistical process control charts (SPCC); also known as control charts
   - Pie charts
   - Bar charts
   - Pareto charts
   - Cause-and-effect diagrams (fishbone or Ishikawa diagram)
   - Scatter diagrams
3. Apply the CASE PDCA model to assess, plan, test, evaluate, and put into action quality improvement effort. Again, the issue needing improvement determined in question 1 may be used.
4. Describe an experience in a cross-functional team. Did the team display the stages of team development? Was the team able to move through all stages? If not, how could the facilitator have assisted with the effort?
5. Write a set of "ground rules" for an improvement team.
6. Practice facilitating each of the decision-making techniques below:
   - Brainstorming
   - Multivoting
   - Nominal group technique
   - Force field analysis
   - Root cause analysis
   - Consensus

Managing Complementary Health Care: A Vision for the Future

We cannot live only for ourselves. A thousand fibers connect us with

our fellow men; and among those fibers, as sympathetic threads, our

*actions run as **causes** and they come back to us as **effects.***

HERMAN MELVILLE

PART IV: IMPORTANT TERMS AND CONCEPTS

Acupuncture
Alexander Technique
Aromatherapy
Auric Field
Autogenic Training
Ayurvedic Medicine
Bioacoustics
Bioelectric Energy
Bioenergy Therapies
Biofeedback
Chinese Medicine
Chiropractic Manipulations
Classical Yoga
Complementary and Alternative
  Medicine (CAM)
Craniosacral Therapy
Creative Visualization
Feldenkrais Therapy
Flower Essences
Guided Imagery
Hatha Yoga
Health
Herbology/Herbal Medicine
Homeopathy
Hydrotherapy
Hypnosis
Law of Similars
Law of Infinitesimal Dose
Magnetic Therapy

Materia Medica
Meditation
Mind–Body Medicine
Musculoskeletal Therapies
Naturopathic Medicine
National Academy of Acupuncture
  and Oriental Medicine
National Institutes of Health (NIH)
Neurolinguistic Programming (NLP)
Nutritional Supplementation
Office of Alternative Medicine
Physiotherapy
Polarity Therapy
Prana
Prevention
Qi
Reflexology
Relaxation Response
Rolfing
Sound Healing
Structural Integration
Therapeutic Massage
Therapeutic Touch
Three Doshas (Vata, Pitta, and
  Kapha)
Traditional Chinese Medicine
  (TCM)
Yoga
Yin/Yang

Complementary and Alternative Medicine (CAM): An Introduction to CAM Modalities

by Janice E. Benjamin, RN, MS, L.Ac., with Suzanne K. Powell, RN, BSN, CCM

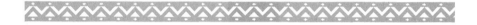

I was passionate,
filled with longing,
I searched
far and wide.
But the day
that the Truthful One
found me,
I was at home.
—Lal Ded, 14th-Century poetess

Modern medicine continues to search far and wide for the perfect drug, the best technology, the purest science, and the illusive road to immortality through genetic manipulation. It seems, however, that the truth has been here at home all along—in the chicken soup your grandmother makes for you when you are sick, in the herbs growing wild in the fields in almost every neighborhood in this country, in the powerful prayer of a loved one when all seems hopeless, in the compassionate touch of a nurse or doctor allowing tears to wash away the fear, in the unrelenting belief of a child or an adult in miracles, and in the open heart of compassion and love that lives in each one of us. The American public made a statement in Eisenberg's 1990 survey about alternative health care (Eisenberg, Kessler, Foster, Norlock, Calkins & Delbanco, 1993). They want to move closer to a quality of medicine that heals them without further injury, that meets them at the place where they are, and that honors the innate healing potential of who they are, not what disease they have. Slowly, but surely, the health care industry is responding.

These next three chapters look at some of the complementary and alternative therapies gaining acceptance in health care delivery systems across the country and explore the role of case management in the successful integration of these therapies into conventional medical care.

Medicine can be simply defined as a therapeutic intervention aimed at treating disease. Complementary and alternative medicine (CAM), in the United States, can be simply defined as any therapeutic intervention not based on conventional, Western, allopathic treatment protocols as taught in medical universities (Milbank, 1998), although that is slowly changing as more universities incorporate studies of CAM in their curricula (Moore, 1998). So, if you have a pain in your back and you do not go to an MD, but you go to your grandmother for her family remedy, or an acupuncturist, or a homeopathic practitioner, or a health food store and pick a remedy off the shelf, or a Feldenkrais therapist, or an aromatherapist, or a spiritual healer, or a massage therapist, or an herbologist, or a practitioner who uses visualization techniques, or your spiritual community for healing prayer—you have used CAM. Dr. Hassan Rifaat, Director of the Alternative Medicine Program at Oxford Health Plans, wrote that the basic concept behind alternative medicine is that it "asks each person to take a broader look at health as a lifetime goal of daily wellness, rather than seeing it as a curing process, or an episodic response to pain/disease" (Rifaat, 1998, p. 54). There is an enormous resource of "other" modalities that can and do provide health care options for preventing and treating disease, and, politics and economics notwithstanding, their use is growing by leaps and bounds in this country.

The definition of *complementary*, as found in *Webster's New World Dictionary*, is "that which completes or perfects." The American public appears to agree with this definition, as Eisenberg's article indicated (Eisenberg, Kessler, Foster, Norlock, Calkins & Delbanco, 1993). There appear to be pieces missing from conventional medicine and, with or without the health care industries' financial blessing, the American public is out in full force looking for that which can complete or perfect their health care needs, be it prevention or active treatment. Case managers need to be prepared to work with their clients to provide knowledgeable direction and support regarding the costs and health benefits of a rapidly growing sector of health care in this country.

In 1992, the Office of Alternative Medicine was created at the National Institutes of Health (NIH), to "...evaluate alternative medical treatments, fund studies to determine their effectiveness, and integrate effective treatments into mainstream medical practice" (Toran, 1996, p. 57). The 1990s have seen a phenomenal increase in awareness and consumer interest in self-care, conventional health care, and alternative health care options for treatment. The Internet has been instrumental in this growth by facilitating instant access to unbelievable amounts of information. The rising costs of health care, even with managed care, have contributed to the need to look for other less expensive and more cost-effective treatment options. The breaking down of barriers between cultures and countries has also created a environment in which new ways and old ways of thinking about health care are blending. Many social, political, and economic forces have come together to create a renaissance in health care. It is a wonderful opportunity for providers and consumers, and it is an enormous challenge for case management.

CAM embraces a large, unmapped territory in the United States. We treat with and insure allopathic medicine because it is familiar. Sometimes, however, the impact of disease on an individual or on a society demands looking into unfamiliar places to find a cure. When I worked with cancer patients at NIH in 1987, physicians often said to patients for whom a treatment protocol had failed, "There is nothing else that can be done." What I always thought should have been said is, "There is nothing else that WE can do." The potential for the human spirit to intervene and overcome incredible odds cannot be confined within the boundaries of allopathic medicine, or any other health care modality. "Once we awaken from the dogmatic slumber of believing that one medicine has all the answers, then we can go on with an open mind to examine the whole range of healing systems that the genius of the human race has so patiently worked out" (Kaptchuk & Croucher, 1987). And the health care consumer has made it clear that they understand this and that they want to be able to choose what works best for them.

Case management is positioned to be of great service to the health care industry and to consumers by providing a resource of knowledge about what CAM modalities are available, what kind of diseases they can best treat, what contraindications can arise when integrating two or more modalities, what a course of treatment involves, what outcome measures can be used, what potential savings can be expected, and how best to choose a provider.

Chapter 10 describes some of the CAM modalities being used by consumers, with references for further study. Chapter 11 describes how some health plans across the country are dealing with the CAM challenge. Chapter 12 looks at how case management can best respond to this evolving CAM phenomena, and some of the concerns about integrating CAM into mainstream medicine.

"It is more important to know what sort of person has a disease,
than to know what sort of disease a person has."

—HIPPOCRATES

When the germ theory of disease was embraced in the mid-nineteenth century, modern medicine was born out of the belief that disease resulted from an assault on the body by an infectious agent outside the body. Metaphors of war developed to describe the intention of modern medicine to respond to this assault—looking for drugs that are "magic bullets," or funding research for the "war on cancer" (Burton, 1997). Certainly there are germs and viruses outside the body that can cause disease, but nothing is designed more perfectly to defend against these organisms than the human immune system. Many CAM therapies believe that treatment aimed at strengthening and supporting our immune system would be more to our advantage. There is a saying in Chinese medicine that "To administer medicine after an illness begins is...like digging a well after becoming thirsty or casting weapons after a battle has been engaged" (Kaptchuk, 1983, p. 134). Treating disease once it has settled in the body is more difficult and more expensive than protecting the body from disease. Prevention is the best medicine, but it has not been a significant part of the focus of treatment in modern medicine.

Most of the time people go to a doctor, not because of an attack by germs, but because of chronic physiologic dysfunctions, such as high blood pressure, low back pain, or migraine headaches. The most frequently used therapy available to physicians for treating chronic complaints is drugs. Unfortunately, as a study presented in the *Journal of the American Medical Association* (JAMA), April 15, 1998, indicated, 100,000 people die every year of complications of prescribed drug therapy. We clearly need to have other options for treating chronic illness. Following are some of the options the American consumer has taken the initiative to incorporate into their personal efforts to prevent and treat illness.

One category of CAM consists of modalities that are considered complete health care systems in themselves. Two of these systems, Chinese and Ayurvedic medicine, are recently transplanted to the United States from other countries. The other two systems, homeopathy and naturopathy, were part of health care delivery early in the history of the United States, but lost favor when allopathic, or modern, medicine began to exert its dominance in the early 1900s. These four systems as a whole tend to focus on prevention and self-care, but also provide therapeutic options for treating acute and chronic illness. For this reason, it is important for consumers to ask practitioners of these systems for evidence of licensure, certification, or appropriate training in their area of expertise.

TRADITIONAL CHINESE MEDICINE

Traditional Chinese Medicine (TCM) has been practiced in China for at least 4,000 years. Acupuncture needles made of bone, dating even further back in history, have been found in archaeological excavations in China (Cheng, 1993). TCM is a philosophy and practice of medicine based on the theory that health exists when the forces of Yin and Yang are balanced within the body-mind-spirit. "Disease represents an imbalance of these forces that leads to excesses or deficiencies of life energy in various organs, resulting in illness if not corrected" (Milbank, 1998, p. 8). TCM prescribes the use of acupuncture, herbs, applications of heat and suction, dietary changes, and massage to achieve this balance. TCM does not recognize a separation between body-mind-spirit, but understands that disease can originate, manifest and/or be healed through any of these three aspects of a human life (Horrigan, 1998). For example, a headache can be the result of excess anger, and can be treated by reducing the anger. Insomnia can result from an imbalance in a person's spirit, and can be treated by calming the spirit. Diagnosis and treatment are unique to each individual, because everyone presents with a unique constellation of symptoms. The whole picture, not just one symptom, is essential for understanding the source of the imbalance that is resulting in the patient's complaint. TCM looks at patterns of symptoms and bases diagnosis and treatment on the whole picture, the whole person (Jacobs, 1997).

"Chinese medicine can only be properly understood in the context of Chinese philosophy" (Firebrace & Hill, 1994, p. 54). TCM is rooted in a culture that values tradition, relationship, and Nature. The most often quoted text that guides the practice of TCM is *The Yellow Emperor's Classic of Internal Medicine,* which was written over 2,000 years ago. Most of the subsequent hundreds of Chinese medical texts are discussions of and expansions on teachings from this classic discourse on Chinese medical philosophy. TCM builds on the experience and wisdom of its ancestors, giving this practice of medicine a very strong foundation.

In TCM, nothing is seen to exist in isolation, and everything exists in relationship. A sunny day is enjoyable when it has been raining for 2 weeks, but not so appreciated if it has not rained for 2 months. So it is in health that a symptom, like a headache or fever, by itself does not reflect the whole picture of that patient's health. It points, through its relationship with other signs and symptoms, to a root cause or imbalance. The emotional and environmental influences on the patient, such as recent loss, stress at a job, local weather patterns, and chemical exposures, are also taken into consideration. Treatment is, therefore, not focused on just the symptom, but also on the imbalance within the whole system that has manifested as a headache, for example.

Much of Chinese medical theory has been based on observations of the cycles found in Nature, and human beings are seen as the place where Heaven and Earth come together (Firebrace & Hill, 1994). Health is considered to be not only harmony within the body-mind-spirit, but harmony with Nature. For example, in Winter the sap of trees goes into the roots and growth slows down;

so it is that human beings also must conserve their energy and slow down their activity during this time of the year. *The Yellow Emperor's Classic of Internal Medicine* discusses what illnesses will manifest in the Spring if this change in behavior is not honored during the Winter. Human beings are seen as a part of Nature and subject to the same laws that manifest in cycles seen in the natural world.

Two concepts essential in understanding how diagnoses and treatments are developed in TCM are the concepts of Qi and Yin/Yang. Qi can be loosely translated as energy (Ryan & Shattuck, 1994). "Neither the classical nor modern Chinese texts speculate on the nature of Qi nor do they attempt to conceptualize it" (Kaptchuk, 1983, pp. 36–37). It is rather understood within the context of its function and can be seen as the vital force that runs throughout the body, animating and supporting the function of different organ systems. There are many forms of Qi, again depending on its function. There is lung Qi, and stomach Qi, and the Qi found in food, for example. Qi is what is manipulated and brought into balance during an acupuncture treatment. It is accessible because it is organized along pathways, called meridians, that weave throughout the entire body, from the surface to deep within the organ systems. The key symptom of a deficiency of Qi is fatigue. If the lungs are deficient in Qi, you will have a cough with fatigue. If the Heart is deficient in Qi, you will experience heart palpitations with fatigue.

The concepts of Yin and Yang are "...a theoretical method for observing and analyzing phenomena" (Cheng, 1993, p. 11). Yin and Yang are the forces that maintain homeostasis in the body-mind-spirit, a balance between catabolism and anabolism, rest and activity, and heat and cold. Yang represents the functional aspect of the body-mind-spirit, and Yin represents the substance of the body-mind-spirit. Examples of Yang phenomena are heat, agitation, rapid movement and the daytime. Examples of Yin phenomena are cold, rest, slow movement and the nighttime. "These qualities are opposites, yet they describe relative aspects of the same phenomena" (Kaptchuk, 1983, p. 8). One cannot exist without the other, nor can one dominate the other. They must work in harmony. The concepts of Yin and Yang help the TCM practitioner understand where imbalances are in the body-mind-spirit and, therefore, where to direct the treatment. For example, if a patient speaks rapidly, has severe headaches that are better with rest, has a rapid pulse, feels hot all the time, and has trouble falling asleep, his Yang energy is in excess and treatment would focus on tonifying the Yin aspect of the body to restore balance. Treating the symptoms alone, for example, giving an aspirin for a headache, can suppress the Yang symptoms, but will not restore the Yin, so the imbalance remains and can manifest later as something potentially more serious.

Treatment in TCM aims to engage the movement and function of Qi to restore the balance of Yin and Yang in the body. Based on the patient's symptom picture and other diagnostic tools, such as pulse taking, the practitioner identifies where the imbalances in the body are originating and works to restore balance. "The Chinese system should be more successful with functional illnesses and those whose lack of associated structural change puts them out of reach of allopathic methods of diagnosis and treatment" (Weil, 1988).

Practitioners of TCM, who graduated from nationally accredited schools and passed a national standards examination for their licensure, have undergone an education that is at least 3 years long and requires at least 800 hours of supervised clinical experience before they can practice. There are 32 accredited schools in the United States that provide training in Chinese medicine, and about 10,000 licensed practitioners, according to the National Acupuncture and Oriental Medicine Alliance. Currently, 34 states regulate the practice of acupuncture or the use of Chinese herbs. The medical and naturopathic physicians' associations and the chiropractic association have developed acupuncture certification programs for their profession, allowing them to practice after only 200 hours or 50 hours of classroom study, respectively. They do not typically use TCM diagnostic methods when treating patients, but match acupuncture points to specific symptoms.

The art and science of TCM is, of course, more complex than can be presented in this chapter, but the effectiveness of treatment based on TCM is rapidly gaining recognition and acceptance in the medical community and among insurance plans (Long, 1998). In November, 1997, the NIH convened a consensus conference to evaluate one aspect of TCM, acupuncture. The panel of doctors and scientists looked at acupuncture's efficacy, its mechanisms of treatment, and directions for further research. They noted a "...paucity of high-quality research assessing (the) efficacy of acupuncture compared with placebo or sham acupuncture" (NIH, 1997, p. 3). They concluded that acupuncture shows promise for the treatment of postoperative pain, nausea and vomiting from chemotherapy, addiction, stroke rehabilitation, headaches, menstrual cramps, tennis elbow, fibromyalgia, myofascial pain, osteoarthritis, low back pain, carpal tunnel syndrome, and asthma.

The professional community of acupuncture and TCM practitioners continues to work on adding to the body of scientific research to demonstrate the mechanisms by which this 4,000-year-old medical system works. In 1996, the National Academy of Acupuncture and Oriental Medicine published a compendium of 71 controlled clinical studies evaluating the use of acupuncture and other TCM modalities (Birch & Hammerschlag, 1996). One mechanism of action that has been researched and suggests why acupuncture is effective in the management of pain is that it stimulates the release of endorphins, the body's natural opiates, into the central nervous system (Pert, 1997).

Other studies have suggested that neurotransmitters, such as serotonin, are released after treatment with acupuncture (Gerber, 1996). A further mechanism to explain how acupuncture works is that the insertion of acupuncture needles in the body, because of the temperature differences between the part of the needle that is in the body and the part that is left exposed, creates an electrical potential gradient that attracts a flow of ions to the local tissue (Jacobs, 1997).

"Studies have reported that acupuncture helps stroke patients, improves exercise performance in young men, and increases uterine contractions in pregnant women who are past their delivery dates" (Milbank, 1998, pp. 8–9). Acupuncture is also growing in acceptance as an effective treatment for drug addiction, both for managing the symptoms of withdrawal and for reducing the rate of recidivism (Brumbaugh, 1993).

When looking for a practitioner, the 34 states that regulate the practice of acupuncture have state associations that can be contacted for a list of licensed professionals in that area. There are two national associations for licensed practitioners of TCM, a national association for medical doctors who use acupuncture in their practice, and the different state associations for chiropractors that can be contacted to locate practitioners in your area who use acupuncture or TCM in their health care practice.

ACUPUNCTURE RESOURCES

National Acupuncture and Oriental Medicine Alliance
14637 Starr Road S.E.
Olalla, WA 98359
(253) 851-6896
www.acuall.org

National Certification Commission for Acupuncture and Oriental Medicine (NCCAOM)
(202) 232-1404
www.nccaom.org

American Academy of Medical Acupuncture (MDs only)
(213) 937-5514
www.medicalacupuncture.org

AYURVEDIC MEDICINE

Ayurvedic medicine has recently come to the attention of the American public through the many popular books of Dr. Deepak Chopra. "Ayurveda is a Sanskrit word, derived from two roots: ayur, which means life, and veda, knowledge" (Lad, 1991, p. 1). Ayurvedic medicine, a 5,000-year-old philosophy and system of practice, teaches people how to live in harmony with all aspects of life by caring for themselves on a day-to-day basis. Ayurvedic medicine is deeply rooted in the ancient culture and religion of the Indian continent and addresses the whole person as body-mind-spirit. "The first question an Ayurvedic doctor asks is not 'What disease does my patient have?' but 'Who is my patient?'" (Griggs, 1995, p. 107). It is out of that soil that the illness grows, and if the soil can be improved, the disease can no longer grow. The tools of Ayurvedic medicine include dietary prescriptions, massage, herbal medicines, meditation, yoga exercises, detoxification, and breathing exercises. The sun is also considered to be a source of higher consciousness, and some level of exposure to the sun is considered to balance the body (Burton, 1997).

Diagnosis and treatment begin with identifying the patient's basic constitution, and this begins with identifying the patient's body type, or dosha, of which there are three—vata, pitta, and kapha. The doshas "govern psychobiological changes in the body and physio-pathological changes too" (Lad, 1991, p. 4). Vata represents dryness, coldness, activity, breath, mental clarity, subtle mood shifts, and astringing functions. A vata body type is thin, has dry skin, has cold hands and feet, can be moody, is very imaginative, tends toward constipation, and is very active.

Pitta represents heat, oily fluids, sharp qualities, light, liquid, and spreading qualities. A pitta body type is of a medium build, has thin hair, a short temper, tends toward ulcers and acne, perspires easily, has a strong appetite and warm skin, likes to read, and is very passionate emotionally. Kapha represents heaviness, slow movement, cool temperatures, static qualities, sweet and salty tastes, and density. A kapha body type is heavyset, has slow digestion, sleeps long and heavy, is affectionate, tends toward high cholesterol levels, tends to procrastinate, is slow to anger, tends to have thick and wavy hair, and has good memory (Lad, 1991).

The three doshas are also found within each individual in specific areas of the body. Vata activates the respiratory and circulatory systems, and is located in the large intestine, pelvic area, thighs, bones, skin, and ears. Pitta regulates the metabolism of food, water, and air, and is located in the small intestine, stomach, sweat glands, eyes, skin, and blood. Kapha regulates the structure of muscles, bones, and fat, and is located in the chest, lungs, and spinal fluid (Burton, 1997).

Each body type is a unique combination of the five elements of creation, which are space, air, fire, water, and earth. The Ayurvedic practitioner looks for where the original balance of that dosha has been disturbed and focuses treatment on restoring balance among the doshas and the five elements. Imbalance can be caused by stress, improper diet, lack of spiritual practice, erratic lifestyles, emotional or physical trauma, and environmental factors (Griggs, 1995).

"Ayurvedic medicine also takes into account how the seasons and time of day influence health. Dietary and other therapeutic suggestions are often prescribed with this in mind" (Burton, 1997, p. 66). Summer is considered to be the time of year when pitta qualities are most prevalent. Autumn is the season when vata types are more susceptible to illness, and winter is the season for kapha.

Ayurvedic medicine places an emphasis on prevention of disease, and diagnoses through observing and questioning the patient, palpating the body, listening to the heart, lungs, and intestines, assessing the quality of the pulse, of which there are six positions on each wrist, looking at the quality of the tongue, and examining the condition of the urine (Burton, 1997).

There are four main tools the Ayurvedic practitioner uses to treat imbalances: cleansing and detoxification, palliation, rejuvenation, and mental–spiritual healing. Cleansing (shodan) is accomplished through a process called pancha karma. It involves the use of herbal massage, sauna baths, enemas, special diet, and purgative teas, all administered daily for a week to eliminate toxins held in the physical and mental body. Palliation (shaman) is used to balance the doshas and is a more gentle form of cleansing for people with a weak immune system or overall depleted constitution. It focuses more on healing at the spiritual level and involves the use of herbs, yoga and breathing exercises, fasting, limited sunbathing, and meditation and chanting. Rejuvenation (rasayana) is a rebuilding program after a cleansing and is said to increase longevity. It uses herbs, yoga and breathing exercises, and diet to tone the body's physiologic systems. Mental–spiritual healing (satvajaya) "...is a method of improving the mind to reach a higher level of spiritual/mental functioning, and is accomplished through the release of psychological stress, emotional distress, and unconscious negative beliefs" (Burton, 1997, p. 69). The tools used for satvajaya include chanting specific sounds, concentrating on specific geometric patterns to alter ordinary patterns of the mind, meditation and directing the flow of energies throughout the body, and the use of certain gems and crystals for their vibrational quality.

Ayurvedic medicine is a complete medical science and can be used in the treatment of any health care problems. The World Health Organization supports the use of Ayurvedic medicine and its integration with modern medicine (Burton, 1997). Deepak Chopra, M.D., through his books and workshops, has taken the American public deeper into the heart of Ayurvedic medicine and its ancient foundations in consciousness. "When you look at Ayurveda's anatomical charts, you don't see the familiar organs pictured in Gray's Anatomy; rather you find astonishing diagrams of where the mind is flowing as it creates the body" (Chopra, 1989, p. 3). Ayurveda was born out of the ancient spiritual traditions of India, and this aspect of healing cannot be separated from treatment.

The "new" paradigm of quantum physics and its exploration into the world of consciousness seems to be a rediscovery of a knowledge that our ancient ancestors understood and on which they built two enduring medical systems— Ayurveda and Traditional Chinese Medicine. What is the spiritual foundation of modern Western medicine? I believe Dr. Chopra's overwhelming popularity addresses a need to return to the awareness that we have the power within us to heal, which is the deeper meaning of the word *ayurveda*.

AYURVEDA RESOURCES

The College of Maharishi
Ayur-Veda Health Center
P.O. Box 282
Fairfield, IA 52556
(515) 472-5866

NATUROPATHY

In the 1920s, there were 22 colleges of naturopathic medicine in the United States. In the 1950s, 26 states offered licensure in naturopathic medicine. By 1955, under pressure from the American Medical Association, only eight states offered licensure, and all of the schools were shut down. As interest in alternative medicine has increased, the profession is also enjoying a resurgence in interest, with three schools now open in the United States and 18 states either offering or working on licensure for naturopathic physicians (Jacobs, 1997).

Naturopathic medicine is a large umbrella that covers the use of many treatment modalities. "Naturopathic medicine grew out of alternative healing systems of the 18th and 19th centuries, but traces its philosophical roots to the Hippocratic school of medicine (circa 400 BC)" (Murray & Pizzorno, 1991, p. 4). About 100 years ago in this country, concepts of public health and hygiene, natural and healthy diets, traditions of Native and European herbology, hydrotherapy and physiotherapy, and the new area of homeopathy developing in Europe came together to form "naturopathy" (Jacobs, 1997). Benedict Lust, a physician who migrated from Germany in 1892, is considered the originator of naturopathy in the United States and opened the first school to train naturopathic doctors in New York City in 1900 (Weil, 1988).

The underlying goal of naturopathic medicine is to strengthen the body's immune system so that it can heal itself. The naturopathic physician "...relies upon the healing wisdom, vital energy and intelligence of the organism to restore normal and healthy function" (Jacobs, 1997, p. 93).

The six principles that define naturopathic medicine are: (1) the body has the ability to heal itself, and treatment is designed to support those natural, innate processes; (2) diagnose and treat the underlying cause of illness, do not suppress the symptoms; (3) do no harm; thus use only natural means and substances to treat; (4) treat the whole person, each person having their unique and potentially unlimited ability to heal; (5) the physician is a teacher who empowers the patient to take more responsibility for their health; and (6) prevention is the best medicine (Burton, 1997).

"Health is viewed as more than just the absence of disease; it is considered to be a vital dynamic state which enables a person to thrive in, or adapt to, a wide range of environments and stresses" (Murray & Pizzorno, 1991, p. 6). Whereas allopathic or modern medicine focuses on treating disease, naturopathic medicine focuses on prevention and support of body systems, so that a person can obtain their optimal level of health. For example, if a person complains of mild but annoying headaches once a month, an allopathic physician would probably recommend aspirin or Tylenol as needed to suppress the pain. A naturopathic physician would see monthly headaches as a sign of a weakness in one of the body systems, or possibly a sign of toxicity in the body, and recommend a cleansing diet and herbs to rebuild the body. In other words, monthly headaches would be seen as not optimal health and the body's way of asking for help to restore itself to optimal health.

Many times symptoms that modern medicine treats with drugs, such as inflammation, are seen in naturopathic medicine as a healing process that the body is using to restore homeostasis. Treatment, therefore, should not be aimed at suppressing these symptoms, such as a fever, or the disease can be driven deeper into the body and can result in chronic illness. Toxemia, or an "...inappropriately high level of metabolic waste products and exogenous toxins in the blood...," is seen as a root cause for many chronic disease patterns (Jacobs, 1997, p. 95). The underlying process for the development of toxemia is seen as improper diet and stress. Stress releases adrenal hormones that reduce the flow of blood to the digestive system, and improperly digested food can result in fermentation within the digestive tract. This fermentation or putrefaction generates bacteria and toxins that can enter into the bloodstream and accumulate in cells and body tissues. The foundational treatment in naturopathic medicine is improvement of the internal environment of the body through proper diet and the reduction of stress (Jacobs, 1997).

Andrew Weil, M.D., states that "...naturopathy can offer a refreshing balance to the aggressive, invasive, and unnatural practices of modern allopathy" (Weil, 1988, p. 139). He suggests, however, that some of their diagnostic tools and treatments need stronger scrutiny by scientific research. Naturopathic medical training in accredited schools in the United States, of which there are three, is a postgraduate level of education. The 4-year programs include 2 years of education in basic medical sciences, 2 years of education in naturopathic philosophy and treatment modalities, and 2 years of supervised clinical experience. There are correspondence programs that confer the degree of Naturopathic Doctor, or N.D., but they do not require supervised clinical experience, and their graduates are not eligible for licensure (Jacobs, 1997).

NATUROPATHY RESOURCES

The Institute for Naturopathic Medicine
66½ North State Street
Concord, NH 03301-4330
(603) 225-8844

HOMEOPATHY

Homeopathy is based on three principles: the Law of Similars, the Law of Infinitesimal Dose, and the Laws of Holism (Burton, 1997). It was developed by a German physician, Samuel Hahnemann, in the late 1700s, and was born out of his dissatisfaction with the practices of medicine at that time. Hahnemann was experimenting with cinchona bark, being used to treat malaria, and discovered that daily ingestion of this drug by healthy individuals reproduced the symptoms of malaria. He then speculated that if large amounts of the drug recreated the symptoms of malaria, perhaps small doses would stimulate the body's immune system to fight the disease (Burton, 1997).

Hahnemann went on to test hundreds of other herbs and substances, and carefully recorded the symptoms they produced in healthy individuals. This testing for symptoms is called a "proving." From these provings, Hahnemann developed what is known as a "drug picture" for each remedy; that is, the physical, mental, and emotional symptoms that match the symptoms of a specific "proving" or homeopathic remedy (Gerber, 1996). The provings and drug pictures developed into and demonstrated the first principle of homeopathy that "like cures like," or the Law of Similars.

The most interesting effect Hahnemann discovered, when first treating patients homeopathically, was that the more he diluted his remedies, the more effective they were in curing patients. The remedies are diluted in a specific manner call succussing, which involves rapidly shaking the solution with each subsequent dilution (Burton, 1997). So Hahnemann began diluting his remedies to the point where there was not a single molecule of the original substance to be found in the remedy. The more diluted the remedy, the more powerful it was in its effect. Rather than the physical structure of substances, he appeared to be capturing the energetic essence of substances in his remedies (Kaptchuk & Croucher, 1987). This led to the second principle of homeopathy that the more dilute the remedy, the greater its potency, or the Law of Infinitesimal Dose.

This second principle of homeopathy is one of the most controversial. Modern medicine is based on effecting cellular changes in the body by the application of drugs with molecular properties. These drugs also treat by effecting an opposite change in the body on a cellular level. For example, if you have a fever, you are given medication that stops the molecular changes in the body that are producing the fever. In homeopathy, if someone has a fever, she is given a remedy that contains no molecule of the original substance and is believed to be able to cause a fever in a healthy individual. Research in Europe, however, is beginning to demonstrate evidence of how homeopathic remedies may be working.

An Italian physicist, Emilio del Giudici, has theorized that water has a molecular structure that allows it to store electromagnetic signals (Gerber, 1996; Burton, 1997). Concurrently, Wolfgang Ludwig, a biophysicist in Germany, has done research that measures the electromagnetic signals given off by homeopathic remedies (Burton, 1997). These research efforts suggest that homeopathic remedies capture and hold the electromagnetic frequencies of specific herbs in a water solution. The remedies are theorized to match biomagnetic frequencies of specific disease processes, and their ingestion stimulates the body's electromagnetic field to throw off the disease. This, however, still requires a paradigm shift to accept, first, that electromagnetic frequencies in the body can be manipulated and, second, that manipulation of electromagnetic frequencies can make a difference in the outcome of an illness (Gerber, 1996).

In 1900, there were almost 100 homeopathic hospitals and 22 homeopathic medical schools in the United States. However, as the American Medical Association (AMA) and the pharmaceutical industry grew in power, homeopathy was systematically discredited and forced out of the mainstream (Brown, 1979; Burton, 1997). On June 30, 1988, the prestigious scientific journal, *Nature,* published the results of a study done by Jacques Benveniste, a medical researcher at a prestigious laboratory in France, in which they were able to stimulate an immune response in basophilic cells in vitro with homeopathic doses of anti-IgE (Davenas et al., 1988). The medical community responded strongly in opposition to this publication, and urged *Nature* to send a team of observers—a magician to detect slight of hand, a medical frauds investigator, and a member of *Nature*—to the laboratory in France to replicate the experiments and prove or disprove their findings. They reported that the study design was flawed, although two other laboratories, one in Italy and one in Israel, were getting similar findings in their experiments with homeopathic doses of drugs (Arnall & Casteris, 1989). Because the apparent mechanism of action of homeopathic remedies cannot be explained by the molecular theory for medicine, its acceptance remains controversial. However, continuing research done by Dr. Benveniste has found that homeopathic remedies exposed to high heat or magnetic fields lose their ability to effect the changes they had demonstrated in prior research protocols. It is this last finding that seems to support the theory that "...homeopathic remedies are indeed energetic medicines with mechanisms different from those of conventional drugs utilized by...pharmacologists and physicians" (Gerber, 1996, p. 566).

The goal of homeopathic therapy is to increase the patient's natural defenses so that the body-mind-spirit can heal itself (Jacobs, 1997). I first discovered homeopathy when my son was 3 years old and developed symptoms of croup. I took him to a pediatrician and was told that there was nothing that could be done because the cause was viral. I remember being amazed that at the end of the 20th century, with computers, men on the moon, and organ transplants, here was a professional health care practitioner telling me nothing could be done. Fortunately, I didn't believe her and went looking for someone who could do something, and found an M.D. who was also a homeopathic physician. He gave my son a remedy that afternoon, and he did not suffer any symptoms that night. The second time my son developed croup, he took the appropriate homeopathic remedy, and the symptoms lasted about 6 hours. The third and last time he developed croup, it lasted about 4 hours. Both of my children were treated by this homeopathic doctor during their entire childhood. And I believe, because homeopathy enhanced their immune system every time it was challenged rather than attacking and suppressing the symptoms, they are healthier and stronger as adults.

Homeopathic practitioners ask many detailed questions of patients to get an accurate and unique symptom picture before selecting a remedy. Homeopathy can be used to treat almost any physical or emotional condition, but the remedy is very specific to that patient. This is the third principle of homeopathy, which is to treat holistically. There is a *materia medica* used by homeopathic practitioners, which is a compendium of thousands of "provings" conducted over the past 200 years. Homeopathic remedies have been Food and Drug Administration (FDA) approved, and their manufacture is closely regulated (Burton, 1997). Homeopathy is practiced by physicians, naturopaths, lay homeopaths with formal education, and often through self-medication. More dilute, thus more potent remedies, can only be secured with a prescription from a practitioner with licensure or credentials. Remedies for the common cold and simple trauma can be found in a lot of pharmacies over-the-counter. My experience with homeopathy is that their effect on the body can be powerful and, for more serious illnesses, I would recommend a practitioner with training rather than self-medication.

HOMEOPATHY RESOURCES

National Center for Homeopathy
801 North Fairfax, Suite 306
Alexandria, VA 22314
(703) 548-7790

MIND–BODY MEDICINE

What has now become an accepted healing phenomenon was once dismissed as the "placebo effect." The ability of a belief or image held in the mind to directly effect a change in the body on a physical, cellular level is now called mind–body medicine and includes such practices as meditation, hypnosis, biofeedback, creative visualization, the relaxation response, autogenic training, and neurolinguistic programming (NLP). All of these modalities make use of the intimate relationship and constant communication between the mind and the body.

Here is a simple example of how that relationship works. Imagine that you are sitting in your home at night, curled up in your favorite chair with hot cocoa and a great book. All the bills are paid, your kids are safe in bed, everyone you love is in good health, and it's been a great week. You feel happy, safe, and content. Suddenly you hear an unfamiliar noise. You start thinking about the evening news report on a convict who escaped from a local prison, and an image comes into your mind of the convict trying to break into your house. Almost instantly your pupils dilate, large quantities of adrenalin are released into your bloodstream, your digestive system shuts down and blood is shunted to your extremities, your bladder wants to empty, your heart rate increases, your blood pressure rises, the erector muscles in your hair shafts contract and goose bumps appear on your skin, saliva flow increases, blood clotting factors increase, and your liver starts dumping glucose into your bloodstream (Achterberg, 1985). Profound physiologic changes happen instantly simply in response to an image or belief that formed in your mind. You soon realize it is only a tree limb knocking against your window as the wind blows, and all the physiologic responses reverse themselves.

In the 1970s, Herbert Benson, M.D., first started exploring the relationship between the body and mind while doing research on the physiologic impact of stress on the body. His early work resulted in the development of what he called the "relaxation response," which can restore homeostasis and allow the body to heal from the physiologic changes that occur as the result of chronic stress. The "relaxation response" is achieved through mental imagery in a meditative state and activates the body's parasympathetic nervous system (Benson, 1996). The stress response, also called the "fight-or-flight" response, is initially an adaptive physiologic response to prepare you to get out of harm's way; but chronic activation of this system, without restoration of nonstress physiology, is believed to be the cause of many cardiovascular and immune dysfunction diseases (Achterberg, 1985). I have taught this technique to patients in hospital settings and seen how, at the very least, it helps them recover a sense of control over the course of their disease and treatment.

Dr. Benson's continued research on the placebo effect, which he calls "remembered wellness," found that in some studies there was a 70% improvement in patients who received treatments that had no medical foundation for their effectiveness, but which the patient believed was a cure. He has concluded that "belief in or expectation of a good outcome can have formidable restorative power, whether the positive expectations are on the part of the patient, the doctor or caregiver, or both" (Benson, 1996, p. 32). What you, the caregiver, believe can affect the outcome. In 1987, I worked with a cancer patient who chose to undergo chemotherapy, along with a macrobiotic diet, creative visualization, and positive imagery. I remember he would not let anyone into his hospital room unless they firmly believed that he was going to have a complete cure. He chased many a doctor and nurse out of his room, but he also had a quick, total response to treatment. I saw him 2 years later, and he was still cancer free and had organized a national support group for cancer patients. He was the cure for his cancer. Chemotherapy was only one of the tools he chose to use. We must be careful not to take this power, inside of each and every one of our patients, away from them.

One remarkable study Dr. Benson quotes in his book took place in 1950 (Benson, 1996, p. 32). Pregnant women suffering from persistent nausea and vomiting were given syrup of ipecac, which normally induces vomiting, and were told that it would relieve their symptoms. In a significant number of women, it relieved their nausea. Their belief overrode a normal physiologic response to a strong drug. Dr. Benson references many similar study results in his book and also cautions that beliefs can have the opposite effect—causing harm. In 1989, I was asked to teach relaxation and guided imagery to a cancer patient having severe pain unresponsive to medication. When I walked into her room, my first impression was that she looked 9 months pregnant. She walked around, got in and out of bed, and in every way carried herself like a pregnant woman. She was resistant to using relaxation and guided imagery, and as I got to know her I found out that she had an elective abortion about 12 years earlier. Further discussion showed that she believed that this cancer was God's punishment for having chosen to have an abortion. She did not respond to my efforts or to the chemotherapy, and she soon died. I can't say her beliefs caused the cancer, but I can say that her beliefs prevented her from accepting an opportunity for relief from her suffering.

"Western medicine still makes serious distinctions between mental, emotional, and physical roots of illness despite the amassing of research that finds that mind and body are so interwoven that such distinctions are not only artificial, they're unscientific" (Benson, 1996, p. 50). Candace Pert, Ph.D., has made significant scientific contributions to our understanding of how the mind–body relationship is mediated through biochemical pathways (Pert, 1997). Dr. Pert's research has identified and mapped the activity of 70 to 80 neuropeptides involved in modulating mind–body communications. These neuropeptides were once believed to have receptor sites only on neural tissue and be responsible for transmitting nerve impulses. Dr. Pert's research has found that there are receptor sites for these neuropeptides on the cell walls of a variety of body tissues, including the lining of the gastrointestinal tract, the kidneys, the pancreas, the heart, and the cells of the immune system. The limbic system, considered the center for emotions in the brain, has been found to be flooded with receptor sites for all of these neuropeptides. The neuropeptide-receptor mechanism on cell wall surfaces is a way for the cell to receive information from other body systems to effect a change in the function of that cell. It appears, therefore, that these neuropeptide messengers keep all of the body's organ systems in communication. "This interlacing of the nervous, endocrine, and immune system surely suggests a unified healing system" (Pert, Dreher, & Ruff, 1998, p. 34). There no longer seem to be any boundaries within the body–mind system, so that emotions of hope and images of faith are able to have direct, biochemical communication with our heart and immune system.

The relaxation response is a prerequisite for creative visualization, or **guided imagery.** "Visualization or imagery is the thought process that invokes an inner mental picture usually using all the senses, which include vision as well as hearing, smell, touch, taste, position and movement" (Jacobs, 1997, p. 174). Using all the senses in guided imagery, called *sensory recruitment,* activates more centers in the brain and increases the likelihood of eliciting the desired effect (Burton, 1997). Guided imagery as therapy was first popularized in the 1980s, when Dr. Bernie Siegel applied this technique in his work with cancer patients. I was working in the field of oncology at that time, and almost every patient came into the hospital for chemotherapy with Dr. Siegel's book *Love, Medicine, and Miracles* packed in their suitcase.

The goal of guided imagery is to enter a deep relaxation state and then visualize a process taking place in your body that alters the course of the disease. For example, a cancer patient might visualize angels coming into her body and surrounding the cancer with radiant light and dissolving the cancer cells. Or a patient with high blood pressure might visualize her blood vessels expanding and relaxing. Given what Dr. Pert has found in her research, as noted above, these images in fact can send biochemical messages to the immune system or blood vessels to attack the cancer or relax the cardiovascular system.

PSYCHOTHERAPY RESOURCES

The Academy for Guided Imagery
P.O. Box 2070
Mill Valley, CA 94942
(800) 726-2070

Guided imagery "...is a proven method for pain relief, for helping people tolerate medical procedures and treatments and reducing side effects, and for stimulating healing responses in the body" (Burton, 1997, p. 247). Its applications are limited only by one's imagination. It is a process that can be directed by a therapist or taught to the patient to do on their own. In either case, it is best for the patient to use the imagery that comes naturally to them, rather than have the therapist chose an image, because the sensory associations are already in place.

Hypnosis is a form of guided imagery, but the role of the therapist is more directive. It is "...an artificially induced state characterized by a heightened receptivity to suggestion" (Burton, 1997, p. 308). It can be used in the treatment of chronic pain, in overcoming addictions, for sleep disorders, and in treating mental health problems. Shrouded in negative publicity for years, hypnosis was accepted in 1958 by the American Medical Association as a viable form of treatment (Jacobs, 1997).

During hypnosis, the patient is put into a deep relaxation state and given suggestions to change a pattern of behavior or physical response to a situation. For example, once in a deep state of relaxation, the therapist might suggest to a patient with insomnia that tonight when they go into their bedroom they will suddenly feel drowsy, and as they are putting on their pajamas they become even more drowsy, and as they put their head on the pillow they are so drowsy they will fall asleep almost instantly. As this is repeated over and over in sessions, the patient will come to truly believe this and will, in fact, fall asleep under these circumstances every night. There are three criteria for successful hypnosis: trust in the therapist, a desire to be changed by hypnosis, and a quiet environment during the session (Burton, 1997).

Meditation, an ancient spiritual practice for achieving spiritual awakening, works by quieting the incessant, random flow of thoughts through the mind (Jacobs, 1997). Based on the work of Dr. Pert noted above, if thoughts engage neuropeptide messengers, then the body is constantly barraged by undisciplined thought processes. Try sitting quietly and not thinking about anything, or not attaching feeling to any thoughts that arise. When I first started practicing meditation, I found it disconcerting that I had no control over my thoughts. "This incessant activity is associated with chronic tension" (Jacobs, 1997, p. 163); as noted above, chronic tension is implicated in many chronic illnesses.

There are several styles of meditation that make use of different postures, different modes of achieving deep relaxation, and different techniques for focusing the mind. Many times meditation will bring up uncomfortable images or emotions that have been pushed deep into the subconscious, but proper training can provide techniques for looking objectively at these issues. Mindfulness meditation is taught in a pain and stress management program developed by Dr. Kabat-Zinn at the University of Massachusetts Medical Center (Burton, 1997). Mindfulness meditation is a form of meditation developed in the traditions of Buddhism and is designed to allow the meditator to be at peace in any experience in which they find themselves. It requires very focused attention and a nonjudgmental attitude (See Box 10-1).

> **Box 10-1**
>
> ### MINDFULNESS MEDITATION TECHNIQUE
>
> Choose a quiet, comfortable place to sit, with your back straight and your eyes closed. Allow a few moments for your body to relax, then begin to focus on your breath. You can focus on the rise and fall of your abdomen as you breathe, or on the gentle feeling of the breath as it passes across your nostrils. As thoughts arise, keep your focus on your breath. If your mind wanders, return your focus to your breath. Gently, without effort. As thoughts come and go, notice how they shift and change, without any attachment to the thoughts as you return your focus to your breath. With your breath as a point of focus, be aware of changes in you body. Without becoming attached to the changes, just acknowledge them and return your focus to your breath. Attend fully to just that moment, with your breath as the anchor for your mind. Practice for 10 to 20 minutes each day, preferably at the same time each day. This practice will help you to be more attentive to the day-to-day experiences of your life, without effort or stress, but with a deeper appreciation of the fullness of life that exists in each moment.

Meditation takes daily practice, preferably at the same time each day, commitment to practice whatever obstacles come up, a quiet place in which to practice, a time when you are not rushed to keep another appointment, and from 15 to 30 minutes out of your day. Avoid pushing yourself beyond what you can do, but do not give up too easily as you are learning. The body also tends to resist the discipline of sitting perfectly still for 15 or 30 minutes, and all sorts of physical aches and pains will manifest until you have mastered the practice (Jacobs, 1997). Perhaps it will help to know that, as a spiritual practice, meditators will sometimes sit from 8 to 10 hours per day.

Biofeedback training uses technology to provide feedback to patients training to gain conscious control over physiologic functions of the body, such as regulation of the heart rate. "Before the 1960s, most scientists believed that autonomic functions, such as heart rate and pulse, digestion, blood pressure, brain waves, and muscle behavior, could not be voluntarily controlled" (Jacobs, 1997, p. 73). Biofeedback has shown that, with practice, people can intervene and regulate the autonomic functions of their body. Research has shown biofeedback to be effective in treating insomnia, asthma, hypertension, irritable bowel syndrome, migraines, muscle pain, and eating disorders (Burton, 1997).

Biofeedback works by hooking the patient up to a machine that measures one or more physiologic functions, such as skin temperature, heart rate, brain waves, muscle tension, blood pressure, and the electrical conductivity of the skin. The patient is then asked to, for example, tell their heart rate or imagine their heart rate slowing down, or their blood pressure decreasing. When a change in heart rate or blood pressure occurs, the machine will flash a light or make a beeping noise. This serves as feedback to the patient, reinforcing whatever conscious or unconscious thought or imagery they were using, and, with practice, trains that person to consciously alter that particular physiologic function.

Autogenic training is a technique for inducing deep relaxation. It was developed in 1932 by Dr. J. Schultz, a neuro-psychologist in Germany. "It consists of a series of simple mental exercises designed to turn off the stressful 'fight–flight' mechanism in the body which causes the release of adrenalin, and turn on the restorative and recuperative rhythms associated with profound psycho-physical relaxation and healing" (Jacobs, 1997, p. 170). Autogenic training can be used for stress management, chronic pain, improving mental concentration, anxiety, phobias, high blood pressure, weight loss, overcoming addictions, insomnia, irritable bowel syndrome, stuttering, palpitations, and as a supplement for almost any health problem to reduce the stress associated with coping with illness or to reduce side effects from medications. Training sessions take from 1½ to 2½ hours, and people with active drug addiction or psychosis, or with a history of epilepsy, are cautioned about using this technique unless closely supervised.

Neurolinguistic programming (NLP) is the study of the relationship between neurology, linguistics, and "programs," or patterns of behavior. The *neurology factor* is not described in a medical sense, but rather refers to how one thinks and feels; the *linguistic component* refers to the use of language as a link between the external environment and subjective experiences of that environment; the *"programming" principle* is based on the hypothesis that one's *subjective* experiences can manifest as real life experiences, almost like a self-fulfilling prophecy. The NLP premise is that this "programming" can be *evaluated* and *changed*—therefore, changing one's life experiences. NLP believes that thinking is tied closely to physiology; thought processes can change the physiologic state. This theory is aligned with many other mind–body concepts. NLP provides a focused map with which to evaluate the current thought processes and then change them. The formal definition of NLP is: *the study of the structure of subjective experience.*

NLP evolved out of cognitive science research (linguistics, psychology, computer science, cybernetics, and anthropology) at the University of California between 1972 and 1981. Originally developed by John Grinder, a professor at the University of California and Richard Bandler, a graduate student, they wanted to know why some psychotherapies appeared to work better than others, and the results were more permanently sustained; they elected to study Milton Erickson, Virginia Satir, and Fritz Perls. Using those techniques in a systematic way, Bandler and Grinder were able to effect rapid and profound changes in human behavior.

My first experience with NLP occurred after a family member shattered his wrist in a horse accident. The nerve involvement caused so much pain that no medication gave relief; after more than 2 weeks of sleeplessness and discomfort, the skin started sloughing off his hand (from nerve damage, according to one physician). A certified NLP specialist came over. For over an hour, I witnessed many questions about such issues as the type of pain, the color of the pain, the sound of the pain, the location of the pain, and the path of the pain's movement. At various intervals, the patient was requested to change the color or move the path of the pain. After the session was completed, the pain was *significantly* decreased—and it never returned to the previous pain scale. Although an anecdotal experience, I was duly impressed.

According to Joel P. Bowman, Ph.D. (*spider.hcob.wmich.edu/bis/faculty/ bowman/nlp.html*), the role of the senses being linked to subjective experience has been around since Aristotle; however, Bandler and Grinder were the first to systematically examine this role in relation to the construction of subjective experience. Our five senses, called *sensory systems* or *sensory modalities* in NLP, are the raw data of experience; this is where the internal and external intersect. Our internal mental maps are constructed out of things we have seen, heard, tasted, smelled, and touched. NLP believes that different people develop a propensity for, and attach greater significance to, information they perceive through preferred senses (visual, auditory, or kinesthetic). For *visuals,* seeing is believing, and these people think in terms of pictures; they may use phrases such as, "I *see* what you are talking about." *Auditories* have internal conversations and use phrases such as "I *hear* what you are saying." *Kinesthetics* prefer the senses of smell, taste, and touch, and measure life by the way things feel to them; they may say, "This does not *feel* right to me." The NLP therapist in the example above assessed the patient's sensory preference, and worked with the individual's primary sense(s).

NLP practitioners use many other verbal and nonverbal cues to assess the way people are experiencing reality, and indicate specific kinds of thought processes: these include eye movements, certain gestures, breathing patterns, voice tone changes, and even very subtle cues such as pupil dilation and skin color changes.

MUSCULOSKELETAL THERAPIES

Musculoskeletal therapies are treatment modalities that bring the patient's awareness to body posture and movement, and manipulate the physical body to facilitate the flow of blood and energy through the muscles, fascia, and skeletal structures. These therapies include the Alexander method, the Feldenkrais technique, craniosacral therapy, rolfing, chiropractic manipulation, yoga, massage, and reflexology.

The **Alexander Method** was developed by F. M. Alexander, an actor in Australia in the late 1800s, who kept losing his voice and, thus, his livelihood. Over a decade of exploration, self-observation, and experimentation, he began to understand that the way he held his head, neck, and back affected the way he breathed, resulting in inadequate support for his vocal apparatus (Jacobs, 1997). Experiments done at Tufts University in the 1970s, "concluded that Alexander's methods could effectively interrupt or inhibit habitual and learned responses that interfere with proper body functioning" (Burton, 1997, p. 100).

"The Alexander Technique focuses on restoring a balanced, dynamic posture, or coordination of the head and the spine" (Jacobs, 1997, p. 104). The goal is to reprogram neuromotor patterns through repetitive musculoskeletal movements or postures. An example of a session might involve the patient repetitively getting from a sitting to a standing position, while the instructor used verbal and touch cues to realign the body as it is engaged in this movement. The Alexander method brings conscious awareness not only to one's body and how it helps or hinders movement, but also to the emotions involved in changes in body posture. Therapists who use the Alexander method do not treat specific medical conditions, but teach patients how to live more comfortably and efficiently in their body. "The Alexander method teaches a more relaxed and natural posture and movement patterns that balance the head while relaxing the neck muscles" (Brody, 1990). The overall goal is to coordinate the interrelated functions of the muscles and skeleton, so that they work together and not against each other.

Feldenkrais is very similar in its goals. "This system combines stretching, exercise and yoga to improve awareness of movement patterns and encourage proper body movement" (Jacobs, 1997, p. 290). The method was developed in the 1940s by Moshe Feldenkrais, a physicist in nuclear research, after he sustained a personal injury. Rather than undergo surgery that was being recommended, he began a study of the human body, exploring the fields of physiology, neurology, psychology, and anatomy. He wrote: "Each one of us speaks, moves, thinks, and feels in a different way, each according to the image of himself that he has built up over the years. In order to change our mode of action we must change the image of ourselves that we carry within us" (Burton, 1997, p. 101). Feldenkrais viewed the body as a complex interaction of many physical, emotional, and mental systems and believed that if we changed dysfunctional postural and movement habits, we could change dysfunctional patterns on all three levels of experience.

There are two approaches to Feldenkrais therapy. Patients can participate in group sessions called *Awareness Through Movement,* or receive one-on-one therapy called *Functional Integration.* The group approach involves a series of movement exercises taught to participants to subtly change postural habits. The one-on-one sessions involve a practitioner using touch to direct the participant's body during movement to move more fluidly. The movements are never imposed on participants, but each person is encouraged to find the relationship with their body that is most beneficial to them (Burton, 1997). This relationship is found, and can often be changed, through the process of consciously participating in the simple changes that happen in your body with movement.

Craniosacral therapy "manipulates the bones of the skull to treat a range of conditions, from headache and ear infection to stroke, spinal cord injury, and cerebral palsy" (Burton, 1997, p. 149). Just as the human body has a rhythm associated with the heartbeat and with the breathing, there is also a rhythm to the ebb and flow of fluid within the cranium and spinal cord generated by subtle pressure changes as fluid enters and exits these spaces. These pressure changes cause movement in the cranial bones, and if this movement is blocked, the fluid rhythm is disrupted, and it is postulated that a wide range of physical problems can result from this disruption. Although there is debate in the medical community about the ability of the cranial bones to move, craniosacral therapists believe that the cranial sutures between each bone are meant by their design to allow movement (Burton, 1997).

There are two approaches to craniosacral work. One is the sutural approach developed by William Garner Sutherland, an osteopathic physician in the early 1900s. Practitioners of this system manipulate the sutures, or joints between the cranial bones, to assure that they move smoothly in relationship to each other and in response to the rhythm of the cerebrospinal fluid. Sutherland called this system the "primary respiratory mechanism" and believed that the skull, spine, sacrum, and meninges all move to accommodate this rhythm. He also believed that this fluctuation in spinal fluid pressure changes generated an electromagnetic energy field that cycled between being positively and negatively charged (Jacobs, 1997).

The mechanism for systemic change through craniosacral manipulation is thought to be the fascial connections that are altered when a therapist adjusts the relationship between the cranial bones, vertebrae, and sacrum. Connective tissue is believed to hold the forces of old trauma through alterations in its shape and in its electromagnetic charge. Craniosacral therapy is especially effective as preventive medicine for infants and children, and can treat a large range of illnesses in adults because of its ability to effect changes in the central nervous system (Jacobs, 1997).

The second approach to craniosacral therapy is called the meningeal approach and was developed in the late 1970s by John Upledger, an osteopathic physician. His understanding of the relationship between the skull bones, sacral bones, meninges, and cerebrospinal fluid pressures is very similar to the first approach. Treatment involves the therapist first detecting where the restrictions in the craniosacral system are located, by sensing changes in the electromagnetic field. The therapist then applies gentle traction on skull bones, positions along the spine, and the sacrum, which "brings about a release by gently tractioning and elongating the meningeal membranes" (Burton, 1997, p. 151).

Rolfing, also called *Structural Integration,* is a form of deep, tissue massage, developed over a period of 25 years by Ida P. Rolf, a biochemist, and first presented to the public in the 1950s. Based on her own experience after an osteopathic manipulation, Dr. Rolf came to understand that "...the body's structure profoundly affects all physiological and psychological processes" (Burton, 1997, p. 102). Rolfers, practitioners who perform Rolfing, manipulate and stretch the body's fascial tissue to release adhesions and relieve restricted muscles and joints.

Rolfing is offered in an initial series of 10 sessions, with each session concentrating on a specific area or function of the body. Usually "before" and "after" pictures are taken of the patient so that they can see the often dramatic changes in the way in which they hold their body. I underwent a series of 10 sessions and can attest to the fact that, for me, the change in my posture was significant. I felt more at home in my body, and movements seemed less stressful. Recent research has shown that Rolfing allows the body to conserve energy more efficiently, contributing to less fatigue; enhances neurologic function in general; reduces lordosis (sway back); and significantly reduces chronic stress (Jacobs, 1997).

The system of **Yoga** was first chronicled 2,000 years ago in India, but is said to have its origins in ancient Hindu teachings almost 4,000 years ago. "Classical yoga is organized into eight 'limbs' that provide a complete system of physical, mental, and spiritual health" (Burton, 1997, p. 469). Some of the yogas focus on developing the mind, some on developing the body, and some on developing the deeper inner life of the spirit. *Hatha yoga* is the yoga of movement and coordinated breath. It is the daily practice of postures, balanced movements, and stretching, in coordination with rhythmic breathing. It is done in a meditative state, that is with a quiet mind, to balance the nervous and endocrine systems, stimulate the internal organs, and promote the smooth flow of *prana,* or energy, throughout the body (Jacobs, 1997).

The benefits of hatha yoga are impressive. They include increased exercise tolerance, increased muscle strength and joint flexibility, increased bone strength, enhanced blood oxygenation, improved cholesterol metabolism, improved cardiovascular function, more efficient respiratory function, balanced glucose metabolism, normalized bowel function, stimulation of the immune system, emotional balance, and increased intellectual function (Jacobs, 1997). Dr. Dean Ornish's Program for Reversing Heart Disease, in Sausalito, California, incorporates yoga practices. The University of Massachusetts Medical School Stress Management Clinic incorporates yoga into the pain management program. Dr. Herbert Benson, at Harvard Medical School, has done research on yoga practices and has found that they can elicit the "relaxation response" for combating the effects of stress (Jacobs, 1997). "The therapeutic results of yoga are starting to make converts of the established medical community, with some insurance companies now covering expenses, thus signaling an acceptance of the economic benefits yoga can bring to the health care system as well" (Burton, 1997, p. 473).

Therapeutic massage is the use of touch to manipulate the soft tissues of the body for the purpose of relieving muscle tension and promoting blood circulation. There are more than 100 styles of massage, which are categorized according to the type of strokes or manipulations used, the depth of the massage, the incorporation of movements with the massage, the body part worked on, and the overall goal of the session. The goals can include relaxation, improved circulation of blood and lymph for detoxification, relief of pain and recovery from injury, emotional release, and stress management (Jacobs, 1997). Swedish massage is the most common style of massage and uses gliding strokes, friction, and kneading, always directed toward the heart, because the overall goal is to improve blood circulation to the musculoskeletal system.

Massage can be used to relieve muscle strain, relieve the pain of arthritis, reduce anxiety, relieve muscle spasms, treat repetitive motion disorders, increase endurance and energy, relieve headaches, reduce swelling around joints or injuries, and reduce the symptoms of depression. Massage therapists are not trained to make medical diagnosis, and most states require therapists to be licensed. Conditions contraindicated for massage include certain skin conditions, late stages of osteoporosis, bleeding disorders, unhealed wounds, and certain circulatory conditions (Jacobs, 1997).

Reflexology is a type of massage that works only on areas of the feet and hands, where there are believed to be "reflex" points that can stimulate the glands and organs in the body. It is thought to have its roots in the practice of acupuncture, and that the "reflex" areas correspond to acupuncture points on the feet and hands (Jacobs, 1997). The therapist sees the whole body superimposed on the bottom of the foot and, based on painful spots on the foot or the symptoms reported by the patient, the therapist works on those areas on the foot. "Practitioners often target the breakup of lactic acid and calcium crystals accumulated around the 7,200 nerve endings in each foot" (Burton, 1997, p. 108). Because these nerve endings have connections with the spinal cord and brain, this is believed to be the mechanism by which the whole body can be affected.

Reflexology has shown to be effective in reducing the symptoms of premenstrual syndrome, hypertension, and anxiety and can be easily taught to patients for self-care at home. There is a certification process for reflexologists who have adequate training.

Chiropractic manipulations, called *adjustments,* are ". . . concerned with the relationship of the spinal column and musculoskeletal structures of the body to the nervous system" (Burton, 1997, p. 134). It is believed that when the spinal column is out of alignment, it interferes with the flow of nerve impulses or messages from the central nervous system. Thus, misalignment can have an impact on every part of the body. The spinal column, that is, the vertebrae, can become misaligned through trauma, poor posture, stress, and muscle tension.

Although evidence of chiropractic has been found to date back thousands of years, it was first developed in the United States in 1895 by David Palmer, a healer in the Midwest. He developed the first college of chiropractic in 1910 and during his lifetime articulated the philosophy on which chiropractic is built. Fundamental to his philosophy was the belief in an "innate intelligence" in the body to heal itself, and the role of the chiropractor was to remove obstacles to that process (Jacobs, 1997). Monthly chiropractic adjustments are recommended for preventive medicine, and chiropractic treatment has been found effective in the treatment of "respiratory conditions, gastrointestinal disorders, sinusitis (inflammation of a sinus), bronchial asthma, heart trouble, high blood pressure, and even the common cold" (Jacobs, 1997, p. 137).

MUSCULOSKELETAL RESOURCES

North American Societ of Teachers of Alexander Technique
(800) 473-0620

The Feldenkrais Guild
P.O. Box 489
Albany, OR 97321
(503) 926-0981

International Rolfing INstitute
P.O. Box 1868
Boulder, CO 80306
(303) 499-5903

International Institute of Reflexology
P.O. Box 12462
St. Petersburg, FL 33733
(813) 343-4811

Upledger Institute
11211 Prosperity Farms Road
Palm Beach Gardens, FL 33410
(407) 622-4706

BIOENERGY THERAPIES

Bioenergy therapies are treatment modalities that work on balancing the patient's energy body, sometimes called the auric field, and include such modalities as polarity therapy, therapeutic touch, magnetic therapy, and sound therapy. During this type of therapy, the practitioner's "energetic system represents a charged battery (at high potential) which is used to energize (or jump start) the subtle energetic system of a sick individual who is at low potential. This flow of healing energy from high to low potential appears to be similar to the flow of electricity, which behaves in a similar manner" (Gerber, 1996, p. 310).

Polarity therapy was originally developed by Dr. Randolph Stone, a physician, chiropractor, and naturopath. His interest in the underlying causes of illness led him to the study of ayurvedic and oriental medicine concepts of the energy field that surrounds the body and resulted in the publication, in the

1940s, of his findings about the human energy field. He wrote that "polarized energy currents precede physical form and are primary factors in well being" (Jacobs, 1997, p. 49). He found that the human energy field could be altered by touch, diet, sound, exercise, emotions, and environmental factors. Polarity therapy promotes the smooth flow of energy along electromagnetic paths around the body by releasing blockages of energy.

The body is viewed as an electromagnetic field, with a positive charge at the top and the right side of the body, and a negative charge at the bottom and the left side of the body (Jacobs, 1997). The therapist uses his or her own polarity to activate the flow of energy around the patient's body. For example, the therapist might place her right hand (a positive charge) on the knee of the patient (a negative charge), then place her left hand (a negative charge) on the shoulder of the patient (a positive charge). This joining of polar opposites creates a flow of energy that allows blockages to be released within the patient and homeostasis to be restored for healing on a physical, mental, and emotional level. "The benefits of polarity therapy can include an enhanced sense of well-being, improvement in physical health, increased energy, and a deeper understanding of oneself. It is useful for all conditions, from excellent health to extreme disease, and Dr. Stone himself specialized in cases that others pronounced as hopeless" (Burton, 1997, p. 112).

Because all living things have an energy field, what you eat is seen as very important in either supporting or undermining your human energy field. Vegetables sitting in a store for weeks will have a different energy field from vegetables fresh picked from a garden. The former can drain energy from your energy field, and the latter can nourish your energy field (Kempner, 1981). Subsequently, the energy of the therapist can promote healing or add to the energetic imbalance. If the therapist is sick or is emotionally upset during a session, her energy will be out of balance and, at the least, treatment will be ineffective. I encourage patients to trust their intuition, so that if they are in a room with a practitioner of any type, including medical doctors, and "feel" uncomfortable in their presence, they should not continue in a healing relationship with that person. More damage than good may result from such a relationship.

In her nursing theory, the Science of Unitary Man, Martha Rogers, Ph.D., also understood the role of the human energy field in providing care to a patient. She viewed the human energy field as the basic unit of a living system, which imposes pattern and organization on the whole. She further admonished nurses to understand that their energy field interacted with that of their patients, and just by walking into a patient's room you could have an impact on that patient's health (Rogers, 1970).

Therapeutic touch was developed by a nurse, Dolores Krieger, Ph.D., R.N., and has been the subject of several research studies. It is a "contemporary interpretation of several ancient healing practices in which the practitioners consciously direct or sensitively modulate human energies" (Burton, 1997, p. 111). Therapeutic touch has been clinically documented as effective and is used by nurses in many hospital settings.

Dr. Krieger first became interested in hands-on healing in 1971, while participating in a research project looking at biochemical changes that could be measured after the laying-on-of-hands by a known psychic healer. The study was repeated again in 1973, and both times the results were positive. Dr. Krieger decided this was important for health care professionals to understand, and she developed a curriculum for nurses. The first therapeutic touch class was taught at New York University to Master's-level nurses and was titled "Frontiers in Nursing: The Actualization of Potential for Therapeutic Field Interaction" (Gerber, 1996).

A therapeutic touch session begins with the practitioner centering, or quieting, himself or herself. Next the practitioner assesses the energy field by placing his or her hands 2 to 6 inches away from the patient's body and, by slowly passing his or her hands over the patient's body, senses or feels where the energy is blocked. Then the practitioner will focus on those blocked areas by placing his or her hands over the area and using energy to restore balance. The session can last for 20 to 30 minutes, and the patient usually experiences a sense of relaxation, although suppressed emotions can sometimes be released (Burton, 1997).

A recent article in *JAMA* (Rosa, Rosa, Sarner, & Barrett, 1998) reported on a study debunking the assertion that therapeutic touch practitioners could sense energy fields. Twenty-one practitioners were blinded to the investigator, who placed his hand over one of their hands and then asked them to identify which hand he was near. Only 44% identified correctly, which is what would be expected by random chance. This was a study done by a 6th-grader for a school project, but was allowed publication in a very prestigious scientific medical journal. Dr. Achterberg responded, in *Alternative Therapies* (Achterberg, 1998), out of concern that many in the medical community were latching onto this study and somehow extrapolating its results to all of CAM. Her article showed that there were no physicians involved in the original study, which is apparently unusual for *JAMA,* the parents of the child who helped with the study were members of an organization called "Quackwatch, Inc.," so their objectivity was in question, and using one study to project a blanket statement about the effectiveness of therapeutic touch, when almost 800 other studies have reported some level of effect using therapeutic touch, was, at the very least, unscientific.

I believe this study and the responses to it bring up an important issue for case managers. CAM is an area of controversy, and practitioners on both sides can be very passionate about their beliefs. As patient advocates, and advocates for quality health care, we need to keep informed about what works, constantly evaluate results, understand both sides of a controversy, and, most importantly, be assured that the patient's health and safety are the goal for all providers involved in the care and management of that patient.

Biomagnetics, or **magnetic therapy:** The earliest use of magnetics is recorded in Chinese writings from approximately 2000 BC, and ancient Hindu, Egyptian, Persian, and Tibetan writings refer to the use of a natural magnet, the lodestone. Magnetic therapy is used extensively in many parts of the world, including India, China, Japan, Russia, Canada, and France. According to some literature, the earth was once surrounded by a much stronger magnetic field than today. Scientists have recorded a decline in the strength of the earth's magnetic field over the past 155 years. The effects of the decline in the magnetic field on human health was realized when early cosmonauts experienced bone-calcium loss and muscle cramps while in space above the earth's magnetic field for an extended time. When artificial magnetic fields were placed in the space capsule, astronauts maintained their health.

In the past several years, magnetic studies have been done around the world. In some orthopedic studies, non-uniting fractures showed improved healing speed when magnets were placed on the area. Other studies indicate that biomagnetic and electric currents can relieve pain. One study has demonstrated the efficacy of bioelectric therapy in treating acute anxiety (Lowenhaupt, 1998). A condition termed magnetic field deficiency syndrome was identified in Japan in the late 1950s. It is characterized by a lack of energy, general aches and pains, frequent headaches, and dizziness; the symptoms were alleviated by the external application of a magnetic field to the human body. Interestingly, these symptoms resemble the more current epidemic of fibromyalgia and chronic fatigue syndrome.

William Pawluk, M.D., is a Board-certified family doctor on the faculty at Johns Hopkins, and has trained in acupuncture, hypnosis, and homeopathy; he has also been successfully using magnets as a CAM modality for several years. According to Dr. Pawluk, magnetic therapy acts on the body in the following ways:

- It is believed that magnetic therapy works on human metabolism mainly through the circulation of red blood cells, primarily because of the iron content in the blood. The adult human body contains 4 to 5 g of iron, which can be traced to all parts of the body; therefore, iron is an available element through which magnets may do their work.

- Europeans have measured increased blood flow in conjunction with magnet use; in some cases, thermograms have been used for measurements. Lay people report this increase in blood flow as feelings of warmth and tingling.
- Magnets are thought to affect chemical processes within and between cells. Chemists use sensitive magnetic equipment to measure simple and complex molecules. Researchers at Harvard have found that saltwater passes through a membrane quicker with a magnetic field.
- Magnets appear to affect nerve signals. High-strength magnets have caused anesthesia in one study; through a principle in physics called the Hall effect, Dr. Robert Becker put salamanders to sleep before surgery with electromagnetics. Some studies indicate that magnets can stop epileptic seizures. They are also used to study and map nerve structures deep in the brain, normally only accessible during brain surgery.
- Acupuncture and magnetic therapy are excellent in combination, especially for pain, fibromyalgia, and strains. However, this is not new; the earliest Chinese writings (2000 BC) spoke about the use of magnets with acupuncture. Dr. Pawluk states that magnets stimulate the acupuncture points and meridians. Many acupuncturists place magnets on the treated points, because they allow treatment to continue after a visit.

Although several studies concluded that magnetic therapy does not cause side effects, there are conditions in which they should not be used or should be used with caution:

- Pregnant women and people with pacemakers or automatic defibrillators are advised to avoid using magnets.
- Do not apply to an acute injury less than 48 hours old.
- Do not apply magnets to an area where a liniment or other chemical has been applied in the last 24 hours.
- Avoid using in an area that has a metal pin or plate implanted.

Again, the consumers have spoken; everyone from professional golfers and football players to the generic low back pain patient sing their praises. Therapeutic magnets can be found everywhere from drugstores to mail order catalogs. More research is needed to determine their value.

"It is worth noting that we commonly use the word 'instrument' in two primary arenas: music and medicine. This is not coincidence. Music is medicine. The human voice, and our conscious use of it, as instrument, is the scalpel of healing our diseased planet profoundly needs."

—THE VEIN OF GOLD: THE KINGDOM OF SOUND
JULIA CAMERON/TIM WHEATER

Sound therapy or **sound healing:** Sound therapy has been around since the advent of mankind. Ancient rituals of healing included singing, chanting, and the percussion of drums and rattles. *Toning,* which is the sustained vocal sounds of vowel tones, has been used for healing for thousands of years. The ancients "knew" that sound could destroy or heal; now, with our current technology and scientifically based research techniques, many are coming to that same conclusion. The current interest in sound healing is not insignificant; an Internet search for "sound healing" yielded over 15 million matches. The connection between sound and health/healing is being researched objectively by a growing number of groups and individuals. This is in response to the considerable evidence that various types of music, in specific keys, and with prescribed rhythms, can have a profound effect on humans.

The human system responds to sound in two related ways: through *rhythm entrainment* and through *resonance* (Burton Goldberg Group, 1997). The process of entrainment, or rhythm entrainment, results when the body matches its rhythm to the tempo of an external rhythm. The concept of entrainment was first noted in 1665 by a Dutch scientist, Christian Huygens. He observed that the pendulums of a roomful of grandfather clocks would begin to swing in unison, even though the pendulums were swinging at different times earlier in the day. This "experiment" was attempted repeatedly, with the same results. Centuries later, physicists ascertained that any atomic matter can be impacted by external pulses.

The power of rhythm comes from the concept of entrainment, as indicated *externally* by feet tapping while listening to upbeat rhythms. However, many believe that entrainment occurs on an internal basis, as external rhythms actually alter the tempo of our *internal* pulse systems. Pulses speed up or slow down to synchronize with an external periodic pulse; brainwaves entrain to the rhythm on a record or the pace of a speaker's presentation; the heart rate, respiration, and brainwave cycles entrain to each other. If we slow the breath, the heart rate and brainwaves will follow. Slowing brainwaves can cause heart rate and respiration to decelerate (Leeds, 1997). Conversely, in the 1960s, studies were performed because it was discovered that young people were having heart arrhythmias that seemed to be linked to certain heavy "rock" music. Erratic rhythms have simulated heart arrhythmias in the physical body, and anxiety can be generated psychologically.

Resonance is a second avenue in which humans respond to sound. Closely related to entrainment, resonance is the transmission of vibrations from one medium to another. The transmission of a resonant vibration requires three conditions. First, there must be an original vibrating energy source, such as sound via musical instruments or voices. Second, there must be a transmitting medium; air is the most common carrier for humans. Third, there must be a receiving agent of the vibration. The principle of resonance is most easily demonstrated through the use of a tuning fork and a piano. If a tuning fork keyed to the tone of 440 Hz (cycles per second) were struck, the "A" (or 440 Hz) string would vibrate on the piano. The vibration of the tuning fork triggered a response of a similar frequency (Andrews, 1992).

Sound and Brainwaves: The brain is an electrochemical organ, and electroencephalograms have been measuring electrical activity of the brain for over half a century. Researchers have divided this electrical brainwave activity into four main categories; ranging from the most activity to the least activity, the brainwaves are as follows (Emond, 1997):

- Beta Brainwaves: Most of our waking moments are spent in the beta frequency, in which our brainwaves pulsate at between approximately 15 and 40 cycles per second. Beta waves are of relatively low amplitude and are the fastest of the four different brainwaves. Beta waves are characteristics of a strongly engaged mind, such as a person in active conversation.
- Alpha Brainwaves: Alpha brainwaves pulsate at 9 to 14 cycles per second; this is the level humans experience when they are in moderate meditation or relaxed and walking in a garden. Where beta represented arousal, alpha represents nonarousal; alpha brainwaves are slower and higher in amplitude than beta brainwaves.
- Theta Brainwaves: Theta brainwaves vibrate at a greater amplitude and slower frequency range, which is between 5 and 8 cycles per second. Theta brainwaves are induced during repetitious activity where the tasks are automatic: running/jogging, freeway driving (when you cannot remember the last 5 miles), taking a shower, etc. Theta states are associated with deeper experiences of creativity, meditation, and daydreaming.
- Delta Brainwaves: When humans are asleep, the brainwaves cycle from 1.5 to 4 cycles per second. Here the brainwaves are of the greatest amplitude and slowest frequency. Lower amplitude (down to zero) is one method to define "brain death." Deep dreamless sleep would take one down to the lowest frequency of approximately 2 to 3 cycles per second.

Researchers have known for years that if humans do not spend enough time in the delta state (sleep deprivation), irritability, agitation, and possible hallucinations are induced. Recently, research has been done on deficiencies of the alpha brainwaves. In 1989, Dr. Eugene Peniston of the VA Hospital in Fort Lyon, Colorado, and Dr. Kulkosky, of the University of Southern Colorado, published a landmark study involving alcoholics and children of alcoholics in relation to brainwave biofeedback. The doctors discovered that many of these individuals shared a glaring deficiency; alcoholics and their children were not producing as much alpha brainwaves as a normal person. Drinking alcohol, however, produced more alpha (Halpern, 1997).

This brings us to the connection between brainwaves, health, and sound/music. The alpha state is a most desirable one because it is the frequency of brainwave that promotes relaxation and alertness; fortunately, there are many ways to induce an alpha brainwave state: biofeedback, meditation, yoga, or practice exercises suggested in Dr. Herbert Benson's landmark book, *The Relaxation Response*. Another method is to use sound, or specific types of music (1997).

Many types of music tend to dominate and override the natural rhythm of the heart by "entraining" it to the rhythm of the drumbeat. Slower, more relaxed rhythms will entrain the body to a more relaxed, meditative state. Scientists have discovered that this is related to a slowing down of the heartbeat and has been measured with micro-motion sensing devices. At the same time, our brainwaves shift from their everyday beta range (approximately 15 to 40 cycles per second) into the deep alpha range of about 9 to 14 cycles per second (1997).

On a more microscopic scale, Sharry Edwards uses tones or frequencies to create a healing effect. Sharry Edwards began her research into sound healing almost 20 years ago. As a young woman, tests showed that Edwards could hear sounds beyond the range of normal human hearing; an audiologist also found she could vocally produce sine waves. This incident led to her first project, which showed the ability to control a person's blood pressure by as much as 32 points using her voice. It was discovered, after years of testing patients' voice patterns, that there was a correlation between "missing" notes or frequencies and specific medical conditions.

The technique is often referred to as *bioacoustics,* which may be loosely described as a cross between music therapy and biofeedback. However, the sounds or frequencies used for this research are 'low-based frequencies,' rather than 'music' as we know it. These low-frequency sounds are presented to elicit specific biologic and emotional responses (Edwards, 1999). The bioacoustic principle hypothesizes that the brain perceives and generates impulse patterns that can be measured as brainwave frequencies; these impulses are, in turn, delivered to the body by way of nerve pathways. "The theory incorporates the assumption that these frequency impulses serve as directives that sustain structural integrity and emotional equilibrium" (1999).

The evolution of technology has allowed voice patterns to be graphed through computer programs, rather than a less technical method. To facilitate the myriad of interested researchers, The Sound Health Alternative & Resource Center International, Inc., was created.

SOUND RESOURCES

Sound Health Alternative & Resource Center International, Inc.
(614) 753-3930
htpp://sharryedwards.com

Janalea Hoffman, author of the book *Rhythmic Medicine: Music with a Purpose,* and a musician with a Master's degree in music therapy, uses music, rhythm, and entrainment in combination with guided imagery to impact health and well-being. Using practical techniques that are being used by health care professionals, she has developed a system of *Musical Biofeedback,* designed to assist patients to control their body rhythms. This music is composed with a rhythm that slows from 80 to 50 beats per minute. The listener learns how to match their heart rate and breathing pattern to the rhythm of the music; this, in turn, helps to lower blood pressure and has also been beneficial in lessening stress-induced heart arrhythmias. This technique was first researched decades ago using baroque music and was documented in Ostrander and Schroeder's landmark book, *Superlearning.* Another technique, called *Musical Acupuncture,* uses a steady cello rhythm of 50 beats per minute and has been useful in treating chronic pain such as arthritis, headaches, and backache. It is based on the idea that music can penetrate painful areas and "move the energy in the pain." The patient is involved, in that they are taught to mentally direct some of the tones into the discomfort, similar to acupressure or acupuncture.

The *Sound Healers Association* is a nonprofit organization founded in 1982. Their purpose is to disseminate information on the therapeutic and transformational uses of sound and music to the general public, including activities such as music and toning groups in hospitals, hospices, holistic centers, and schools. A research component investigates various techniques of sound and

---

SOUND RESOURCES

Rhythmic Medicine
P.O. Box 6431
Leawood, KS 66206
(913) 696-1990 (phone)
(913) 696-1994 (fax)

American Musical Therapy Association (AMTA)
8455 Colesville Road — Suite 930
Silver Spring, MD 20910
(301) 589-3300

---

music to objectively study their effects. The Sound Healers Association has an International Directory of Sound Healers, promotes national conferences, and distributes a newsletter featuring articles/announcements of workshops and concerts related to sound, music, and well-being.

SOUND RESOURCES

Sound Healing Association
P.O. Box 2240
Boulder, CO 80306
Phone: (303) 443-8181
Fax: (303) 443-6023
http://www.healingsounds.com/sha/shabout.html

There is so much activity and research in sound and healing that it would take a volume to describe. *The Tomatis Method* was developed by Dr. Alfred A. Tomatis, an *ear,* nose, and throat specialist. Simplistically, the Tomatis Method "reawakens" and balances hearing. Dr. Tomatis considers sound a nutrient, and, like others, believes that when the full spectrum of sound frequencies cannot be "digested" by the ear, health and psychological problems can occur. *The Monroe Institute* has done investigative research into the relationship of sound patterns and mental states for decades. The basis for the research is to find frequencies that balance the hemispheres of the brain through a process known as "Hemi-Sync."

Various components that make up sound and music, and play integral parts in the healing process, are being researched all over the globe. When a mother sings a lullaby, she hopes to "entrain" the agitated child with a soothing *melody*. *Harmony*, the relationship of one tone to another, is thought to alter, raise, lower, transmute, and shift energies. Pitch, the highness or lowness of a tone determined by the speed at which the tone vibrates, has well-known consequences. Psychoanalyst Roberto Assagioli states that "sound has great power over inorganic matter. By means of sound it is possible to cause geometric figures to form on sand and also to cause objects to be shattered. How much more powerful, then, must be the impact of this force on the vibrating, living substance of our sensitive bodies." Sound wave technology is being used in all phases of life, from medicine to space travel. Sound is accepted for diagnosis of many conditions through ultrasound technology. The "new" sound technicians claim that diagnosis can occur through individualized assessment of a person's sound/voice pattern. The future will likely prove the accuracy of this hypothesis; and it will catapult sound as a treatment and method of healing.

Flower essences are considered to be a form of "vibrational" medicine. Much like homeopathy, flower essences contain the energetic pattern of a flower, rather than its molecular structure. Energetic patterns around living things have been demonstrated through Kirlian photography and were first discovered in the 1940s. "Kirlian photography is a technique whereby living objects are photographed in the presence of a high frequency, high voltage, low amperage electrical field" (Gerber, 1996, p. 53). Using this technique, the electromagnetic field around living objects can be captured on a photographic plate held behind the object. These electromagnetic fields are considered to be the template or pattern that directs the growth of the physical, cellular structure of that object.

Flower essences are believed to work by affecting the energetic patterns of the body, rather than working directly on the cellular structures of the body (Scheffer, 1988). Edward Bach, a homeopathic physician in England in the early 1900s, is considered to be the father of the modern use of flower essences for healing. In his practice as a physician, Dr. Bach became increasingly interested in the role emotions played in contracting disease, and he began looking for simple, natural ways for patients to recover emotional balance. Bach "...felt that illness was a reflection of disharmony between the physical personality and the Higher Self or soul" (Gerber, 1996, p. 244). Abandoning a lucrative practice in London, he retired to his country estate, where he worked with flower essences and, before his death in 1936, eventually developed 38 flower essences with their indications for use on specific emotional imbalances.

Bach himself wrote: "The action of these remedies is to raise our vibrations and open up our channels for the reception of the Spiritual Self; to flood our natures with the particular virtue we need, and wash out from us the fault that is causing the harm" (Scheffer, 1988). Flower essences are used to change physical problems by working on the emotional and psychological imbalances in the body.

Flower essences are prepared in a very specific manner. The flowers need to be picked in the early morning, placed in a bowl of spring water, and left in the sun for 3 hours. The flowers are removed, and the flower water is poured into sterile bottles half filled with brandy. This bottle is considered the "Mother Essence," and only a few drops of this mixture are added to other bottles of spring water and brandy to prepare a remedy for a patient. Combinations of different flower essences can be put into one remedy (Burton, 1997).

Flower essences are typically included as part of another therapy, such as massage or psychotherapy, or the patient may be self-educated and have chosen to add this form of treatment to his or her healing efforts. Conditions con-

---

BIOENERGY RESOURCES

Polarity Wellness Center
10 Leonard Street, Suite A
New York, NY 10013
(212) 334-8392

Nurse Healers—Professional Associates, Inc.
175 Fifth Avenue, Suite 2755
New York, NY 10010
(212) 886-3776
Therapeutic Touch Resource

Bach Flower Remedies
The Dr Edward Bach Centre
Mount Vernon, Bakers Lane
Sotwell, Oxon
OX10 0PX, UK
Telephone: +44 (0) 1491 834678
Fax: +44 (0) 1491 825022

sidered to be affected by flower remedies are physical conditions that are made worse during stress, and any illness in which an unresolved emotional trauma is suspect as contributing to the symptoms (Burton, 1997).

Aromatherapy: Anyone who has ever smelled a rose in full bloom on a warm summer day, knows that the sense of smell can elicit a response in parts of the body other than the nose. When something is inhaled, "...the vapor travels immediately to the limbic system of the brain, which is responsible for the integration and expression of feelings, learning, memory, emotions, and physical drives" (Jacobs, 1997, p. 209). Aromatherapy uses the aroma from essential plant oils to stimulate a healing response. As well as being used for their scent, essential oil extracts can be applied topically.

Literature on the use of essential oils goes back to Egyptian times, but the name *aromatherapie* was coined in 1937 by Rene Gattefosse. In 1910, while experimenting with essential oils for treating war wounds, Mr. Gattefosse sustained severe burns to his hands during a laboratory experiment. He applied the essential oil of lavender "...to the burns and documented an abrupt arrest of the gasification of tissues and subsequent rapid healing of the wounds" (Jacobs, 1997, p. 206).

Many factors effect the preparation of essential oils, including the time of year the plant was picked, the condition of the soil the plant was growing in, and the pressure and temperature at which the oil was extracted. Essential oils, being lipid soluble, can penetrate every cell in the body and easily cross the blood–brain barrier. They have not been approved by the FDA for internal use and are most frequently used in massage oils, in bath water, by direct topical application, and by inhalation of the aroma (Higley, Higley, & Leatham, 1998).

Essential oils can be inhaled to effect an emotional response in the body, either to stimulate or relax a patient. Some commonly treated problems include acne, muscle pain, sinusitis, dandruff, depression, headaches, insomnia, nausea, stress, varicose veins, and eczema (Jacobs, 1997). Aromatherapy "...is most often used to promote relaxation, increase productivity, reduce stress, and lower blood pressure" (*Case Management Advisor,* 1997). Some of the chemical components of essential oils have the properties of bactericidals, immune stimulants, sedatives, nervous system stimulants, antivirals, digestives, antidepressants, and analgesics. Topical applications are absorbed into the skin and, therefore, will reach deeper tissues and organ systems.

Because some essential oil components also can be toxic, the use of essential oils, whether by a therapist or by self-medication, requires careful consideration of this fact. "There are no legal standards or aromatherapy training, certification, or licensure in the United States as there are in Great Britain, although there are many schools and individuals offering aromatherapy training" (Jacobs, 1997, p. 210). Often professionals licensed in another field, such as psychiatry or massage, will incorporate the use of essential oils into their practice.

When working with a provider who uses aromatherapy in their practice, ask for some evidence of training or experience in the use of essential oils, or if working with a patient who is self-medicating, assess their level of knowledge about the potential toxicity of some oils. This, however, is a relatively inexpensive therapy that lends itself easily to self-care, and there are many books on the market that the case manager can reference for the patient to safely incorporate aromatherapy into their health care.

AROMATHERAPY RESOURCES

National Association for Holistic Aromatherapy
P.O. Box 17622
Boulder, CO 80308
(303) 258-3791

CAUTION: Certain essential oils are toxic if taken internally. Some essential oils also may cause allergic skin reactions. Consult a certified practitioner or a reliable text before using any essential oils.

HERBAL AND NUTRITIONAL MEDICINE

"**Herbal Medicine** is the use of whole plants, or parts thereof, for the treatment of disease and the maintenance of good health. It is the oldest form of medicine known and has been practiced [around the world] for thousands of years" (Jacobs, 1997, p. 68). It is still the only form of medicine used in many primitive cultures, and it is also the most accessible medicine available to American consumers who are interested in alternative treatment for prevention or disease management. Just witness the plethora of herbal remedies found in health food stores across the country. *Time* magazine's cover story for November 23, 1998, entitled "The Herbal Medicine Boom," reported that one third of all Americans have used herbs for a variety of health-related reasons, and now some of the giant pharmaceutical companies are gearing up to compete in the herbal formula market (Greenwald, 1998).

Herbal medicine is an integral part of Chinese and Ayurvedic medicine, but the most commonly used herbs in the United States are from the European and

Native American traditions of herbal medicine. "The Greek physician Hippocrates left a list of 400 plants, many of which, including Elder, Garlic, Hawthorn, Henbane, Juniper and Thyme, are still in use today" (Jacobs, 1997, p. 69). Galen, a Roman physician around 150 AD, developed a more rigid system of prescribing herbs and created the first division among physicians— those who followed his classification of herbs and those who prescribed herbs based on experience handed down from Hippocrates. In the 15th century, the German physician Paracelsus introduced inorganic poisons, such as lead and mercury, into medical treatment, and herbal or plant medicine began to lose favor among physicians (Jacobs, 1997). Herbal remedies, however, remained an inexpensive and easily accessible medicine for the common folk.

Britain has a strong history of herbal medicine based on the native traditions of the Druids, to which they added the herbal knowledge brought by Greek and Roman explorers. A British apothecary, Nicholas Culpeper, published a materia medica of herbs in 1652, creating a stir among physicians. His book translated the herbs and their indications for use from Latin into English, thus making it more accessible to the public. Unfortunately, it was at this time that the Church of Rome began its 300-year persecution of "witches," which included persons using natural herbs for healing, so much of the knowledge about herbal healing was lost. Interestingly, many of the superstitions of that time, such as gathering herbs during a full moon, have gained scientific support. "It has been discovered that the alkaloid activity of many plants can fluctuate during the moon's cycle or even over a 24-hour period" (Jacobs, 1997, p. 70). Thus, picking plants at certain times of the day or month assures they are in their most potent state.

Herbal medicine made a revival in the 18th century in England, perhaps spurred by the inclusion of herbs learned from Native Americans during their voyages to the New World. "Today, herbal medicine is a blend of tradition and modern science" (Jacobs, 1997, p. 70). However, at best we have knowledge of only 2% of Nature's pharmacopeia. "There are an estimated 250,000 to 500,000 plants on the earth today (the number varies depending on whether subspecies are included). Only about 5,000 of these have been exclusively studied for their medicinal applications" (Burton, 1997, p. 254). Because from 60% to 70% of modern medicine's apothecary consists of drugs derived from plants (Weil, 1988), there is so much more we have to learn.

Modern drugs are made by extracting from plants that ingredient in the chemistry of the plant that is considered to be the "active" biochemical affecting the symptom being treated. Herein lies the argument for using the whole plant as medicine. Herbalists contend that by extracting the "active" ingredient only, the other ingredients naturally found in the whole plant are lost, and

Nature put these other ingredients in to prevent the side effects so often seen with drug therapy. Unfortunately, the economics is such that patents cannot be taken out on naturally occurring herbs, so time and money spent in research and marketing may not be recouped (Burton, 1997).

Herbs work in very much the same way that drugs work. They have biochemical components that can interact on the cellular level to effect change in human physiology, and they are classified by how they affect the body. For example, diuretics promote the flow of urine, stimulants increase metabolism, and antispasmodics ease muscle cramping. Herbs can come in the form of a loose tea, tablets, capsules, tinctures, essential oils, and ointments. There are no licensing bodies in the United States for herbalists, but naturopathic physicians have a firm background in plant medicine. Practitioners of Oriental and Ayurvedic medicine are qualified to recommend herbs from their tradition, and there are courses that offer certification in herbology (Burton, 1997).

Herbal medicine can be used for a wide range of conditions that can be self-medicated, such as the common cold, insomnia, constipation, headaches, menstrual cramps, minor pains, and skin rashes (Burton, 1997). For more complex or serious conditions, consult with a trained practitioner. A recent concern among health care providers that has developed with the increased use of herbs by consumers is their interactions with prescribed drugs. There are resources (see insert) for keeping informed about the latest research in this area, and it would be wise to encourage patients to share with the medical team what over-the-counter herbal formulas they are using.

HERBAL MEDICINE RESOURCES

American Botanical Council
P.O. Box 201660
Austin, TX 78720
(512) 331-8868

Nutritional supplementation, or vitamin therapy, is another burgeoning aspect of CAM in which self-prescription plays a big role. It is estimated that 46% of Americans take vitamin and mineral supplementation on a daily basis (Burton, 1997). Jeffrey Bland, Ph.D., a biochemist and nutrition expert, believes that "overconsumptive undernutrition," or the overeating of foods with little or no nutrition—junk foods—is the leading nutritional problem in the United States. Studies have shown that two thirds of the average American diet consists of fats and sugars (Burton, 1997). Rather than change their diets, American consumers are spending millions of dollars a year on vitamin supplements.

The government's Recommended Daily Allowance (RDA) for vitamins and minerals is based on what is necessary to prevent severe nutritional deficiencies. However, research today shows that the RDAs may be too low, and many Americans are suffering from mild deficiencies, with symptoms such as "...nervousness, insomnia, mental exhaustion, improper immune function, or proneness to injury" (Burton, 1997, p. 387). Nutritional supplementation can be a complex challenge, however, because most vitamins and minerals work synergistically and often require a combination of nutrients and nonnutrients to be effectively used (Jacobs, 1997). It is always wise to ask a patient what kind of and how many nutritional supplements he is taking, because improper supplementation can cause side effects. Meeting nutritional needs through a healthy diet is the best way to assure that the appropriate nutrients are combined.

A large part of naturopathic medicine is devoted to proper dietary recommendations and the use of nutritional supplementation, not only to prevent illness but to treat many chronic conditions (Murray & Pizzorno, 1991). Naturopathy has always seen the direct correlation between diet and health. But now more and more medical doctors are recommending supplementation as the research builds to support the important, essential role vitamins and minerals play in maintaining good health. As their popularity grows, there is much controversy about how much regulation should take place on the part of the government. Many people have had good success in treating chronic illnesses because they had the freedom to explore the use of large doses of vitamins or minerals, and they would not like this freedom taken away from them (Greenwald, 1998). As long as research continues on nutritional supplements, and consumers keep themselves educated on these findings, nutritional supplementation can be a good, relatively inexpensive adjunct for prevention of disease and maintenance of health.

The Integration of CAM

by Janice E. Benjamin, RN, MS, L.Ac.

CLINICAL INTEGRATION OF CAM

Eisenberg's 1990 survey estimated that 22 million people in the United States had visited a complementary and alternative medicine (CAM) provider during the previous year (Eisenberg, Kessler, Foster, Norlock, Calkins, & Delbanco, 1993). It was further estimated that more visits were made to CAM providers during that year than were made to primary care physicians (Milbank, 1998). And, most remarkably, it noted that consumers were willing to pay for these services out-of-pocket. "Five surveys conducted since 1990 report frequent use of CAM ranging from 30 to 73% by patients suffering from conditions such as cancer, arthritis, acquired immunodeficiency syndrome, multiple sclerosis, and acute back pain" (Pelletier, Marie, Drasner, & Haskell, 1997, p. 112).

The publication of these results has sent a shock wave throughout the medical establishment, and, in response, the medical professions and the insurance industry have been working to develop ways to integrate CAM into their treatment options and plan benefits. Leading the way for the insurance industry, in 1996, "Washington State required all health insurers to add coverage of CAM treatments to their coverage of standard medical care" (Milbank, 1998, p. 1). The medical profession responded and, by 1998, added elective courses on CAM to the curriculum of 27% of the medical schools in the United States (Milbank, 1998). "As part of their course agenda many faculty members who teach CAM classes promote a mutual respect between conventional medicine providers and alternative practitioners" (Moore, 1998). All evidence suggests that CAM is a growing phenomenon, and its use represents a shifting paradigm in health care delivery.

The most frequently cited reasons for increased consumer interest in the use of CAM therapies are:

- Dissatisfaction with limited options for treatment within allopathic medicine
- Perceptions of being treated too impersonally by medical doctors and hospitals

- Increased exposure to medical practices from other countries; increase in research indicating that many CAM therapies work
- An emphasis on wellness by the baby boomer generation
- A growing concern over the side effects of allopathic drugs
- An increase in support for CAM by nationally known figures (Pelletier, Marie, Drasner, & Haskell, 1997)

"Managed care, with its focus on patient involvement, preventive care, and health promotion, would seem a natural fit for alternative therapies. But until now, that has not been the case" (Toran, 1996, p. 57). Oxford Health Plans in Norwalk, Connecticut, has identified the following measures that will be necessary to achieve success in integrating CAM and conventional allopathic medicine:

- Doctors and hospitals must accept and offer alternative treatments.
- Doctors must be trained in alternative practices.
- Providers of alternative medicine must be credentialed.
- Studies of alternative medicine clinical outcomes must be undertaken.
- Insurance companies must offer access to alternative medicine providers to their members (Rifaat, 1998).

Personal interviews and a search of the literature indicated that all of these issues are being thoughtfully addressed and implemented in a variety of settings across the United States.

Health Plans

In 1997, **Oxford Health Plans** was one of the first major managed care companies to develop a CAM program within their health care network. "One of the main reasons Oxford decided to offer alternative medicine was in response to our members demands" (Rifaat, 1998). Following Eisenberg's 1990 survey, a survey done within the Plan network indicated that 33% of their members had accessed a CAM provider in the previous 2 years, and that the plan members were paying for these services out-of-pocket. Based on these results, Oxford Health Plans first identified five issues they believed would need to be addressed to successfully build a CAM program within their existing network of providers:

1. A network of credentialed CAM providers would need to be developed.
2. A CAM supplement to their regular benefits package would have to be provided.

3. They would need to offer a mail order service for their members to be able to purchase CAM-related products.
4. An information service to educate members about CAM modalities would have to be made available.
5. An ongoing CAM research program would need to be supported.

Oxford Health Plans then set up their own advisory boards to develop standards and credentialing guidelines for a variety of CAM modalities. The CAM modalities initially chosen to be offered through the Health Plan were acupuncture, massage, chiropractic care, nutritional counseling, naturopathy, and yoga (Rifaat, 1998). Consideration is currently being given toward offering reflexology, aromatherapy, Tai Chi, Alexander technique, Reiki, and Feldenkrais in the near future (Milbank, 1998). The requirements for CAM providers' participation in their network mandated that "alternative medicine providers meet state licensing requirements; meet clinical experience requirements; have a specialty certification (where applicable); undergo a site visit; have minimum malpractice levels; and commit to continuing education in their discipline" (Rifaat, 1998, p. 54). Their network currently includes approximately 2,500 CAM providers, and their members can access these providers directly without a physician referral. Oxford Health Plans also "offers an alternative medicine 'rider' that allows commercial groups to purchase insured coverage for certain alternative providers" (Rifaat, 1998, p. 54).

Oxford Health Plans addresses the need for consumer education by providing an ongoing seminars program for its members and an on-line medical guide. Their website, www.oxhp.com, offers information to all interested parties, but only their members can access the Conventional and Alternative Remedies Encyclopedia (CARE) found at this website. The Plan also has a research arm, with current studies being conducted both in collaboration with Beth Israel Deaconess/Harvard Medical School (Cromell, 1998) and within the Oxford Health Plans' network alone (Rifaat, 1998). Oxford Health Plans has provided some clear direction on how to successfully integrate CAM into an already existing health care delivery model, and is starting to generate the studies needed for other health plans to take the step to respond to consumer demands for CAM.

The **Arizona Centers for Health and Medicine** in Phoenix, Arizona, first opened in 1996 and currently has two clinics in their metropolitan area. The following information was provided during a visit to one of their clinics in September, 1998. The clinic is based on an integrative health care model and is staffed by medical doctors, osteopathic doctors, acupuncturists, and naturopathic physicians. The CAM modalities being offered include acupuncture, osteopathic manipulation, guided imagery, homeopathic medicine, herbal medicine, Feldenkrais, and naturopathic medicine. They will refer patients to yoga and Tai Chi services outside of the clinic, if indicated. The medical doctors, as primary care physicians (PCP), get referrals for medical care from outside of the clinic, but the bulk of the referrals for CAM are made from within the clinic network. Most of the CAM services are paid for out-of-pocket; however, they reported that a recent patient was able to get services reimbursed through her private insurance plan because of successful negotiations by the case manager who had initially referred the patient to their facility for chronic digestive problems.

When a patient first accesses the Arizona Centers for Health and Medicine, they are assigned a PCP who assesses what, if any, CAM modalities would be appropriate for their condition. They are then advised what will and will not be covered by insurance, and it becomes their choice whether to try the CAM modalities suggested. It was reported that most of the patients will choose to try the CAM recommendations, even though they know it will be a self-pay. The patient population was described as mostly patients with chronic health conditions that have not responded to conventional medicine who are already educated about the benefits of CAM before coming to the clinic. The clinic provides ongoing educational offerings on CAM for the general public and maintains a pharmacy that offers homeopathic remedies, Chinese herbal formulas, Western herbal formulas, and books and tapes on a variety of alternative medicine topics.

The physicians who staff the clinics and the patients who use the clinics for health care do not find it difficult to move between conventional medical care and CAM. They are trying to become a specialized clinic rather than a primary care facility, and the biggest obstacle to integration of these services is the willingness of insurance companies to consider reimbursement for CAM services. The Arizona Centers for Health and Medicine actively markets their services to local and national insurance plans, but they have found that the limitation in literature and research demonstrating cost benefits makes it difficult. They are not participating in research at this time.

In an interview with Jerry Whitworth, Director of the CAM program at **Columbia Presbyterian Medical Center,** in New York City, he indicated that they initiated CAM services for their patients about 4½ years ago. He noted that they started by introducing noninvasive services, such as Tai Chi, Qi Gong, yoga, meditation, and guided imagery, because there was literature to support their effectiveness in eliciting the relaxation response (see Chapter 10 on the relaxation response), which has demonstrated through research specific health benefits. Initially, it was accepted that, at the very least, CAM could help with quality of life issues associated with pain management, depression, and limited mobility.

The program was first introduced through the Department of Cardiology at the hospital, because the initiators of the CAM program were trained in that area of medicine; other departments interested in using these CAM modalities would refer patients to the cardiology department. Mr. Whitworth indicated that the CAM program has been designed and grown through careful consideration of the medical doctors' concerns, and they have tried to keep the indications for these services based on current research within the medical community. They regularly consult with the heads of the various departments to address their concerns, needs, and objections, and try to look at which CAM modalities, when joined together, can work for a greater number of disease pictures. The program is viewed as a tool for disease management, and, as the program is becoming more accepted among their clinical providers, they are working on developing policy and procedure manuals for the use of CAM modalities throughout the hospital.

The program is currently called the Department of Complementary Medical Services, and they are doing clinical trials, and empirical and outcomes-based studies within the hospital to evaluate the effectiveness of CAM. To minimize risks and assure acceptance of CAM, the hospital administration provides oversight for QA and QI issues, which also allows the hospital to have input into the standards of care they want for their specific institution. Mr. Whitworth identified five aspects of the CAM program that needed to be developed and maintained for integration with conventional medicine to be successful:

1. Ongoing inpatient and outpatient research.
2. Follow-up patient care to assure compliance with treatments initiated in the hospital.
3. Building and maintaining a data bank to support the efficacy of CAM treatments.
4. Tracking trends and setting future goals as the program grows.
5. Ongoing education for both patients and providers.

The average patient stay at Columbia Presbyterian Medical Center is five to seven days, so education, as well as intervention, is important to assure compliance and follow-up. The patients can access the CAM services through either self-referral or referrals made by nurses, or other health care providers interfacing with the patient during their hospital stay. The patient, depending on their specific needs, is assessed by a nurse specialist, and a personal CAM treatment is designed for them. The key to the initial assessment is to identify any physical obstacles to the patient's participation in the program and to design a treatment that honors the patient's point of reference. The patient is then taught some techniques to reduce stress, which might include guided imagery, hypnosis, massage, or music. Acupressure is also available for some specific indications, such as arthritis. On discharge, the patients are sent home with teaching handouts and exercises to continue to support the initial objectives for CAM. Mr. Whitworth indicated that changes in lifestyle and in beliefs is an important part of stress reduction, and this is where most of the resistance is met. More invasive techniques, such as acupuncture, are being looked at for introduction to the hospital at a later date.

The staff that does patient teaching and follow-up are trained through the Department in the CAM modalities being provided and in the goals of the program. Part of the Department training requires that the staff remain neutral as they provide and teach these techniques, to more scientifically evaluate the impacts. The providers are considered to be senior practitioners and must have licensure in a Western modality and certification or licensure in a CAM modality. For example, a registered nurse who is also certified as a massage therapist or a physical therapist who is also certified in hypnosis can become a part of the Department. Mr. Whitworth noted that many of the hospital staff who support the program have indicated that they do not necessarily believe in a physiologic impact from the interventions, but they can acknowledge an improvement in the quality of life for their patients. Currently, private philanthropies are underwriting the development and growth of the program.

Mr. Whitworth identified some of the obstacles to integration of CAM at Columbia Presbyterian Medical Center as reimbursement by insurance companies, resistance by conventional practitioners, and patients' lack of knowledge about CAM. They address the concerns of the insurance industry by keeping their studies focused on disease outcomes and patient benefits, which can best be translated into decreased health care costs. The outcomes measures used are ones currently available in the research community, such as the Beck depression scale and some commonly used quality-of-life scales. The program tries not to create an "either/or" atmosphere, but encourages flexibility of services to address the needs of all parties involved. The educational tools are kept neutral in their language, and patient feedback is encouraged. The program is looking at other hospitals and clinics to develop collaborative relationships in research and in developing standards.

Joan McKenzie, of **McKenzie Case Management Services,** Redding, California, specializes in workers' compensation case management. She noted in a telephone conversation that in her experience family practitioners and rehabilitation physicians are most likely to refer patients to CAM, and many times the request to try CAM comes from the injured worker. She has been in case management for 15 years and sees more and more members of the medical community embracing the use of CAM alongside conventional medicine. Although workers' compensation insurance in California does not pay for any CAM modalities, she finds that patients are willing to pay out-of-pocket if there is evidence that a particular modality can be effective.

Ms. McKenzie maintains a file of articles and information about research and outcomes in the use of CAM, so that she can have a body of evidence about CAM modalities when she approaches a patient or a physician about incorporating CAM into an existing treatment protocol. She believes that as more studies with outcomes are made available, the insurance companies will start covering CAM. She finds most physicians open to discussing a referral to CAM, but also recognizes that the lack of practice standards and guidelines for most CAM modalities makes it difficult to provide direction about how to incorporate a particular modality into a medical treatment plan. When looking for a CAM provider, she noted, make sure that he or she is certified in their field.

Ms. McKenzie's recommendations for providing case management for CAM included the following:

1. Educate yourself and have some evidence of the effectiveness of a modality before recommending its use.
2. Talk to practitioners of CAM in your community to understand what they do and what success they have had with various medical problems.
3. Consider opposing views; be objective and avoid any practitioner that suggests they can cure everything.
4. Negotiate flat rates for stated objectives; sometimes you can get CAM covered under this umbrella.

Ms. McKenzie indicated that she asks for a 6-week trial of CAM when she makes a recommendation, before deciding whether it will work for that patient.

Dianne Hice, with **Presbyterian Hospital's Health Plan,** Albuquerque, New Mexico, noted that they have contracts with acupuncturists and chiropractors through their health plan. They have in-house credentialing criteria and require the CAM practitioners to be licensed by the state. CAM modalities not regulated by the state, therefore, are not currently being considered for inclusion in the plan's network. The Health Plan initiated acupuncture services for their members in response to public demand, and the inclusion of chiropractic services was mandated by the state.

Ms. Hice indicated that the Director of the Health Plan is involved in national efforts to integrate CAM into conventional medicine, although this was not necessarily the position of their Executive Board. They are evaluating the successes and failures of other plans in incorporating CAM into their services and waiting for more results from outcome studies being done at various medical centers in the United States. As evidence becomes more available, they will consider the incorporation of other CAM modalities. There are no obstacles to members accessing the two modalities now being offered, but there are liability concerns about providing further services without some basis in research or documented evidence of efficacy. With this concern in mind, the Health Plan is moving carefully in their efforts to include CAM in their network of services.

Members access CAM on recommendation from their PCP. They have no educational programs in place for their members at this time, but handle each request on an individual basis. Ms. Hice related a case of a woman with a long history of migraine headaches that often necessitated visits to the emergency department. She was not responding to conventional treatment and was referred through their in-house case manager for acupuncture treatments. At the time of our interview, Ms. Hice reported that the patient had been free of headaches for 6 months. Her recommendations for case management of CAM was to refer according to diagnoses that have evidence of efficacy through research and to coordinate the ongoing care with the conventional medical team.

Rebecca Gudorof, Director of the Mind–Body Institute at **St. Joseph's Pain and Complementary Medicine Center** in South Bend, Indiana, indicated that they have been offering alternative therapies at their pain management center since 1974 and using acupuncture for 14 years. She attributed their successful use of alternative therapies in their pain management program to the neurosurgeon who first opened the clinic. He had a personal interest in alternative therapies and incorporated biofeedback, electrical stimulation, stress management, relaxation training, and art therapy into the early treatment plans.

Ms. Gudorof reported that 3 years ago there was a top organizational decision at St. Joseph's to look into CAM therapies to see whether they might be incorporated into their current medical services. To that end, their medical director traveled to other facilities already using CAM, including Dr. Andrew Weil's clinic in Tucson, Arizona, Dr. Deepak Chopra's center in San Diego, California, and Dr. Herbert Benson's Mind–Body Center at Harvard Medical Center. The medical director returned with recommendations for St. Joseph's board, and, based on these recommendations, an internal task force was developed to assess:

- The level of physician interest or acceptance within St. Joseph's Medical Center.
- The level of consumer interest within the local community.

- The number and types of CAM resources already available in the local community.

The Medical Director was particularly impressed with Dr. Benson's program at the Mind–Body Center, and the task force was eventually sent to his facility to participate in a series of educational programs on mind–body medicine. It is this model for health care delivery that St. Joseph's has decided is the best fit for their patient and professional community, and their institution, and the long-term goal is to integrate this model of care as the practice standard for their facility.

Mind–body medicine is a model for assessing, treating, and looking at outcomes (see Chapter 10 on mind–body medicine). Mind–body medicine is research based, and continues to be researched through Dr. Benson's Mind–Body Center at Harvard Medical School and its affiliated clinics. In August 1997, St. Joseph's converted their outpatient cardiac rehabilitation unit to the mind–body model, and in June 1998, they opened an outpatient mind–body cancer program. They are in the process of converting aspects of the pain program to the mind–body model, currently use the mind–body model for their smoking cessation and weight management programs, and are developing a women's health clinic based on this model. Acupuncture is also offered in the pain clinic, but it is not considered part of the mind–body medicine model, and coverage varies depending on the patient's insurance plan.

Ms. Gudorof identified one of the obstacles to successful integration of CAM into conventional medicine as the need for further education about CAM concepts and modalities, for both health care practitioners and consumers. The Mind–Body Institute has in-house case managers who help educate the patients and direct them into the CAM clinics as indicated, as well as educate the staff about mind–body medicine. Referrals to CAM are made by the primary care physicians, except for acupuncture, which can be a self-referral by the patient. The Institute participates in research as an affiliate of Dr. Benson's Mind–Body Center in Boston, Massachusetts.

A survey of physicians' attitudes about CAM was done at **Hennepin County Medical Center** in Minneapolis, Minnesota, in 1997. "The medical center was one of the first in the United States to open an alternative medicine clinic on campus" (Boucher & Lenz, 1998, p. 59). The clinic offers massage, herbal remedies, and acupuncture, and serves about 700 patients per month. The medical center also supports a research department studying the use of CAM for treating addictions and hypertension. The survey was done to add to the body of surveys done so far to assess the level of acceptance of CAM within the medical community. Results of other surveys have indicated that 36% to 93%

of physicians have referred patients to CAM, attended lectures on CAM, or participated in training for at least one CAM modality.

The survey at Hennepin County Medical Center was done by sending a written questionnaire to all physicians who work at least 20 hours a week at the medical center. The questionnaire addressed both general knowledge and acceptance of CAM and more specific knowledge about CAM therapies for those physicians with more experience using CAM. Forty percent, or 109, of the physicians queried responded to the questionnaire. The results indicated that:

- Most physicians supported the integration of CAM into the practice of allopathic medicine.
- Consumer interest in CAM was the driving force behind the physicians' interest.
- All the physicians together had knowledge of more than 40 CAM therapies.
- The physicians believed that integration of CAM with conventional medicine would have a positive effect on health care delivery.

My overall impression from interviews and a reading of the literature is that the medical community is more than ready to take seriously the integration of CAM within the current health care delivery system. The main issues are (1) the need to have more research-based evidence regarding the efficacy of specific modalities and (2) how best to fund these efforts. A significant move was made toward addressing at least the first issue when the American Medical Association "...recently issued a proclamation to all members encouraging them to become involved in the scientific evaluation of alternative medicine" (Boucher & Lenz, 1998, p.65).

ST. JOHN'S WORT CAN EVEN MAKE HMOs HAPPY

According to the American Botanical Council, one Oklahoma-based HMO has begun prescribing herbal medicines based on a report by a member-doctor showing a potential annual savings of $500,000 to $750,000. The report compares the costs of scientifically tested herbs such as St. John's Wort ($9 per month) with those of popular drugs such as Prozac ($72 per month). The member-doctor estimates that the indirect cost savings, from fewer emergency room and clinic visits, for example, will drive the actual savings even higher. "In today's managed care environment," the member-doctor says, "the language is that of cost savings" (*Let's Live*, August 1998, p. 18).

The Milbank Memorial Fund offered seven recommendations to assure that there is accountability for the safe integration of CAM into conventional medicine (Milbank, 1998):

1. Consumers need to keep themselves well informed of the benefits and risks of CAM modalities.
2. Physicians need to keep themselves well informed about CAM treatments and research being done in that field.
3. Physicians who incorporate CAM into their practice need to be clear with their patients about their changing role.
4. CAM practitioners have to allow evaluation of their treatments by scientific scrutiny.
5. Medical educators need to keep themselves and their students abreast of the latest research in CAM.
6. Health plans should be prepared to clarify their decisions regarding coverage of CAM and be more involved in evaluating the benefits of CAM.
7. State licensing boards need to be more accountable for the regulation of all health care providers.

Insurance Issues

Insurance company policies are often identified as a significant obstacle to the integration of CAM into the health care delivery system in the United States. "However, until there is clear scientific proof of the efficacy of particular CAM therapies, each insurance company is left to decide for itself whether the effectiveness may exceed the cost of covering a particular therapy" (Pelletier, Marie, Drasner & Haskell, 1997, p. 115). "Insurers also worry that they might have to pay for CAM treatments in addition to MD-DO treatment, thus incurring higher costs" (Milbank, 1998, p. 6). Even as the medical community moves aggressively ahead to integrate CAM, it is still a very gray area for insurance providers.

In 1996, Stanford University School of Medicine's Complementary and Alternative Medicine Program of Stanford (CAMPS) conducted a comprehensive literature review and database search on insurance coverage of CAM, and interviewed 18 insurance companies about their policies regarding coverage of CAM. Nine of the companies were known to already offer coverage for some CAM therapies, and the other nine were randomly chosen (Pelletier, Marie, Drasner & Haskell, 1997). The literature review found that the proponents of insurance coverage for CAM most often cited three reasons why the insurance industry would be able to demonstrate cost savings if they decided to include CAM coverage within their benefits:

1. A limited number of studies have shown that visits to CAM providers are less expensive than visits to allopathic physicians.
2. Some surveys indicate that people attracted to CAM are often healthier to begin with, so users of CAM benefits are at lower risk for costly medical care needs.
3. Many CAM providers offer preventive medicine, which can decrease the potential cost for expensive medical care in the future.

Box 11-1

SAMPLE OF INSURERS/PLANS THAT OFFER SOME FORM OF COVERAGE FOR CAM MODALITIES

- HealthPartners Health Plan, Phoenix, AZ
- BlueCross of Washington & Alaska's AlternaPath, Seattle, WA
- American Western Life Insurance Company's Prevention Plus, San Mateo, CA
- Suburban Health Plan, Inc., Shelton, CT
- Kaiser of Northern California
- Sloans Lake Managed Care, Denver, CO
- Complementary Healthcare Plans, Portland, OR
- Minnesota's HealthPartners
- Blue Shield's Lifepath, Phoenix, AZ
- Mutual of Omaha
- Prudential Health Insurance
- St. Augustine Health Care HMO, Tampa, FL
- Kaiser Permanente, Oakland, CA

Of the 18 insurance companies interviewed, 12 said that "...market demand was their primary motivation for offering coverage of CAM" (Pelletier et al., 1997, p. 116). All of the 18 insurance plans offered coverage for at least one CAM therapy (see Box 11-1 for a sample of insurers covering CAM modalities). The most frequently covered therapies were:

- Chiropractic and osteopathy (covered by 18 plans)
- Acupuncture (covered by 17 plans)
- Biofeedback (covered by 16 plans)
- Preventive medicine (covered by 15 plans)

- Nutritional counseling (covered by 12 plans)
- Massage therapy (covered by 11 plans)
- Hypnotherapy (covered by 10 plans)
- Acupressure (covered by 9 plans)
- Homeopathy (covered by 8 plans)
- Naturopathy (covered by 7 plans)

Other modalities covered to a lesser extent included herbal medicine, guided imagery, meditation, yoga therapy, Ayurveda, craniosacral, reiki, Rolfing, the Ornish heart program, support groups, Qi Gong, Alexander technique, and reflexology (1997).

Some of the ways that CAM is being incorporated into existing benefit packages include:

- Stand-alone plans through which health plans or employer groups contract with a speciality health plan for their CAM coverage
- Riders and supplemental plans that offer some CAM services for a little higher premium and co-pay
- Discount programs that provide access to a network of CAM providers who have agreed to discount their services to members of a specific health plan (Gelonek, 1998)

Reimbursement for CAM services is dictated by a variety of issues, including the current market rate for a service; the practitioner's license or level of education; internal decisions made by a particular health plan; and the Current Procedure Terminology (CPT) code being used. Insurers recognize that some CAM services are being offered under CPT codes not designed for that procedure, and some insurance companies are developing "dummy codes" for their CAM providers to use. It was found that insurers will consider a specific CAM procedure if it can be determined to be medically necessary, if there is any evidence in the literature that this therapy has some efficacy, and if the CAM provider has licensure or certification in that state and has malpractice insurance (Pelletier, Marie, Drasner & Haskell, 1997). This is clearly an area in which case management can intervene and negotiate CAM services for a patient by establishing medical necessity and assuring that the CAM provider is appropriately licensed or certified in his or her field and adequately insured.

To address the concern about finding credentialed CAM practitioners, a "...number of insurers and managed care organizations are beginning to establish their own credentialing criteria for network providers" (Toran, 1996, p. 61).

Research Issues

*"What we observe is not nature itself, but
nature exposed to our method of questioning."*

—W. HEISENBERG

I was working at the National Institutes of Health (NIH) in 1992, when the first rumors began quietly circulating that a new office at NIH was being formed—the Office of Alternative Medicines (OAM). I was thrilled and filled with hope for the future of CAM and promptly called the OAM to see whether I could find a job with them as a nurse with a research background. I was told that their budget could barely cover more than a secretary to field calls. Today, 6 years later, the OAM has been elevated to the status of the National Center for Complementary and Alternative Medicine (NCCAM), and given a budget of $50 million for fiscal year 1999. This represents a 250% increase from the OAM budget for 1998 (Muscat, 1999). These changes have occurred because of legislation passed by the Congress and Senate in Washington, DC.

The NIH is the medical research arm of the federal government's Department of Health and Human Services, and it consists of 25 institutes and centers that focus their research dollars on specific categories of disease (for example, the National Institute for Cancer, and the National Institute on Aging). This new status within the NIH gives the NCCAM more authority to conduct research, issue grants, and appoint advisory panel members to set future directions for research. The NCCAM currently supports 13 medical centers across the United States doing research on CAM treatments for geriatrics, HIV/AIDS, asthma, cancer, cardiovascular disease, addictions, pediatrics, allergy and immunologic disorders, women's health, general medical conditions, stroke and neurologic conditions, and several areas of research on pain (Integrative Medicine Consult, 1998).

The November 11, 1998, issue of the *Journal of the American Medical Association* (*JAMA*) was devoted wholly to the discussion of CAM and the study of outcomes research that has been done with CAM therapies. "It marked the first such effort by a mainstream U.S. medical journal and was an attempt to meet doctors' need for high-quality scientific information on treatments that more and more patients are trying...." (Okie, 1998). This also represents significant recognition by the established medical profession that CAM is here to stay and that they are ready to embrace its study within the scientific model of investigation. The big question, however, that is debated in the literature is, "Does CAM lend itself to investigation using the same scientific guidelines that are used to study the efficacy and safety of allopathic treatments?"

CAM practitioners do have some basis for being wary of scientific scrutiny, because it was once used to prevent them from participating in mainstream health care (Milbank, 1998). The often-given rejection of CAM modalities, because they do not have "scientific" evidence for their use, has holes in it on closer scrutiny. Some of allopathic medicine's standard treatments have also not been scientifically proven (1998). It is time for all aspects of health care to be revisited and looked at with new eyes.

The three basic criteria that have needed to be met when designing research in allopathic medicine are objectivity, reproducibility, and predictability. The protocol design best suited to meet these criteria is the double-blind, random-ized, controlled clinical trial. "Double-blind" means that neither the study subject nor the researcher knows who is getting the real treatment/drug and who is getting a placebo. "Controlled" means that one group of subjects is randomized to get the active treatment/drug and the control group is ran-domized to get a placebo, but no one knows to which group they have been randomized (DePoy & Gitlin, 1994). This design was developed because it works so well for an allopathic model that does not believe consciousness or bioenergy systems can have any impact on the intended effects of their treatment interventions. For example, if you have high blood pressure and you take a "proven" anti-hypertensive drug, it should work irrespective of your lifestyle, your belief system, your emotional state, or your interper-sonal or professional relationships. CAM practitioners object to this model for scientific research because it is too impersonal and does not allow for mul-tiple levels of experience to come into play in the healing process (Dossey, 1995). It is these multiple levels that can be hard to control, reproduce, and predict.

As an example, neurolinguistic programming (NLP) (see Chapter 10) is a fascinating CAM modality that could have many medical and psychological implications. As research in this area becomes more scientifically based, the case manager may be able to learn to "read" their patient's cues to better assess their needs. However, according to Stever Robbins, it is difficult to "prove" that NLP works using traditional methods. Some research problems include (Robbins, 1998):

1. The practice of NLP takes intensely detailed perception and skill. Interven-tions must be performed smoothly and "congruently" or the intervention will not work. It is difficult to find experimenters who are trained in these skills and are also objective enough to do credible research.
2. There is not a credentialing process or quality control in NLP. Two well-trained NLP practitioners should reach an identical diagnosis, and be able

to tell you exactly how they reached it, down to the eye movement. Research based on poor practitioners will yield poor results.

3. As stated above, the standard model of research does not allow for multiple levels of experience to come into play in the healing process, because they are hard to control, reproduce, and predict. NLP integrates so many levels of experience, isolating and controlling one piece may be a formidable challenge.

4. NLP interventions are based on a very individualistic diagnosis. Two people with a similar diagnosis/symptoms may have different cognitive structures; they may therefore react very differently to the same NLP intervention.

In CAM, a continuum of therapies are available to patients. Some therapies would lend themselves to the double-blind study model, such as taking herbal medicine for a specific condition; whereas, at the other end of the spectrum, interventions such as prayer or reiki or sound therapy will require a different set of theories about their mechanism of effect and how to measure their impact on a disease process. The underlying belief that seems to drive the interest in CAM is that a human being is so much more than anatomy and physiology, and one's consciousness or mind plays a much more important role in health than allopathic medicine has entertained in its study of disease. And what about energy fields? These perspectives on the human condition do not easily fit into objective, reproducible, and predictable little boxes (Dossey, 1995). We need to know that a health care practice is safe and that it has some theoretical foundation for its methods, but research also can be about redefining and finding new and unexpected outcomes. As allopathic and alternative practitioners continue to work side-by-side and become more integrated in clinical settings, research itself will be changed.

Another myth about CAM and research is that there is very little of it available. However, CAM has been an accepted part of health care in Europe for many years, and their research institutions have collected a good body of evidence for many CAM modalities (Cromell, 1998). The dilemma CAM researchers face in the United States has been access to research dollars. "In order to receive grants for medical research and be published in the major medical and scientific journals, physicians and researchers are compelled not to stray far from conventional views" (Burton, 1997). This, however, is slowly changing, and the NCCAM is playing an important role in getting money out into the community of CAM practitioners and researchers. There are good resources (see Chapter 12) for finding reliable references to current research on all kinds of CAM therapies, and the future looks bright for improving not only CAM through new research efforts, but improving conventional medicine as well.

Legal Issues in CAM

A newly forming concern among health care providers and insurance plans is their legal liability when choosing to incorporate a CAM modality into their practice or benefits package, or when referring a patient to a CAM practitioner. Equally of concern is not referring to a CAM practitioner when emerging literature is indicating that a particular CAM therapy is proving to be beneficial for certain conditions.

The first issue encompasses two aspects of referral liability. One aspect is the licensure or legal standards under which a CAM practitioner is providing treatment. If a CAM practitioner does not practice under any state regulation, that is, if he or she has no license or certification because it is not required by the state, such as a lay homeopath, is the physician liable for referring to someone practicing medicine without a license? Or, if the CAM practitioner is licensed or certified but provides a treatment that is out of their scope of practice, is the referring physician liable? The answer to these questions may vary from state to state. Even if no harm is done, a complaint to a state medical board that frowns on the practices of CAM, for example, can lead to a finding that a physician is liable for referral to a person practicing without a license and the CAM practitioner can be liable for practicing medicine without a license (Cohen, 1999).

There is not much in the literature addressing the legal issues surrounding the integration of CAM and conventional medicine. M. H. Cohen, J.D., in his book *Complementary & Alternative Medicine: Legal Boundaries and Regulatory Perspectives,* comprehensively addresses the legal concerns that are developing and would be a good resource for a case manager working with CAM services being integrated with allopathic services.

CAM Implications
for Case Managers

by Janice E. Benjamin, RN, MS, L.Ac., and Suzanne K. Powell, RN, BSN, CCM

Case management can be seen as an opportunity to bring balance into what is often a tense and complicated relationship. Figure 1 depicts the health care delivery system without the element of case management. In this situation, the patient is at risk of becoming the object of a tug-of-war between the insurance plan/benefits and the medical providers. The patient's world is unstable, and the patient is pulled from one end of the delivery system (insurance) to the other (medical providers); as CAM therapies move into the health care setting, this will be intensified. Figure 2 shows the transition that can occur when case management is added to the delivery system. The case management influence allows the patient to be the center of health care and opens up the dimensions shown in the three circles, so that all aspects of the patient's experience-of-self can be incorporated into the holistic care of the patient:

- Body-mind-spirit
- Family/friends/personal support system
- Religion/culture/economic influences

Too often the medical and insurance partners in a relationship are looking at the patient's situation from a limited perspective. The insurance companies have their statistics, actuarial tables, guidelines, and expected outcomes on disease-specific processes. Physicians have an opportunity to bring holistic considerations into the relationship with the patient, but they also have their bottom lines based on the disease process that is being treated, the financial pressures and the risk contracts they have agreed to, and their own knowledge of CAM modalities.

The case manager is in a unique position in this relationship, in that case management looks at the patient (or disease population) from a whole-picture perspective. It is imperative that the case manager look at *all* options that will impact the final outcomes of the patient's health. If the case manager is aware of alternative modalities that may positively affect the patient's health, he or she has an ethical obligation to inform those involved with the care of this infor-

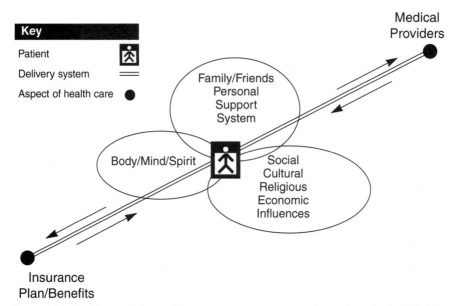

Figure 12-1. Health care delivery without case management. (By Janice E. Benjamin, RN, MS, L.Ac.)

mation. There is also an obligation to evaluate and inform about insurance benefits (or lack thereof) for the alternative modality. When someone's quality of life (or life itself) is at stake, all information must be provided so that the health care team can make an informed choice. The case manager is often the "balance" between opposing forces and must be astute in negotiating win–win outcomes for all parties involved in the delivery of care. Again, the case manager's "bottom line" is to focus on the patient.

CAM modalities can be a rich resource from which to draw tools for achieving a win–win outcome that best meets the needs of the patient. Depending on the setting in which the case manager is employed—acute inpatient, outpatient, HMO, workers' compensation, private payor—the initiative for incorporating CAM into the treatment plan may originate from:

1. The patient or one of their family members
2. The physician or a member of the medical team
3. A representative of the payor or plan
4. The case manager

Once a CAM consult has been requested, one of the first steps a case manager will need to take is to identify the rationale behind the request to incorporate CAM into a treatment plan. The case manager also must assess what the

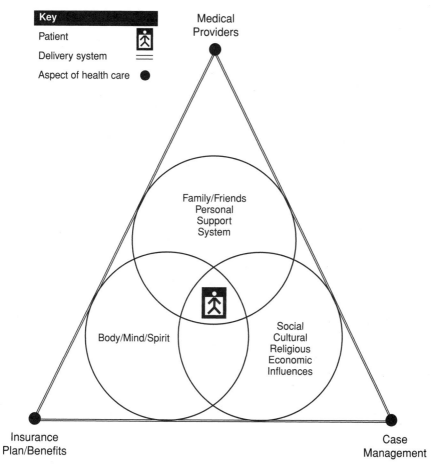

Figure 12-2. Health care delivery with case management. (By Janice E. Benjamin, RN, MS, L.Ac.)

expected outcomes are for the CAM modality that was chosen. "Patients who turn to alternative therapies want something the traditional care model is not giving them" (Lowenhaupt, 1998, p. 30). A relevant issue that Eisenberg's 1990 survey revealed was that most consumers using CAM were not telling their treating physician about the modalities they were using (Eisenberg, Kessler, Foster, Norlock, Calkins & Delbanco, 1993). Current literature is identifying some concern that, especially in the case of many herbal supplements, this can put the patient at risk for adverse interaction between conventional and alternative treatment modalities (Greenwald, 1998). This is an area where case management can be of invaluable service to both the patient and the health care team. If a case manager discovers that a patient they have been working with is already using CAM, and the medical team and health plan are unaware that another form of treatment is being used that could be having an impact on the expected medical outcomes, the case manager has an opportunity to align the two through education of all parties involved.

There are several challenges, and several opportunities to educate, that are being addressed as CAM comes into the medical arena like rolling thunder. The CAM concern mentioned above is primary. Others cited in the literature include:

1. Lack of availability of practice guidelines and standards of practice for CAM practitioners
2. Lack of scientific evidence supporting the efficacy of most CAM modalities
3. Finding a reliable source for understanding the indications and contraindications for CAM modalities
4. Locating credentialing guidelines and services for CAM providers
5. Locating or creating outcomes measures for evaluating treatments with CAM
6. Facilitating acceptance of CAM by insurance companies, physicians, and other health care providers
7. Educating CAM providers about managed care and insurance concepts
8. Educating consumers about the indications and contraindications of using CAM
9. Educating consumers about insurance coverage issues
10. Identifying which of the many CAM modalities are appropriate for each patient

Some of these concerns are addressed in Dr. David Eisenberg's strategy of discussion points between the patient and the practitioner (Eisenberg, 1997). In the absence of practice guidelines, standards of care, and empirically reliable resources, a formal discussion about patient preferences and expectations, followed by a strategic monitoring and follow-up care plan, becomes even more essential. Dr. Eisenberg recommends that a discussion about alternative therapy should not occur until the patient (1997):

- Has undergone a complete conventional medical evaluation, including diagnostic assessment and, where indicated, referral to consultants
- Has been advised of conventional therapeutic options
- Has tried or exhausted conventional therapeutic options or refused these options for reasons documented in their medical record

Using a low back pain patient as an example, the following approach can be considered for integrating CAM and conventional medicine. This hypothetical patient has already had the following treatments fail: nonsteroidal anti-inflammatory medications, physical therapy, regular exercise, and avoidance of heavy or improper lifting.

1. Ask the patient to identify the principal symptom (1997). Low back pain is the principal symptom.
2. Maintain a symptom diary (1997).

   This diary will be used for baseline assessment and evaluation of subsequent alternative (or conventional) therapeutic interventions. A 1 to 10 scale is recommended, where 1 equals "no back pain," and 10 equals "the worst pain imaginable."

3. Discuss the patient's preferences and expectations (1997).

   This is a critical piece, and requires several areas of focus:

   - What modality does the patient wish to attempt; what modality does the patient think may help the problem (remember the mind–body connection, or even the placebo effect)?
   - If the patient lacks preferences for specific therapy, or lacks knowledge about existing options, then investigating further options and shared decision making is important.

4. Review issues of safety and efficacy (1997).

   Physicians are obligated to monitor therapies with potential of documented toxicity, including herbal mixtures, dietary and supplemental formulas, medicinal agents delivered by injections or intravenous infusion (such as chelation therapy), and certain forms of spinal manipulation (1997). Ongoing discussions with the patient are necessary to evaluate any self-directed changes (deletions, additions, or tweaks in the protocols) by the patient.

5. Identify a licensed provider (1997).

   As insurance benefits mandate credentialing of CAM providers, this task may get easier. Check to see whether there is a state association for the therapy you are interested in and whether there are any certification or licensing requirements for that state. Look into national associations and see what national standards have been set for that profession (see Chapter 10 for references to some national associations).

6. Provide key questions for the alternative therapy provider during initial consultation (1997).
   a. Is the provider's belief in the effectiveness of the therapy based on clinical experience with similar patients?

    b. What will the therapy include?

    c. How much time will pass (or how many treatments) before the patient and practitioner have decided that the treatment is/is not helping?

    d. What is the cost per session? Is there insurance assistance?

    e. What are the potential side effects (if any)?

    f. Will the CAM provider communicate diagnostic findings, therapeutic plans, and follow-up with the primary care provider (PCP)?

7. Schedule a follow-up visit or telephone call to review the treatment plan with the patient (1997).

    Dr. Eisenberg suggests the following topics during this follow-up session:

    a. What were the CAM practitioner's responses to the questions in number 6?

    b. What are the potential risks or toxicities of the treatment recommended?

    c. Are there any recommendations that directly conflict with the conventional physician's treatment plan, such as the postponement of surgery in a potentially treatable malignant cancer (1997)?

8. Follow-up to review the response to treatment after a reasonable period (usually 4 to 8 weeks) (1997).

    Assess whether the patient's condition has improved. If positive outcomes have been observed, then there is anecdotal evidence that the treatment (or the CAM practitioner) is beneficial for future similar patients. If there are no positive outcomes, the physician and patient need to "go back to the drawing board" and re-evaluate what options exist.

9. Provide documentation (1997).

    As in all medical records, documentation is critical. Document clinical encounters, conversations, advice that led to treatment decisions, and refusal of any treatments of discussion.

LACK OF AVAILABILITY OF PRACTICE GUIDELINES AND STANDARDS OF PRACTICE FOR CAM PRACTITIONERS

Practice guidelines and standards of practice result from mature endeavors. After scientifically based outcomes measurement studies and continuous quality improvement projects have determined which of the many protocols are most effective, guidelines can start to be developed and standards of practice can be formalized. Although many CAM modalities have been around for hundreds or thousands of years, they have not been scrutinized by today's scientific methodologies. Therefore, accepted practice guidelines are a thing of the future.

There are a few guidelines available now, and, like allopathic guidelines, they will be updated and revised as new information is obtained. Several years ago, the American Chiropractic Association (ACA) adopted formal guidelines designed to manage chiropractic patients in the most efficient and effective manner (Toran, 1996). The goal for the guidelines for Chiropractic Quality Assurance and Practice Patterns is to assist payors and chiropractors to evaluate the treatment given to the patient. These guidelines have been distributed to insurers and utilization review companies (1996). Others are also creating standards and guidelines; the Integrative Medicine Program at the University of Arizona is working with HealthPartners Health Plan to develop standards for rating alternative practitioners (Cromell, 1998). The resources at the end of this chapter and those listed in Chapter 10 are a starting point for reference. As insurance coverage expands to include CAM modalities, coverage protocols will be written. These will have to correspond to evidenced-based research, which is still in its infancy for CAM modalities.

In 1995, a panel convened by the Office of Alternative Medicine (OAM) of the National Institutes of Health decided that "CAM practices currently are unsuitable for the development of evidence-based practice guidelines, in part because of the lack of relevant outcomes data from well-designed clinical trials" (Milbank Memorial Fund, 1998). Another challenge in developing CAM guidelines relates to the fact that, by its very nature, CAM treatment is very individualized; this contradicts the goal of standard guidelines, which attempt to reduce variations in practice (1998).

The NCCAM panel (the OAM has been elevated to the status of the National Center for Complementary and Alternative Medicine [NCCAM]) has more recently published three recommendations to help in the evolution of CAM treatment (1998):

1. Initiate well-designed clinical studies of CAM.
2. Include CAM among the treatment options considered by groups that develop practice guidelines for conventional medicine.
3. Set standards for evaluating the competency of CAM practitioners.

Another issue related to standardized guidelines is that of utilization review criteria for CAM modalities; these, too, must be established and peer-reviewed by those in the profession. Like allopathic utilization review, case managers and others who "manage" the resources of patients must have a template to work with. Carve-out companies who manage chiropractic services have developed some criteria for various back and neck problems. And it may evolve to where, rather than the CAM modality becoming the focus of utilization review criteria, the disease state will be the focus, with the CAM modality being one of the medical treatment options.

LACK OF SCIENTIFIC EVIDENCE SUPPORTING THE EFFICACY OF MOST CAM MODALITIES

During my years as a case manager on the medical-surgical unit of a large metropolitan teaching hospital, I had many HIV/AIDS (human immunodeficiency virus/acquired immune deficiency syndrome) patients in my charge. These people were often readmitted at fairly regular intervals, and I had the opportunity to speak with them about the various healing modalities they were using. A local clinic was available that provided alternative treatment free of charge to people with AIDS. Perhaps because the clinic was so proximal to the hospital, at least 50% of the AIDS population that I case managed used various CAM modalities. The range of treatments included "alternative" intravenous solutions, vitamins, minerals, enzymes, herbs, prayer, guided imagery, homeopathic remedies, acupuncture, and even crystal therapy.

Over the years I was stricken time and again with an anecdotal observation: those AIDS patients who did not use CAM modalities had a long, agonizing terminal curve. Those who used CAM modalities had an enhanced quality of life (in comparison to the non-CAM users), and, when death was imminent, there was a quick decline.

Scientifically, there are too many variables and no real controlled studies to support my observation. But serendipity occurs when no one is looking; and this could be the challenge that some astute (and bold) researcher may tackle. Certainly, anecdotally humans have for centuries "felt better" while using various herbs, acupuncture, chiropractic, massage, and forms of meditation. Conversely, our world demands scientific proof—and outcomes management studies on CAM modalities has already begun. However, it must be realized that, as of this writing, the outcomes studies are in their infancy; and until tangible data are produced, credible guidelines cannot be developed.

Slowly, the effectiveness of some CAM modalities are being confirmed. A Consensus Statement endorsing benefits of acupuncture was produced by an independent panel of experts under the Office of Alternative Medicine (OAM) (now the National Center for Complementary and Alternative Medicine - NCCAM) of the National Institutes of Health (NIH). The statement says, "There is clear evidence that needle acupuncture is efficacious for adult postoperative and chemotherapy nausea and vomiting and probably for the nausea of pregnancy. . . acupuncture may have a more general effect on pain" (Anonymous, p. 16, 1998). Acupuncture was also deemed an "acceptable alternative" to conventional treatments for many other conditions, including headache, low-back pain, tennis elbow, carpal tunnel syndrome, fibromyalgia, menstrual cramps, asthma, stroke rehabilitation, and addiction. Also noted was that there was considerable evidence that acupuncture causes the release of natural pain-relieving substances (endorphins) (Weil, 1998).

In November 1998, the *Journal of the American Medical Association* (*JAMA*) dedicated an entire "theme issue" to CAM treatments; this was an attempt to meet physicians' need for high-quality scientific information on alternative treatments that more people are trying every day. Six alternative therapies were studied using the classical research design of randomized clinical trials in which one group receives a treatment, and another group receives a placebo.

In one study, moxibustion was used to turn fetuses from a feet-first position to a head-first position before delivery. Moxibustion is a traditional Chinese therapy that burns the herb artemisia vulgaris at an acupuncture point (in this case near the toe). The results were impressive. After 2 weeks of therapy, 75% of the fetuses in the moxibustion group turned over; only 48% of the control group changed fetal position. Although no one is sure how or why this works, one thought is that the acupuncture point changes the nerve stimulation to the uterus. Another study using Chinese herbs helped to relieve abdominal pain, constipation, or diarrhea in people with irritable bowel syndrome (Okie, 1998).

In a survey of insurance companies, responses were tallied for the major obstacles to incorporating CAM into mainstream health care. The number one obstacle cited was the need to do more research on efficacy of the therapies (Pelletier, Marie, Dresner, & Haskell, 1997). There are some challenges with doing research on CAM modalities, as stated in Chapter 11. However, unless there is "proof" that these therapies improve quality of life and decrease costs over the long run, "token" CAM benefits will be all many insurance companies will offer. Furthermore, by only offering a small amount of benefits, there is a likelihood that these members will not fully benefit from the CAM care (which often takes time to see results); this, in turn, may lead to a domino effect of both members and payors in concluding that CAM modalities have little or no effect on medical conditions. Only scientific-based research will conclusively answer questions such as (1997):

- What constitutes a clinically defined, effective course of therapy versus what is allowed or limited in the CAM policy?
- What constitutes an adequate length of care for chronic pain with acupuncture?

- How effective is homeopathy versus antibiotics for children with otitis media?

FINDING A RELIABLE SOURCE FOR UNDERSTANDING THE INDICATIONS AND CONTRAINDICATIONS FOR CAM MODALITIES

Finding sources of information on CAM modalities, including indications and contraindications, is not difficult. International resources can be found on the Internet; books on various alternative treatments are proliferating; oldies, but goodies (for example, the *Physician's Desk Reference* (PDR) has a "PDR for Herbal Remedies"); articles on the subject can be found in every magazine from *Better Homes and Gardens* to case management journals. The difficult part is discerning what is reliable and credible information. Some suggestions include:

- Look for comprehensive literature citations, including research and clinical trials in books and articles.
- Research the Internet, using respected and credible sites (such as the NIH website for alternative medicine).
- Ask questions of CAM practitioners who are appropriately licensed and credentialed.
- Obtain information from the universities that are integrating CAM into their mainstream medical internship programs; as of this writing, approximately 53 medical schools offer some type of education about CAM modalities.

The philosophy of the Integrative Medicine Program at the University of Arizona is that by training doctors to combine the best of conventional and alternative therapies, the care plan will yield more cost-effective health care on a long-term basis. This program is supervised by such physicians as Dr. Andrew Weil, a well-known advocate of alternative healing methods. These types of programs are training interns to answer the questions about not only indications and contraindications of various therapies but also possible interactions between conventional therapies and CAM modalities. This program has a 2-year fellowship that includes a curriculum in 12 subject areas such as nutritional medicine and mind–body medicine, mastering the practice of guided imagery, medical acupuncture, homeopathy, and osteopathic manipulation. Part of the program trains the doctors to establish similar programs around the country. Lastly, these medical students do much of their internship in the Integrative Medicine Clinic, rather than the conventional clinics typically seen (Cromell, 1998).

Research is an integral part of this program and others like it. Scientifically based research studies have been done in places such as Germany (especially on herbal medicines). And these universities have made it a priority; a long-term research goal for the Integrative Medicine Program is to develop an agenda to determine which alternative treatments are most effective for specific conditions and circumstances (1998). Credible information is here if the case manager knows where to look. This search will become easier as programs such as the one described become more mature.

LOCATING CREDENTIALING GUIDELINES AND SERVICES FOR CAM PROVIDERS

As the managed care industry agrees to include CAM modalities into their benefit designs, they are mandating that CAM providers go through a credentialing process much like the physician networks. There are already some credentialing organizations that have added the specialty of alternative, or CAM, providers to their marketing list. In the mid-1990s, this may not have been worth the price to the CAM providers to participate in these credentialing organizations; now, they will be wise to "join up" because insurance companies will look for this protection.

When Oxford Health Plans, Inc., became one of the first major health plans to launch a comprehensive alternative medicine program, it was done with much thought and planning to the credentialing component. In an effort to provide members with the same quality of care they receive in the conventional program, Oxford set up alternative medicine boards that helped to set up credentialing standards for their CAM network, which includes approximately 2,500 acupuncturists, massage therapists, nutritionists, naturopathic physicians, and yoga instructors. Oxford's biennial requirements of their CAM network providers resemble any good credentialing program and include the following elements that may be a template for others to follow when credentialing CAM providers. CAM providers must:

- Meet state licensing requirements
- Meet clinical experience requirements
- Have a specialty certification (where applicable)
- Undergo a site visit
- Have minimum malpractice levels
- Commit to continuing education in their discipline (Rifaat, 1998)

Licensing of CAM providers is another growing field. Using acupuncture professionals as an example, various "levels" of education can be acquired to qualify one to perform acupuncture. At this time, there are approximately 10,000 acupuncturists in the United States; approximately 3,000 M.D.s also perform acupuncture. However, the M.D. may or may not have the extensive background as someone with a Master's degree, which is the national standard for the practice in the United States. As mentioned in Chapter 10, in some states M.D.s and D.C.s are credentialed by their own national association, which requires fewer hours of study. It is not unlike the different educational levels in which a nurse may enter the field: diploma course, associate degree in nursing, baccalaureate of nursing, Master's level, etc. Thirty-three states now have licensure standards in which the minimum requirement mandates that those who practice on patients must pass national acupuncture boards. This is growing slowly state-by-state.

Licensing and certification for other CAM practitioners is receiving legislative attention in many states. States now regulate over 1,100 professions and occupations in health and other fields, with approximately 600 of them through licensure; however, one-half of the states regulate fewer than 60 professions, according to the Council on Licensure, Enforcement and Regulation, an association of state and provincial officials from the United States and Canada. Chiropractors are the only CAM practitioners at this time that require a license in all states; as of 1996, 33 states regulate acupuncture, 22 states have massage therapy laws, and nine states regulate the practice of naturopathy (Toran, 1996).

Most national alternative organizations can supply lists of licensed individuals in the states in which the case managers practice (for example, homeopathic associations, acupuncture associations, etc.). As consumers become more savvy (and they are already), they should review the license and professional credentials of any CAM provider they are considering.

One question is: Is it possible to adequately credential or license all forms of CAM modalities? Certainly invasive, or hands-on, techniques such as acupuncture, herbology, or chiropractic require some method to protect the public from poorly trained individuals. Again, this is a growing field; it is unknown whether all CAM modalities, such as yoga teachers or aromatherapy, will also be scrutinized and tested.

The credentialing component of CAM modalities is still in its infancy. Word-of-mouth with satisfied patients is one method to find a practitioner. Another method is to contact national organizations; there are resources in Chapter 10 and at the end of this chapter. However, there are also questions one can ask so that educational choices can be made. As an initial screening, ask the practitioner (Weil, 1998):

1. What training do they have in the applications of the therapy?
2. How long have they practiced?

3. Have they had experience in treating your particular condition?
4. Can they refer you to patients who have been treated by the practitioner with similar conditions?

LOCATING OR CREATING OUTCOMES MEASURES FOR EVALUATING TREATMENTS WITH CAM

Research in the field of CAM is being addressed. Chapter 11 discusses some of the research taking place, and inherent in that research will be the creation of outcomes measures and the subsequent evaluation of the various therapies. The NIH has an starter fund of $50 million for the NCCAM. The recent "theme issue" of *JAMA* demonstrates the power of this change in conventional medicine. Not all of the six studies showed evidenced-based improvement in the condition being treated; but that is why research is done—to establish "best practices," whether the therapies are all "conventional," all "alternative," or a combination of both.

Many countries are more advanced in the study of CAM modalities than the United States. Herbal medicine has been widely used in Europe and Asia for centuries. The research and pooled studies that brought St. John's Wort into the limelight were from all over the globe. Chinese medicine and therapies are centuries old; acupuncture is routinely used in lieu of anesthesia for surgeries from cesarean sections to brain procedures. Ayurvedic practitioners have been treating people from India for centuries. The *Physician Desk Reference for Herbal Medicines* is based on the work conducted by the German Federal Health Authority's Commission E and Jöerg Gruënwald, Ph.D. Germany and the United Kingdom cover many CAM modalities in their national health payment systems. And consider the extensive use of CAM throughout the world (Milbank Memorial Fund Report, 1998):

Country: Britain
Prevalence: 1 in 10 persons uses CAM
Most Popular Types of CAM Modalities: acupuncture, chiropractic, osteopathy, homeopathy, herbal medicine, and hypnotherapy

Country: France
Prevalence: one third of the population uses CAM
Most Popular Types of CAM Modalities: homeopathy

Country: Norway
Most Popular Types of CAM Modalities: homeopathy, acupuncture, aromatherapy

Country: Russia (legalized alternative medicine in 1993)
Officially Recognized CAM Modalities: reflexology, chiropractic, home-
    opathy, a breathing method

Country: Japan
Prevalence: two thirds of the population uses CAM
Most Popular Types of CAM Modalities: herbal medicine, acupuncture,
    and acupressure (shiatsu); over 600 herbal medicines are available under
    the national health insurance system.

Country: Australia
Prevalence: one third of the population regularly visits a natural therapist,
    and two thirds regularly take vitamins and use other "natural" treat-
    ments
Most Popular Types of CAM Modalities: chiropractic, naturopathy, mas-
    sage, herbal medicine, and homeopathy

CAM modalities did not appear on national health systems without efficacy
studies. It is likely that outcomes measurements/research studies can be found
worldwide, and case managers who have access to the Internet can obtain information through that media. Seminars, videos, and texts on CAM modalities
are proliferating, and many discuss research studies that can be used (in whole
or in part). Researchers interested in CAM efficacy are predicting that evaluating standards for uniform reporting of outcomes, such as those in the National
Committee for Quality Assurance and the Health Plan Employer Data and
Information Set, will increasingly include areas of prevention and CAM therapy outcomes standards (Pelletier, Marie, Drasner & Haskell, 1997).

FACILITATING ACCEPTANCE OF CAM BY INSURANCE COMPANIES, PHYSICIANS, AND OTHER HEALTH CARE PROVIDERS

The primary care physician (PCP) of the future will ideally be well versed in
CAM modalities. That does not mean that this physician will have all the
answers or be proficient in all medical techniques. PCPs make referrals—to the
best of their diagnostic ability—when a patient requires a neurologic specialist
or a cardiac specialist. The newer evolution of PCP will also have the ability to
refer their patients to a credible acupuncturist, herbalist, or chiropractor within
the patient's insurance network. If PCPs do not take it on themselves to expand
their medical referral system, then the trend of patient self-referral to CAM
providers will continue—and so will the trend of not telling the PCP about
these visits and supplementation.

To facilitate acceptance of CAM by insurance companies, physicians, and other health care providers, the case manager will need to be both creative and objective. The task will become easier as more credible and evidenced-based research is performed. At this time, several insurance companies are providing some CAM therapies, although the major reason for offering the benefits is in "response to our member demands" (Rifaat, 1998, p. 54). Consumers are using the therapies, and willing to pay billions in out-of-pocket dollars, if necessary. Providing CAM benefits is being seen as a ticket to marketing success. The upside of this is that their membership will also likely have a higher satisfaction level—and perhaps even improved health status.

Case managers cannot expect full acceptance from the health plans until further research is accepted. Health plans are responsible for the health of defined populations; they are accountable for the use and misuse of all medical treatments (conventional and CAM). A recent court decision in Arizona held that the medical director of a health plan is accountable to the state medical board for decisions about patient care, which includes benefit coverage (Milbank Memorial Fund, 1998). That ruling may slow the acceptance of any therapy that does not have the seal of evidence-based research upon it. The expert panel who wrote the Milbank Memorial Fund report (see references) concluded that the following are important considerations when regulating the accountability of alternative medicine (1998):

1. Members of the public, conventional physicians, business and government purchasers of care, health plan leaders, regulators, and legislators are often confused about alternative therapies.
2. Protecting patients from being harmed by alternative treatments is a high priority for public policy, private purchasers, health plans, individual professionals, and discerning consumers.
3. Decisions about which therapists to license and which treatments to reimburse are mainly political decisions to be made on a state-by-state basis.
4. Scientific evaluation and dissemination of the research to the public is essential.

Numbers 1 and 4 demonstrate an essential need for education at all levels of health care and society, from the patient and the physician, to the regulators and legislators. Number 2 shows a concern for patient safety. Ironically, it is the very reason of safety that catapults consumers to alternative treatments. However, the point is well taken; and as patient advocates, the case manager is in a natural position for this task. Number 3 is, even now, the topic of much debate. Acceptance by health care providers may not come easily; but medical university programs will offer much in the way of education to providers, payors, patients, and case managers.

EDUCATING CAM PROVIDERS ABOUT MANAGED CARE AND INSURANCE CONCEPTS

Educating alternative providers about managed care rules and insurance concepts is very much like what the early case managers did with non-CAM practitioners in the 1980s: It was done on a one-by-one basis. As each patient required services, case managers explained utilization review criteria, assisted with moving patients through the managed care maze, built bridges over gaps in coverage, and became trusted collaborators on the multidisciplinary team.

Many CAM providers are all too familiar with managed care principles and methods from the point of view of the stepchild, who has been ignored and ridiculed. Now they are being investigated and analyzed. Case managers can help by explaining to these providers what guidelines, standards, utilization management, PCPs/the gatekeeper concept, and case management are all about. The more difficult concepts will be those that are poorly defined in managed care, such as "medical necessity" or "in a timely manner." Furthermore, if current procedure terminology (CPT) codes are developed for CAM therapies in the future, case managers may be helpful in educating CAM providers in their optimum use. With the patient's permission, and without breaking any confidentiality issues, the CAM providers also must understand their patient's:

- Insurance benefits and limitations
- Medical history
- Prescription medications
- Financial limitations
- Other important aspects of the case

CAM providers will need to understand the insurance company's motives and perspectives before they cover a specific modality. In a study cited in the *American Journal of Health Promotion,* the primary three factors in determining CAM coverage decisions were (Pelletier, Marie, Drasner & Haskell, 1997):

1. Consumer interest. Insurers stated that market demand was their primary motivation for offering coverage of CAM
2. Proof of clinical efficacy as indicated by randomized controlled trials in peer-reviewed journals, or consultation with regional and national experts
3. State-mandated coverage of CAM

As research becomes more scientifically based and as state mandates become more pervasive, several CAM modalities will likely be as commonly covered as chiropractic is today. Case managers are the link between the patient's PCP, physician specialists, and the CAM providers. As in all patient care management, the case manager collaborates and enhances communication with all providers; this is merely another type of specialist on the case.

EDUCATING CONSUMERS ABOUT THE INDICATIONS AND CONTRAINDICATIONS OF USING CAM

It is a common misconception that alternative, or "natural," remedies are always safe to use. This is not true and must be addressed. There are known cautions—and perhaps as many that are still unknown. Herbs and vitamin supplementation provide the easiest examples. White willow bark may have been the first "aspirin" in Adam and Eve's garden and is considered quite safe on its own; yet, with other blood thinners, such as feverfew, gingko, and coumadin, it can be dangerous. Digitalis and foxglove are related, as are valium and valerian. "Advise patients that the absence of documented toxicity for herbs, supplements, or chemical preparations does not equal safety" (Eisenberg, 1997, p. 4). Until recently, no one was aware that a patient on calcium channel blockers should not take them with grapefruit juice. Combining tyrosine (a common amino acid) and the prescription drug Nardil can push blood pressure dangerously high.

Some therapies have more obvious potential for toxicity: herbal mixtures, some diets, supplemental formulas, and specific medicinal agents delivered by injections or intravenous infusion, such as chelation therapy. Others are more low-risk, including homeopathy, most forms of massage, prayer, or guided imagery. However, there are two cautionary notes. Any therapy can cause "indirect toxicity" if:

1. It results in a delay of a proven treatment, or
2. There is a risk for perceived blame and failure among patients, who, expecting a "cure" as a result of mental or spiritual practices, do not experience the desired result (Eisenberg, 1997).

A case manager or physician may, at times, encounter a patient who places them in an uncomfortable position. The patient may be:

- Diagnosed with a particular condition, and refuses any "conventional" attempts or "integrative" approaches; they only want "alternative" therapy
- Opting for a treatment that the case manager or physician does not believe is safe or in the patient's best interests

In those instances, the case manager or physician should not feel obligated to support referrals under certain conditions (1997). Sometimes education is needed. A patient may have heard horrible stories about side effects of conventional treatment (and who has not?) and wonderful cures of CAM modalities. A well-stocked library of articles and patient handouts is essential. Sometimes, taking time to evaluate the shock and fear at the condition will get to the root of the problem. Always take time to evaluate the reasons behind the decisions; it is often enlightening.

Because there are so many new research studies about the efficacy, indications, and contraindications of everything from acupuncture points to single herbs, patients may inquire about a modality or treatment where the jury is still out. For example, the Food and Drug Administration is studying the long-term effects of creatine for building muscle mass. Whether the inquiry is about creatine as an adjunct to recovering from major surgery, or for a teenager's use for body building, sometimes the answer is unresolved. At this time, there is no reliable information on long-term side effects for many supplementals. When this is the case, the patient should be told. If the patient knows of further scientific evidence "for-or-against," ask for a copy of the study and add it to your files or database; research studies are going on worldwide, and no one can be aware of it all. In general, most patients do not read outcomes research, and case managers will be one major avenue for education and resources.

Insurance companies or case managers can produce educative handouts about commonly used CAM therapies and their indications and contraindications. Some journals produce ready-made information sheets that can be used for education purposes; check copyright information with the publisher before they are used. Oxford Health Plans, Inc., prioritized that education of CAM was an important part of their program and established an Alternative Medicine Educational Seminar Program. This program, whose goal is to assist members to make informed choices about CAM provider types and CAM modalities, is led by their credentialed CAM providers. They also provide an on-line medical guide free to their members, the Conventional and Alternative Remedies Encyclopedia, which gives information about medical conditions and both traditional and alternative therapy choices (Rifaat, 1998). In the future, large CAM networks and other insurance companies will likely provide similar informative offerings.

EDUCATING CONSUMERS ABOUT INSURANCE COVERAGE ISSUES

Case managers have been educating patients about insurance coverage issues since we were born. This is no different. As in any insurance benefit, CAM benefits may necessitate consideration of:

- An added premium
- Co-payments
- Deductibles
- Maximum coverage
- Provider networks
- Types of therapies that are included/excluded

As an example, one managed care organization provides its customers with an optional "Alternative Medicine Rider." The following charges and conditions have been assessed:

- An Added Premium: The beneficiary will pay $7.00 per month for the "Alternative Medicine Rider."
- Co-Payments: There is a $20.00 per visit co-payment.
- Deductibles: The annual deductible remains for this benefit/rider.
- Maximum Coverage: Insureds are covered for up to $500.00 per year.
- Provider Networks: The managed care company furnishes a list of credentialed CAM providers.
- Types of Therapies That Are Included/Excluded: Included therapies: acupuncture, chiropractic, Chinese medicine, Ayurvedic medicine, herbal medicine, massage therapy, and homeopathy. Exclusions: all other CAM modalities

Given these conditions, it is up to the patient if he or she wishes to enroll in the extra rider. The case manager must evaluate whether the patient has a "preferred" practitioner; is that practitioner in the allowed network? This particular example is not very enticing (when all the premiums, deductibles, copayments, etc. are added up). However, other plans have more generous benefits, and still others cover no CAM benefits.

Although not specifically an "exclusion," some companies also have "red flags" to indicate that a patient may be either overusing a particular benefit, or is not being helped by that treatment. If your patient, or the provider, are displaying these tendencies, education may be in order. However, consider that any of these "red flags" also may be clinically acceptable protocol under certain circumstances. Some utilization review "red flags" for various modalities may include:

- There is no evidence that treatment is not tapering after 12 treatments.
- The patient displays noncompliant tendencies by not following through with treatment recommendations, but the clinician continues to treat (rather than discharge the patient).
- Multiple clinicians are seeing the patient; there is evidence of duplication of services.

- A clinician prescribes treatment that has previously been tried and has been ineffective.
- Preexisting condition(s) are not addressed.
- Documentation is not adequate.
- Passive treatments are overly used; there is little patient participation. For example, a patient with low back pain uses chiropractic treatment (a passive treatment) for a lengthy period, without results. Physical therapy has not been attempted (an active treatment).
- Several concurrent modalities are scheduled for each session (massage, chiropractic, acupuncture).
- The diagnosis changes several times.
- The clinician submits multiple diagnosis and extensive coding for the same condition.
- X-rays (or other diagnostic testing) are performed repeatedly, or are views of areas not included in the initial diagnosis.

What if the patient has done research on a medical condition, the PCP agrees that this approach may benefit the patient, but the insurance company denies the request? Is all lost? No! There are a few more activities that a case manager can suggest. They will require the medical team's approval and support, and the patient taking on the challenge. One avenue is the appeals process. Every insurance company has an appeals process. It must be followed closely. In addition, more states are requiring appeals processes that include an external, independent review option. This is where an independent third party evaluates the grievance when a denial of services is in effect.

There are also community agencies that can help the patient. If there are problems with insurance coverage, the Medical Care Volunteer Ombudsman Program in Bethesda, Maryland, will assist in finding an independent medical expert to review the case for free. Their phone number is (301) 652-1818. If your patient is unfamiliar with his/her condition and the options, the American Self-Help Clearinghouse can be reached at (973) 625-3037. This is a clearinghouse for self-help groups. Do not overlook the knowledge of the CAM providers; they may be the best resource for peer-reviewed literature that can be used for justification for a case.

An increasing number of states have legislative mandates requiring third-party reimbursement for such CAM modalities as chiropractic or acupuncture. However, the benefits may only cover the treatments under certain circumstances: that it is recommended by the primary physician, it is performed by a licensed provider or one that is in the insured's network, and that it is "medically necessary."

IDENTIFYING WHICH OF THE MANY CAM MODALITIES ARE APPROPRIATE FOR EACH PATIENT

As the research previously listed in all the other sections of this chapter becomes supported by repeat studies, this "challenge" will get easier to answer. Currently, alternative treatments for specific conditions are getting clearer. Decades ago, herbal books indicated that saw palmetto berries could be helpful in a wide range of genitourinary problems, especially those that pertained to men. Now, they are commonly used for relief of prostate symptoms. St. John's Wort was hardly mentioned in the old herbal "classics." Now it is almost a household word, and its use for conditions of nervousness and depression increased 1000% after studies determined its efficacy in these circumstances. Perhaps in a few years, acupuncture/moxibustion will be common practice to turn fetuses because of the study in *JAMA*. Or as more research is completed on specific herbs, their uses will become clearer. At this point, the case manager and primary physician must be aware of, and educate others about, the potential uses and cautions of CAM modalities to their patients.

Each CAM therapy has its uses and its cautions. And some of the less studied and common modalities must still be tried with care. Sound therapy, for example, is still "ahead of its time" and is looked on as hocus-pocus in the eyes of many medical providers (and surely insurance plans). However, those who have used and studied its benefits know the power of sound for healing, and cautions that some tones should not be used on people with a history of seizures must be respected.

The challenge of correctly matching the CAM modality to each patient is not easily met. Each patient has a different set of medical and psychological needs; therefore, CAM modalities cannot be easily identified in "black and white." In fact, many CAM modalities look more to habits and psychological ways a patient copes than at physical symptoms (*e.g.,* homeopathic remedies and Bach Flower Remedies). When I was a case manager at a large teaching hospital in Phoenix, I worked extensively with new interns and all types of residents. In the middle 1990s I noticed a change in some of the interns and residents; they were knowledgeable about CAM modalities and appeared accepting of the benefits. These people were from the University of Arizona College of Medicine. The Program in Integrative Medicine was turning out individuals who were being trained to integrate natural remedies and therapies such as acupuncture into standard health care. This group is also participating in NIH-funded controlled studies on such therapies as the use of acupuncture for major depression (Weil, 1998). Collaborative medicine in the future must meet all the needs of the patient—and this will require expertise from a wide range of professionals.

THE CASE MANAGEMENT PROCESS AND CAM

The integration of CAM modalities with conventional medicine will require additional skills and time for the practitioner. And that is where the case manager steps in. All phases of the case management process can include attention to CAM modalities; furthermore, all phases should include CAM, because studies have shown that only about 40% of people who use alternative therapies tell their physicians. It is estimated that as many as 15 million people who take prescription drugs, for example, also use high-dose vitamins and herbs, which raises concerns about side effects from drug–herb and drug–vitamin interactions (Okie, 1998). Many of the discussion questions above can be determined, and monitored, by qualified case managers with CAM knowledge and experience. Consider the case management process:

1. Case selection
2. Assessment/problem identification
3. Development and coordination of the case plan
4. Implementation of the plan
5. Evaluation and follow-up

Case selection can begin before the patient enters the provider's arena; many patients have been using CAM modalities for years. Because CAM treatment is often a patient-referral model, the second phase of the case management process becomes even more essential.

As in traditional case management, the **assessment stage** is the link between the problem and the treatment plan. One of the first CAM assessment responsibilities is a thorough and accurate description of all CAM modalities in use by the patient. This may take some investigative work or persuading, because many people have been rebuffed by conventional physicians in the past and are not willing to go through that again.

Case managers are familiar with assessment tools. A few tools are starting to address potential alternative treatments; this must become more commonplace. Start with very concrete questions on the assessment tool:

- Do you take any herbal supplements?
  — Which ones?
  — In what dose?
  — How often?
  — What is the reason(s) for taking this herb(s)?
  — What results have you seen so far?

- Do you take any nutritional supplements?
  — Make a checklist of those that are commonly encountered: any vita-min/mineral (list); supplements for weight loss; supplements for sleep; supplements for digestion; ask for further explanation of anything listed. Have a place for "other."
- Have you seen any of the following CAM providers? When? What were the results?
  — Acupuncturist
  — Ayurvedic physician
  — Chiropractor
  — Herbologist
  — Homeopathic physician
  — Hypnotherapist
  — Massage therapist/reflexologist/Rolfer
  — Musculoskeletal practitioner (*e.g.,* Feldenkrais, Alexander technique)
  — Naturopathic physician
  — Traditional Chinese medicine practitioner
  — Other

The remaining stages of the case management process (as it relates to CAM) are not unlike the discussion and practice activities prescribed by Dr. Eisenberg at the beginning of this chapter. The safe integration of CAM into conventional medicine may entail more attention and time than today's physician has. Much of the assessment, follow-up, continuous monitoring, reassessing, and reevaluation can be done by the case manager. Based on the findings, the physician and patient can plan the best medical strategy to optimize patient outcomes and quality of life.

In the development and coordination of the case plan, it is critical to discuss the patient's preferences and expectations. Research is indicating more and more the connection between what a patient thinks and feels may help the condition, and what actually does help. Another important focus is the patient's expectation of how much the therapy may help. If the patient thinks this "may be the ticket," or conversely, "nothing will help," then a self-fulfilling prophecy may occur.

Reviewing issues of safety and efficacy may be a shared case management/ physician task. Basic information can be provided to the patient with preprinted material, discussion, or through a video. The case manager also may assist in finding an appropriate provider that is in the patient's network, and in helping the patient articulate key questions for the alternative therapy provider during their initial consultation visit.

Implementation of the plan is the next step. Once a credentialed and licensed provider is identified, that professional should work with the case manager/physician in educating the patient. The case manager should be a communication link between the primary physician and the CAM provider for several aspects of care:

- What is being done?
- What is the patient's response to the treatment?
- Are there any knowledge deficits noted by the CAM provider?
- Are changes in either the conventional or complementary therapies warranted?

Before any therapy, the patient should be given a template for a symptom diary that will be used for baseline assessment and **evaluation** of subsequent alternative (or conventional) therapeutic interventions. The case manager will need to teach the patient how to use it and discuss important points to note in the diary. What is important to note in the diary will depend on the condition being treated and the CAM provider chosen. For example, if the condition is back pain, a pain scale is essential. The patient should also record exercises done at home and in therapy, visits to the CAM therapies (chiropractic, massage, acupuncture, etc.), and the response to the therapies. If, however, a homeopathic physician is recommended for depression, the diary would be used quite differently. Mood scales may be used in place of pain scales. The homeopathic physician will likely ask about dreams remembered; these should also be noted in the diary.

The case manager may schedule a **follow-up** visit or telephone call to review the response to treatment with the patient. As in any case management experience, evaluation and follow-up must be done periodically to review the patient's symptom diary. CAM modalities often work more slowly than some other modalities; therefore, 4 to 6 weeks may be a good timeframe. Has the patient's condition improved, deteriorated, or remained the same? And as in any case management experience, document.

THE TRUTH ABOUT "ALTERNATIVES"

Every truth passes through three stages before it is recognized:

First it is ridiculed.
Then it is opposed.
And finally, it is regarded as self-evident.

Not too many years ago, health maintenance organizations (HMO) were spoken of as "alternative delivery systems." Now they are mainstream. Washing hands before delivering babies was considered unnecessary. And think of some of the "alternative" ideas that are now "self-evident":

- Vitamin C, zinc, and echinacea for colds
- Folic acid to prevent neural tube defects in the developing fetus
- A low-fat, high–fruit/vegetable diet to prevent heart disease and some forms of cancer
- Saw palmetto for prostate problems
- Vitamin E for heart protection and postmenopausal symptoms
- St. John's Wort versus Prozac
- Full-spectrum light for seasonal affective disorder
- The relationship between homocysteine and heart disease
- Each person's own unique "I swear by . . . "

Three decades ago, all of the above were considered quackery (as I was told many times!). Suddenly, seemingly overnight, CAM is a sensation; it is almost as though everyone came "out of the closet" at once; perhaps it was an idea whose time had come. Certainly, many of the success stories are "anecdotal." However, that makes them no less "successful," especially when the mind–body connection is proving to be so vital. For case managers, one prime motive is to improve the quality of life; yet "quality of life" too, is subjective and "anecdotal." What is quality life to one may be unacceptable to another. One hemodialysis patient commits suicide; another hemodialysis patient feels "so much better!" So where does the definition of "quality of life," or "wellness," lie? Perhaps the answer lives somewhere in the synapses of the mind-body-spirit connection.

CASE STUDIES IN CAM

These two case studies illustrate the fact that case managers can have a significant impact on the integration of allopathic and CAM practices. Case Study 1 can be used for discussion about "problem patients" and for evaluation of our attitudes in similar scenarios. It is likely that, with more CAM modalities being offered, many patients will be asking questions, seeking answers that allow them to participate more fully in their care plan, and becoming more assertive. Case Study 2 illustrates that, even with the initial reluctance and resistance to alternative treatment, claims payors can save dollars and improve the quality of life by listening to the expertise of case managers educated in CAM.

C A S E   S T U D Y   1

Mr. K. was admitted to the oncology research unit with lymphoma. He was a young man, 36 years old, and had never been sick a day before in his life. His girlfriend was at his side day and night and was very instrumental in helping him make decisions about his care and in supporting him 100% in all decisions he made. When I sat through report the first morning I met him, he was characterized as being a "problem patient," because he and his girlfriend asked too many questions. The staff knew of my interest in alternative medicine, so I was asked to be his primary care nurse.

The way that Mr. K. and his girlfriend approached decision making was to be as informed as they could be about every aspect of the disease process and treatment options. They were both well-educated people, so their questions could be quite extensive and detailed. In the course of reading up on cancer, they naturally came across literature about alternative approaches to treatment, and there were very few medical professionals they could talk to about what they read. I was someone in the hospital they could talk to, and they contacted other organizations outside the hospital as well. For example, Mr. K. called as many people as he could find who had been diagnosed with the form of cancer he had and were surviving 2, 3, or more years after diagnosis. He also called authors of various books he read about alternative treatments for cancer.

The final outcome was that Mr. K. decided to undergo chemotherapy and radiation therapy in conjunction with a macrobiotic diet and relaxation/positive imagery techniques. After his decision, he had to find another doctor to work with because his original doctor objected so strongly to the macrobiotic diet. He also frustrated many members of the medical team during his hospital stay because he continued to ask to be fully informed every step of the way. For example, if a nurse came in to draw blood, he wanted to know what parameters they planned to measure and how they related to his treatment. It became clear to me from this experience how so many aspects of allopathic medicine require a patient who is very submissive. I thought Mr. K. was a wonderful example of a patient empowered to educate himself about his options and then choose the best of what health care modalities were available, rather than becoming a passive recipient of whatever was fed to him. The more we learn about mind–body connections, the more important it is that patients participate on all levels in their care. The directive for healing ultimately comes from within the patient.

Mr. K. not only responded unusually quickly to the chemotherapy without the toxicity that can occur if a large tumor reduces too rapidly, but he underwent chemotherapy and radiation therapy with very minimal side effects. Everyone remarked on how smoothly the whole process went for him and the medical team. It was wonderful as a nurse not to have to see and manage all the painful side effects that can come with chemotherapy. I saw Mr. K. 2 years later at an alternative medicine lecture, and he remained cancer free and had started a national support group for cancer patients wanting to use alternative therapies with conventional medicine.

C A S E   S T U D Y   2

Mr. A. was a 55-year-old gentleman from India who sprained his back while doing his job as supervisor of a school district maintenance crew. I was brought in for case management for this workers' compensation claim after the patient had reportedly "failed" physical therapy and a trial of chiropractic treatments. The PCP was now discussing surgery. When I interviewed the patient and his wife, I learned that they believed the chiropractic therapy had been helpful, they very much liked the practitioner, and they felt that their benefits were cut off too soon. They indicated that they did not like the physical therapy treatments because they did not feel they were "listened to" by the therapists. It was also apparent that they believed this was related to differences in culture.

It was clear that Mr. A., who had been employed for 8 years with the school district, enjoyed his job, had worked his way into a supervisory position, and wanted to return. He was also concerned that all of the treatment options had not been exhausted, and he knew of others who had undergone back surgery and did not get relief from their pain. They asked about the possibility of acupuncture treatments being covered by insurance, and, if not, they wanted to continue with the chiropractor who had treated Mr. A. for 2 months.

I discussed the known benefits of acupuncture with the claims payor, providing literature to that effect, but he was adamant that the plan would not cover this modality. I then discussed with him the option of resuming chiropractic treatment, if he could get additional benefits for the patient. I told him I would work closely with the chiropractor, get a treatment plan with very specific, time-limited goals, and assure compliance of the patient. The claims payor agreed. The chiropractor and I developed a good working relationship, he and I reinforced the goals set with the patient, the patient was renewed in his commitment to heal because he was being listened to, and his wife verbalized a significant reduction in stress in her husband. We all know how stress only makes any condition worse.

The outcome was a significant reduction in low back pain, success with weight loss by the patient, and learned skills for coping with the residual low back pain that persisted, including a home exercise regimen to protect him from further injury. The chiropractic treatments came to an end after meeting their goals, the patient was able to return to work, and, of course, the plan saved the expense of surgery. I believe the outcome also could have been successful working with a licensed acupuncturist, but the claims payor was not willing to risk making a decision that has not yet become natural for the insurance industry.

PART IV: REFERENCES, RESOURCES, AND BIBLIOGRAPHY

Achterberg, J. (1985). *Imagery in healing.* Boston: New Science Library.

Achterberg, J. (1998). Clearing the air in the therapeutic touch controversy. *Alternative Therapies, 4*(4), 100–101.

Andrews, T. (1992). *Sacred sounds.* St. Paul, MN: Llewellyn Publications.

Anonymous. (1998). NIH: Effectiveness of acupuncture confirmed. Managed Healthcare News, 14 (1), 16.

Anonymous. (1998). Is alternative medicine really an alternative? *Managed Care Interface, 11*(3), 34.

Arnall, B., & Casteris, C. (1989, February). *East West* pp. 43–47.

Benson, H. (1996). *Timeless healing: The power and biology of belief.* New York: Simon & Schuster.

Birch, S., & Hammerschlag, R. (1996). *Acupuncture efficacy: A compendium of controlled clinical studies.* Tarrytown, NY: National Academy of Acupuncture and Oriental Medicine.

Boucher, T.A., & Lenz, S.K. (1998). An organizational survey of physicians' attitudes about and practice of complementary and alternative medicine. *Alternative Therapies in Health and Medicine, 4*(6).

Brody, J. (1990). Personal health: The Alexander technique. *The New York Times,* June 21.

Brown, E.R. (1979). *Rockefeller medicine men: Medicine and capitalism in America.* Berkeley, CA: University of California Press.

Brumbaugh, A. (1993). Acupuncture: New perspectives in chemical dependency treatment. *Journal of Substance Abuse Treatment, 10,* pp.35–43.

Burton Goldberg Group. (1997). *Alternative medicine: The definitive guide.* Tiburon, CA: Future Medicine Publishing, Inc.

Case Management Advisor (1997, January). pp. 18–22.

Cheng, X., Ed. (1993). *Chinese acupuncture and moxibustion.* Beijing, China: Foreign Language Press.

Chopra, D. (1993). *Ageless body, timeless mind: The quantum alternative to growing old.* New York: Harmony Books.

Chopra, D. (1989). *Quantum healing: Exploring the frontiers of mind/body medicine.* New York: Bantam Books.

Cohen, M.H. (1999). Referral to complementary and alternative providers: A physician's liability. *The Integrative Medicine Consult, 1*(5), 44–45.

Cowley, G., King, P., Hager, M., & Rosenberg, D. (1995). Alternative medicine OK by insurers. *The Phoenix Gazette.*

Cromell, C. (1998, January). Alternative, complementary or nontraditional? *Phoenix Home and Garden,* pp. 100–104.

Davenas, E., et al. (1988, 30 June). Human basophil degranulation triggered by very dilute antiserum against IgE. *Nature, 333,* 816–818.

DePoy, E., & Gitlin, L.N. (1994). *Introduction to research: Multiple strategies for health and human services.* St. Louis: Mosby-Year Book.

Dossey, L. (1982). *Space, time & medicine.* Boston: Shambhala.

Dossey, L. (1995). How should alternative therapies be evaluated? *Alternative Therapies, 1*(2), 6–10.

Edwards, S. (1999). Breaking the sound barriers of disease. [On-line]. Retrieved 1999 from the World Wide Web: http://sharryedwards.com/aboutus.html.

Eisenberg, D., Kessler, R., Foster, C., Norlock, F., Calkins, D., Delbanco, T. (1993). Unconventional medicine in the United States: Prevalence, costs, and patterns of use. *New England Journal of Medicine, 328*(4), 246–252.

Eisenberg, D. (1997). Advising patients who seek alternative medical therapies. *The Integrative Medicine Consult, 1*(1), 4–5.

Emond, L. (1997). What is the function of the various brainwaves? Scientific American: Ask the Experts: Medicine. Retrieved 1999 from the World Wide Web: http://www.sciam.com/askexpert/medicine/medicine31/medicine31.html

Firebrace, P., & Hill, S. (1994). *Acupuncture: How it works, how it cures.* New Canaan, CT: Keats Publishing, Inc.

Gelonek, M., & Chow, S. (1998). Maximizing your return by introducing alternative care benefits. Retrieved 1999 from the World Wide Web: www.landmarkhealthcare.com/articles

Gerber, R. (1996). *Vibrational medicine.* Santa Fe, NM: Bear & Co.

Greenwald, J. (1998, November 23). Herbal healing. *Time,* pp. 58–69.

Griggs, B. (1995). The ancient art of Ayurveda. *Country Living* 106–111.

Halpern, S. (1997). Why musically induced alpha brainwaves are good for you. Retrieved 1999 from the World Wide Web: http://www.innerpeacemusic.com/monthly/alphawaves.htm

Higley, C., Higley, A., & Leatham, P. (1998). *Aromatherapy A-Z.* Carlsbad, CA: Hay House, Inc.

Hoffman, J. (1998). *Rhythmic medicine: Music with a purpose.* Leawood: Jamillan Press.

Horrigan, B. (1998). *Alternative Therapies in Health and Medicine, 4*(3), 80–87.

Insurance Update. (1997). Insurance reimbursement and chiropractic use. *The Case Manager, 8*(3), 10.

Integrative Medicine Consult (1998). *An update from the Center for Alternative Medicine Pain Research and Evaluation (CAMPRE),* Vol. 1, No. 1, p. 6.

Jacobs, J., Ed. (1997). The Encyclopedia of Alternative Medicine. Boston: Carlton Books Ltd.

Kantor, J. (1999). Proofs and explanations within complementary and alternative medicine: An expanded perspective on research. *Managed Care Interface, 12*(1), 62–64.

Kaptchuk, T.J. (1983). *The web that has no weaver: Understanding Chinese medicine.* New York: Congdon & Weed.

Kaptchuk, T.J., & Croucher, M. (1987). *The healing arts: Exploring the medical ways of the world.* New York: Summit Books.

Kempner, K. (1981, March/April). The polarity system: River of life. *Whole Life Times.*

Lad, V. (1991). Introduction to Ayurveda. Retrieved 2/18/99 from the World Wide Web: http://www.ayurveda.com/ayurveda-intro.html.

Leeds, J. (1997). Entrainment harnessing rhythm. Retrieved 1999 from the World Wide Web: http://www.appliedmusic.com/entrainment.html

Long, D. (1998). Varieties of insurance entering alternative medicine market. Retrieved 3/20/99 from the World Wide Web: http://www. ahc pub.com/ambr0998.html.

Lowenhaupt, M.T. (1998). Helping patients decide about alternative therapies. *Strategic Medicine, 2*(5), 30–36.

Managed Care Market. (1997). Research on alternative medicine outcomes. *The Case Manager,* p. 17.

Managed Care Market. (1998). MCOs adding alternative care. *The Case Manager, 9*(2), 18.

Milbank Memorial Fund Report. (1998). *Enhancing the accountability of alternative medicine.* New York: Milbank Memorial Fund.

Moore, N. (1998). A review of alternative medicine courses taught at U.S. medical schools. *Alternative Therapies, 4*(3).

Murray, M., & Pizzorno, J. (1991). *Encyclopedia of natural medicine.* Rocklin, CA: Prima Publishing.

Muscat, M. (1999). OAM elevated to Center status. *Alternative Therapies in Health and Medicine, 5*(1), 24–25.

National Institutes of Health (NIH). (1998). Alternative medicine research using medline. Retrieved 4/20/99 from the World Wide Web: http://altmed.od.nih.gov/oam/what-is-cam/medline.shtml.

NIH Consensus Statement on Acupuncture. (1997 November 3-5); 15(5).

Okie, S. (1998, November 11). 4 in 10 Americans trying alternative health treatments. *The Arizona Republic.*

Pelletier, K.R. (1977). *Mind as healer, mind as slayer.* New York: Dell Publishing.

Pelletier, K., Marie, A., Drasner, M., & Haskell, W. (1997). Current trends in the integration and reimbursement of complementary and alternative medicine by managed care, insurance carriers, and hospital providers. *American Journal of Health Promotion, 12*(2), 112–123.

Pert, C., Dreher, J.E., & Ruff, M. (1998). The psychosomatic network: Foundations of mind-body medicine. *Alternative Therapies, 4*(4), pp. 30–41.

Pert, C. (1997). *Molecules of emotion.* New York: Scribner.

Rifaat, H. (1998). How alternative medicine works in managed care. *Managed Healthcare News, 14*(4), 54.

Robbins, S. (1998). Thoughts on "Proving" NLP. Retrieved 1999 from the World Wide Web: http://www.nlp.com/NLP/random/sciprove.html.

Rogers, M.E. (1970). An introduction to the theoretical basis of nursing. Philadelphia: F.A. Davis.

Rosa, L., Rosa E., Sarner L., & Barrett S. (1998). A close look at therapeutic touch. *JAMA, 279,* 1005–1010.

Ryan, M., & Shattuck, A. (1994). Treating AIDS with Chinese medicine. Berkeley, CA: Pacific View Press.

Scheffer, M. (1988). *Bach flower therapy: Theory and practice.* Rochester, VT: Healing Arts Press.

Seligson, S. (1998). Melding medicines. *Health 12*(4), 64–70.

Simonton, S., & Sherman, A. (1998). Psychological aspects of mind-body medicine: Promises and pitfalls from research with cancer patients. *Alternative Therapies, 4*(4), pp. 50–64.

Toran, M.R. (1996, July/August). Alternatives in the mainstream. *The Case Manager,* pp. 55–62.

Villaire, M. (1998). More health plans add alternative medicine coverage. *Alternative Therapies, 4*(3), 27.

Weil, A. (1988). *Health and healing.* Boston: Houghton Mifflin.

Weil, A. (1998, April). Acupuncture: New uses for an ancient art. *Self Healing,* pp. 2–3.

Zahourek, R.P., Ed. (1988). *Relaxation & imagery: Tools for therapeutic communication and intervention.* Philadelphia: W.B. Saunders.

Resources

(Also see Resource Boxes in Chapter 10)

American Holistic Nurses Association (AHNA)
PO Box 2130
Flagstaff AZ 86003-2130
1-800-278-AHNA
www.ahna.org

Alternative Therapies in Health & Medicine
www.healthonline.com/altther.htm

Practical Review in Complementary & Alternative Medicine
(monthly cassettes) 1999 price: $330.00/year

Holistic Health Promotion & Complementary Therapies
Publisher: Aspen Reference Group
(updates/inserts periodically)

National Center for Complementary & Alternative Medicine
http://altmed.od.nih.gov/nccam

The Integrative Medicine Consult: The Essential Guide to Integrating Conventional & Complementary Medicine (newsletters every 3 weeks)
www.onemedicine.com

Resource for information, current research, lists of certified practitioners, and links to further professional associations.
www.acupuncture.com

www.altmedicine.com

PART IV: STUDY QUESTIONS

1. Plan a complementary and alternative medicine program in your facility or organization. Use the principles and issues for disease management, continuous quality improvement (CQI), team development, and project development.

2. Describe a previous personal experience with CAM modalities. What were the outcomes?

3. Study or take a short course in a CAM modality that is interesting to you. Include any outcomes research that has been done internationally on the subject. Share your experience with others through a written or verbal report.

4. Evaluate a chronic problem that bothers you, a friend, or family member. Discuss this problem with a CAM practitioner. Are there alternatives (other than those suggested by allopathic medical providers) that were suggested? Would you try them? Why or why not?

(continued)

5. If you are starting a new CAM modality, keep a diary as suggested by Dr. David Eisenberg.

6. Research to find practice guidelines on a CAM modality. Tip: Outcome studies have been performed internationally on CAM modalities for many years.

7. Choose an herbal supplement. Research indications and contraindications for the herb.

8. Assess patients for use of CAM modalities. Are their primary physicians aware of the use of alternative medicine? Why? Are there any contraindications that you are aware of? If so, what would you (as a case manager) do about it?

9. Which CAM providers must be licensed or credentialed in your state?

10. Are there any CAM modalities (other than chiropractic) that are included in your insurance benefits or in your patients' plans? Which ones? Assess the benefit: does it encourage the use of CAM modalities, or is it a "token" benefit?

Glossary of Terms

abstraction. The collection of the data.

accountability. Responsibility for one's actions and for achieving defined goals.

acupuncture. Acupuncture is a treatment modality based on the concepts of traditional Chinese medicine, that involves the placement of very thin, stainless steel needles into specific points on the body with the intention of maintaining or restoring the smooth flow of energy, or Qi, along specific pathways, or meridians, that travel along the surface of the body and enter deep into the body to connect with all the organs. Qi is considered a vital energy necessary for the body to function.

Agency for Healthcare Policy and Research (AHCPR). A part of the U.S. Department of Health and Human Services, AHCPR is the lead agency charged with supporting research designed to improve the quality of health care, reduce its cost, and broaden access to essential services.

Alexander technique. Focuses on restoring a balanced, dynamic posture, or coordination of the head and the spine, by reprogramming neuromotor patterns through repetitive musculoskeletal movements or postures.

algorithm. A format for presenting a clinical practice guideline that consists of a structured flowchart of decision steps and preferred clinical management pathways. An algorithm prescribes what sequence of steps to take given particular circumstances or characteristics (AHCPR).

aromatherapy. Uses the aroma from essential plant oils to stimulate a healing response. It is believed that the aromatic vapor travels immediately to the limbic system of the brain, which is responsible for the integration and expression of feelings, learning, memory, emotions, and physical drives.

auric field. A person's energy body.

autogenic training. A technique for inducing deep relaxation. It consists of a series of simple mental exercises designed to turn off the stressful "fight-flight" mechanism in the body that causes the release of adrenalin, and turn on the restorative and recuperative rhythms associated with profound psychophysical relaxation and healing.

Ayurvedic medicine. A 5,000-year-old philosophy and system of practice that teaches people how to live in harmony with all aspects of life by caring for themselves on a day-to-day basis. Ayurvedic medicine is deeply rooted in the ancient culture and religion of the Indian continent, and addresses the whole person as body-mind-spirit. The World Health Organization supports the use of Ayurvedic medicine and its integration with modern medicine.

bar chart. A CQI tool for process improvement that depicts the frequency distribution of data to show the shape and spread of what is being measured. A histogram is a form of bar chart.

baseline data/baseline measurement. Data that are collected before a change in the process has been initiated.

benchmark. A level of quality of care that is set as a goal to be attained, and (possibly) surpassed.

best practices. Practices that have been determined to produce the most favorable outcomes; these practices have been gleaned from comparative quality measurements.

bioacoustics. A cross between music therapy and biofeedback. Similar to sound therapy, bioacoustics uses low-based frequency sounds to elicit biologic and emotional responses.

bioenergy therapies. Treatment modalities that work on balancing the patient's energy body, sometimes called the auric field, and include polarity therapy and therapeutic touch.

biofeedback. Uses technology to provide feedback to patients training to gain conscious control over physiologic functions of the body, such as regulation of the heart rate.

brainstorming. A method of engaging all team members in sharing ideas, suggestions, and options in an open, nonjudgmental environment.

case management. Case management is a collaborative process that assesses, plans, implements, coordinates, monitors, and evaluates options and services to meet an individual's health needs through communication and available resources to promote quality cost-effective outcomes. (definition from *Standards of Practice for Case Management* [CMSA]; Case Management Society of America).

CMSA. Case Management Society of America.

cause-and-effect diagram. A CQI tool for process improvement used to help identify the multiple causes of any outcome or problem. Also known as a fishbone diagram (because it looks like a fishbone), or Ishikawa diagram (after the man who developed this tool).

CAM. Complementary and Alternative Medicine—Any therapeutic intervention not based on conventional, Western, allopathic treatment protocols.

CASE © PDCA. PDCA stands for Plan, Do, Check, Act. It is a CQI model for planning and problem solving of process improvement; the acronym "CASE" is added to the planning stage for case management process improvement activities.

clinical practice guidelines. Systematically developed statements to assist practitioners' and patients' decisions about health care to be provided for specific clinical circumstances (AHCPR).

Chinese medicine. See traditional Chinese medicine.

chiropractic manipulations. Are concerned with the relationship of the spinal column and musculoskeletal structures of the body to the nervous system. It is believed that when the spinal column is out of alignment, it interferes with the flow of nerve impulses or messages from the central nervous system. Thus, misalignment can have an impact on every part of the body.

classical yoga. Yoga that is organized into eight "limbs" that provide a complete system of physical, mental, and spiritual health. Some of the yogas focus on developing the mind, some on developing the body, and some on developing the deeper inner life of the spirit.

common cause variation. Variation in processes that is statistically predictable, random, naturally occurring, and caused by chance.

comparative feedback. Data from several peer groups that is "blinded" and "fed back" to the collaborators in a project. Comparative feedback appears to hasten improvement efforts.

competitive benchmark. Comparisons with the best external competitors in the field.

component management model. In this model, "components" are the various providers that a patient may require along the continuum. Each component, separately and episodically, may strive for cost-effective, quality care. However, in reality, the patient may suffer from the fragmentation because of the providers viewing care from their own perspectives.

continuous quality improvement (CQI). An array of formal quality improvement techniques based on the collection and analysis of data generated in the course of current clinical practice in a defined clinical setting to identify and solve problems in the system (AHCPR).

control group. In experimental and quasi-experimental designs, the control group is the one that is not exposed to the independent variable.

CQI tools for process improvement. Tools that enable teams to focus on problems, collect data, identify root causes, select and test improvements, and monitor changes. Some of these tools include flowcharts, cause-and-effect diagrams, Pareto diagrams, brainstorming techniques, and scatter diagrams.

control chart. A CQI tool for process improvement used to demonstrate trends over time. Control charts add preestablished, statistically determined upper and lower control limits, which provide a visual cue of the degree of variation. Variation exceeding the upper or lower control limits suggests a "special cause" for the variation; variation within the control limits suggests a "common cause" for the variation.

consensus. A method of decision making whereby team members openly express their views and come to an agreement. Consensus indicates support of the decision; it does not always mean that all team members were in unanimous agreement. Coming to a consensus often requires negotiation and mediation skills.

craniosacral therapy. This technique manipulates the bones of the skull to treat a range of conditions, from headache and ear infection to stroke, spinal cord injury, and cerebral palsy. Just as the human body has a rhythm associated with the heartbeat and breathing, there is also a rhythm to the ebb and flow of fluid within the cranium and spinal cord generated by subtle pressure changes as fluid enters and exits these spaces.

creative visualization. See Guided Imagery.

criteria. The standard or principle by which something is judged or evaluated.

cross-functional team. A team in which two or more areas of the organization are charged with addressing an issue that will have an impact on the operations in all areas represented.

customers. Whoever receives the products or services of an organization. See internal customers and external customers.

data. Facts (often numerical) used to make a judgment.

demand management. The use of self-management and decision support systems to enable, educate, and encourage people to improve their health and make appropriate use of medical care.

descriptive design. An evaluation design whose purpose is to describe a population or target area.

disease state management. This is a model of delivering care to whole populations of patients. This model seeks to prevent complications (as in high-risk pregnancy) or disease progression (as in chronic illnesses); maintain high quality of life; prevent future need for high medical resources. Disease management uses an integrated approach that includes pharmaceutical care, continuous quality improvement principles, practice guidelines, and case management.

data abstractor. The person collecting the data.

data collection/analysis. Gathering facts on how a process works or how a process is working; analysis examines the data collected.

demographic data. General information about the patient, such as name, address, phone number.

doshas (vata, pitta, and kapha). The doshas govern psychobiologic changes in the body and physiopathologic changes.

encounter data. Description of the diagnoses made and services provided when a patient visits a health care provider under a managed-care plan.

Encounter data provide much of the same information available on the bills submitted by fee-for-service providers (AHCPR).

evaluation. An essential step in any improvement process. This step examines the reasons to improve, and the method of making that improvement.

evidenced-based methods. Methods that explicitly link public health or clinical practice recommendations to the underlying scientific evidence demonstrating their effectiveness.

experimental design. An evaluation design that examines "cause-and-effect" relationships by comparing one or more experimental groups exposed to a treatment with a control group that has not been exposed to the treatment.

exploratory design. An evaluation design in which the purpose is to examine something new about an experience, event, or process.

external benchmarks. See Competitive Benchmarks.

external customers. Those outside the boundaries of the organization.

Facilitator. A person who has developed special expertise in the quality improvement process and serves as a coach and a guide.

feasibility. Capable of being done, executed, or effected in a practical way.

Feldenkrais therapy. This system combines stretching, exercise, and yoga to improve awareness of movement patterns and encourage proper body movement.

fishbone diagram. See cause-and-effect diagram.

flowchart. A CQI tool for process improvement used to create a picture or step-by-step description of a process.

flower essences. Flower essences are considered to be a form of "vibrational" medicine. Much like homeopathy, flower essences contain the energetic pattern of a flower, rather than its molecular structure.

force field analysis. A CQI tool for process improvement that depicts how competing forces interact when implementing change.

generic benchmark. Benchmarks drawn from the best performance of similar processes in other industries.

goal. A broadly stated or long-term outcome written as an overall statement relating to a philosophy, purpose, or desired outcome (NAHQ).

guided imagery. A.k.a. visualization, is the thought process that invokes an inner mental picture, usually using all the senses, which include vision as well as hearing, smell, touch, taste, position, and movement.

guidelines. See practice guidelines.

hatha yoga. The yoga of movement and coordinated breath.

hard savings. Savings that can be supported by hard dollar data and therefore can be calculated and trended.

health. The World Health Organization's definition of health is "a state of complete physical, mental and spiritual well being, not merely the absence of disease."

health risk appraisal (HRA). (also known as Health Risk Inventory or Health Risk Assessment) This type of survey identifies lifestyle behaviors that may put a patient at medical risk (such as smoking, no use of seat belts (etc.); it also may identify genetic risk (such as male, bald, short).

health status. Information on various domains of health such as physical functioning, mental and emotional well-being, cognitive functioning, social and role functioning, and perceptions of one's peers.

Health Status Survey (SF 12/36). This survey is a SELF assessment tool that measures the patient's PERCEIVED quality-of-life issues; it has proved to be a PREDICTIVE tool that may indicate a patient's potential for illness or hospitalization within 6 months to 1 year.

Health Care Financing Administration (HCFA). The federal agency that oversees Medicare and also oversees the individual state's management of Medicaid.

Health Plan Employer Data and Information Set (HEDIS). A set of standardized measures of health plan performance. HEDIS allows comparisons between plans on quality, access, and patient satisfaction; membership and utilization; financial information; and health plan management. HEDIS was developed by employers, HMOs, and the National Committee for Quality Assurance (AHCPR).

herbology/herbal medicine. The use of whole plants, or parts thereof, for the treatment of disease and the maintenance of good health. It is the oldest form of medicine known and has been practiced for thousands of years.

homeopathy. A healing technique based on three principles: the Law of Similars, the Law of Infinitesimal Dose, and the laws of Holism.

hydrotherapy. Therapies using water for healing.

hypnosis. An artificially induced state characterized by a heightened receptivity to suggestion; a form of guided imagery.

indicator. See quality indicator.

integrated delivery systems. An entity that usually includes a hospital, a large medical group, and an insurance vehicle such as an HMO or PPO. Typically, all provider revenues flow through the organization.

internal benchmark. A benchmark that is derived from similar processes or services within an organization.

internal customers. Customers inside the boundaries of an organization; those who receive products and services before they reach external customers or those outside the organization.

interrater reliability. A monitoring method to ensure that the data collected is correct and reliable. Simply, the goal of interrater reliability is for two abstractors to obtain the same answers.

interventions. What is done; actions intended to have an effect on outcomes.

Ishikawa diagram. See cause-and-effect diagram.

"just in time (JIT)" training. Training that is delivered to quality improvement teams on an "as-needed" basis.

key processes. Those processes that are particularly important because of their impact, cost, or relevance.

materia medica. Used by homeopathic practitioners, this book is a compendium of thousands of "provings" conducted over the past 200 years.

mean. The arithmetic average of the values of a sample variable.

medical review criteria. Systematically developed statements that can be used to assess specific health care decisions, services, and outcomes. (AHCPR)

meditation. An ancient spiritual practice for achieving spiritual awakening, which works by quieting the incessant, random flow of thoughts through the mind.

mindfulness meditation. A form of meditation developed in the traditions of Buddhism and designed to allow the meditation to be at peace in any experience in which they find themselves. It requires very focused attention and a nonjudgmental attitude.

mind–body medicine. The ability of a belief or image held in the mind to directly effect a change in the body on a physical, cellular level is now called mind–body medicine, and includes such practices as meditation, hypnosis, biofeedback, creative visualization, the relaxation response, and autogenic training.

MDS. Minimum data set.

multidisciplinary team. A team that consists of various disciplines. Each one provides needed information so the best outcome can be realized.

multivoting. A CQI selection process used by teams to reduce a long list of options to a reasonable number.

musculoskeletal therapies. Treatment modalities that bring the patient's awareness to body posture and movement, and manipulate the physical body to facilitate the flow of blood and energy through the muscles, fascia, and skeletal structures. Therapies include the Alexander method, the Feldenkrais technique, craniosacral therapy, rolfing, chiropractic manipulation, yoga, massage, and reflexology.

National Committee for Quality Assurance (NCQA). A nonprofit organization that performs quality-oriented accreditation reviews.

naturopathic medicine. The underlying goal of naturopathic medicine is to strengthen the body's immune system so that it can heal itself. Treatment modalities include the use of Western herbs, high-dose vitamins, homeopathic remedies, hydrotherapy, counseling, minor surgery, diet and lifestyle changes, detoxification regimens, and physical medicine modalities such as massage.

NIH. National Institutes of Health.

nominal group technique. A CQI process used to generate ideas within a team and choose the best one.

nutritional supplementation. Vitamin/mineral therapy; may also include the use of herbs.

objectives. Specific action-oriented statements written in measurable and observable terms that define how the goals will be attained (NAHQ).

OAM: Office of Alternative Medicine. Was created to evaluate alternative medical treatments, fund studies to determine their effectiveness, and integrate effective treatments into mainstream medical practice.

operational definition. A description in quantifiable terms of what to measure and the steps to follow to measure it consistently. They are developed for each critical aspect of a project before data are collected. According to Deming, a good operational definition includes (1) a criterion to be applied, (2) a way to determine whether the criterion is satisfied, and (3) a way to interpret the results of the test.

outcomes. The results and consequences achieved through a particular health care service; outcomes also result from care that was NOT received. Desired outcomes include improved functionality, health status, satisfaction, and lower cost of treatment.

outcome indicator. Measures the result of care or services provided, which may be desirable or undesirable.

outcomes management. Seeks to produce desirable outcomes in a clinical setting and is the application of outcomes research into practice.

outcomes measurement. The process of measurement that demonstrates improvement in health care results. This is done through modification of practices in response to information gleaned through outcomes reviews. Three types of outcomes measurements include clinical outcomes, financial outcomes, and patient outcomes.

outcomes research. A term originally used to describe a particular line of health services research that focused on identifying variations in medical procedures and associated health outcomes (AHCPR).

outliers. Cases that are substantially different from the rest of the population. With regard to hospital payment, these are classified as cases with extremely long lengths of stay (day outliers) compared with others in the same DRG. Hospitals receive additional PPS payments for these cases (AHCPR).

paradigm. Fundamental beliefs that underlie the way things are done. A "paradigm shift" depicts a fundamental transformation in beliefs and behavior.

pareto diagram. A CQI tool for process improvement similar to a bar graph. It is used to prioritize action, by distinguishing between the "vital few and the trivial many."

PDCA cycle. A CQI model for planning and problem solving of process improvement; PDCA stands for Plan, Do, Check, Act. PDSA is a similar model: Plan, Do, Study, Act. Also known as the Deming cycle or the Shewhart cycle.

PDSA cycle. See PDCA cycle.

performance improvement. The continuous study and adaptation of functions and processes of a health care organization to increase the probability of achieving desired outcomes and to better meet the needs of those who use health care services.

performance improvement team. See Quality Improvement Team (QIT).

performance indicators. Also sometimes called report cards, performance indicators are measures that can be used to rate providers, insurers, or health care plans according to their performance along several criteria. Common indicators include mortality rates, cost, rates of specific procedures, or rates of hospitalization for preventable diseases (AHCPR).

performance measures. Methods or instruments to estimate or monitor the extent to which the actions of a health care practitioner or provider conform to the clinical practice guideline (AHCPR).

"physician champion." A consultant on the health care team who is a well-respected and dedicated "champion" to the "cause" or process being improved.

pie chart. A CQI tool for process improvement that depicts the percentage that each category of values contributes to the total of all categories.

pilot project. A test project on a small scale.

polarity therapy. Promotes the smooth flow of energy along electromagnetic paths around the body by releasing blockages of energy.

population. The group of people, events, or observations from which the study sample will be chosen.

practice guidelines. (a.k.a. clinical practice guidelines) are defined by the Institute of Medicine as "systematically developed statements to assist practitioner and patient decisions about appropriate health care for specific clinical circumstances."

practice parameters. Strategies for patient management, developed to assist in clinical decision making.

prana. Life force, or energy that occurs throughout the body.

preventive care. The concept designed to prevent disease, or to detect and treat it early, or to manage its course most effectively. Examples of traditional preventative care include immunizations, Pap smears, mammograms, or cholesterol screening. Alternative therapies such as herbal remedies and various CAM modalities are important forms of preventative care.

problem statement. Also called an opportunity statement and is a concise description of a process in need of improvement.

processes. Those activities performed that will achieve a certain end result or outcome.

process indicator. Measures the care activity or services provided.

process improvement team (PIT). See quality improvement team (QIT).

project team. See quality improvement team (QIT).

protocols. Standing orders that prescribe diagnosis or procedure specific activities that have traditionally required a written order in the medical record.

qi. The vital force that runs throughout the body, animating and supporting the function of different organ systems.

quality. (1) As defined by the Institute of Medicine, is the degree to which health services for individuals and populations increase the likelihood of desired outcomes and are consistent with current professional knowledge. (2) The ability to meet or exceed customer expectations with minimum of waste, unnecessary complexity, or rework.

quality action team (QAT). See Quality Improvement Team (QIT).

quality council. A team that usually consists of senior leadership and is responsible for planning, strategy development, monitoring, promoting, and training of the CQI process.

quality improvement. See continuous quality improvement (CQI).

quality improvement projects. Projects that focus on the process of quality improvement. The team could improve a condition of patient care, or a process within an organization.

quality improvement team (QIT). A specially constituted working group to address a specific opportunity for improvement. These teams consist of those people who have regular contact with the process being examined.

quality indicators (QI). Disease-, condition-, or situation-specific statements that represent areas of consensus and are related to processes/outcomes of care. These can incorporate guidelines, standards of care, or practice parameters and must be grounded in literature where available. Quality indicators are measurable and can monitor and assess the quality of important aspects of patient care or services.

quasi-experimental design. An evaluation design that studies the behavior of a population by approximating the conditions of a true experiment in a setting that does not allow the control or manipulation of all relevant variables.

random sample. A group selected for study that is drawn at random from the universe of cases by a statistically valid method.

reflexology. A type of massage that works only on areas of the feet and hands, where there are believed to be "reflex" points that can stimulate the glands and organs in the body.

relaxation response. Achieved through mental imagery in a meditative state and activates the body's parasympathetic nervous system; can restore homeostasis and allow the body to heal from the physiologic changes that can occur as the result of chronic stress.

reliability. The extent to which the data measured are reproducible over time.

report cards. See performance indicators.

risk adjustment. The process used to adjust payment to plans to compensate for differences in health status of enrollees across plans (AHCPR). Risk adjustment is also a technique used in performance improvement projects to "level the playing field" by evaluating issues such as comorbidities, complications, age, gender, etc.

Rolfing. A form of deep, tissue massage. Rolfers, practitioners who perform Rolfing, manipulate and stretch the body's fascial tissue to release adhesions and relieve restricted muscles and joints.

root cause analysis. A CQI tool for process improvement in which the principal cause of a problem or process is exposed.

run chart. A CQI tool for process improvement that graphs data over time, therefore identifying trends.

sample. The subset of a population or the group of cases to whom a performance measure will be applied.

scatter diagram. A CQI tool for process improvement that graphs relationships between two variables (a.k.a. scattergrams).

sensitivity. How well an indicator can detect all cases in which actual quality of care problems exist. Indicators that lack sensitivity may miss cases in which actual quality of care problems exist. Conversely, if an indicator is too sensitive, it may include cases that do not need to be included (JCAHO).

sentinel event. An unexpected occurrence that involves death or serious physical or psychological injury (JCAHO).

Shewhart cycle. See PDCA cycle.

soft savings. Those savings that cannot always be supported by hard dollar data. Case management impacts patients' lives in many ways; therefore, soft savings should also be captured.

special cause variation. Variation in processes that are from uncommon, non-random systematic circumstances.

stages of team development. The stages that teams undergo include forming, storming, norming, and performing.

Statistical Process Control Chart (SPCC). See control chart.

steering teams. See quality council.

Short-Form 36 (SF-36, SF-12). See Health Status Survey.

sound healing/therapy. Sound uses vibrational tones to elicit biologic and emotional responses to promote healing.

standard of care. That degree of care, skill, or learning expected of a reasonable, prudent health care provider in the profession or class to which he or she belongs within the state acting in the same or similar circumstances.

standards of quality. Authoritative statement of (1) minimum levels of acceptable performance or results, (2) excellent levels of performance or results, or (3) the range of acceptable performance or results (AHCPR).

statistical significance. Refers to the results of a statistical test, expressed as a probability, and greater than could be explained by chance occurrence alone. If the size of a population or sample is inadequate, the data may not be statistically significant.

structural integration. See Rolfing.

study design. Refers to the approach and methods used to organize and conduct the study and evaluate the case management interventions.

therapeutic massage. The use of touch to manipulate the soft tissues of the body for the purpose of relieving muscle tension and promoting blood circulation. There are more than 100 styles of massage, which are categorized according to the type of strokes or manipulations used, the depth of the massage, the incorporation of movements with the massage, the body part worked on, and the overall goal of the session.

therapeutic touch. A form of hands-on healing, although often the practitioner's hands are 2 to 6 inches from the patient.

total quality management (TQM). A management theory of quality improvement based on (1) involving the total organization, (2) using statistical quality control, (3) seeking to raise the average performance rather than eliminate outliers, and (4) continuously reevaluating performance after interventions to plan further interventions if needed (AHCPR).

traditional Chinese medicine (TCM). A philosophy and practice of medicine based on the theory that health exists when the forces of Yin and Yang are balanced within the body-mind-spirit.

trend chart. See Run Chart.

validity. The extent to which data measure what they are supposed to measure.

value. The combination of quality, cost, and productivity.

variable. A characteristic or factor that is measured.

variance data. Variances are deviations from expected care. Four types of variances include provider variances, patient/family variances, institution variances, and community variances.

variation. The inevitable difference between actual performance and expected performance. Variation requires further analysis to determine the cause of the variation (special or common causes).

yoga. See classical yoga.

yin/yang. The forces that maintain homeostasis in the body-mind-spirit, a balance between catabolism and anabolism, rest and activity, and heat and cold. Yang represents the functional aspect of the body-mind-spirit, and Yin represents the substance of the body-mind-spirit. Examples of Yang energy are heat, agitation, rapid movement, and the daytime. Examples of Yin energy are cold, rest, slow movement, and the nighttime.

Index

Page numbers in *italic* denote figures; those followed by t denote tables.